# The Curriculum and the Hearing-Impaired Student

Advisory Editor:

**Daniel Ling, Ph.D.**
Dean, Faculty of Applied Health Sciences
University of Western Ontario
London, Ontario

# THE CURRICULUM AND THE HEARING-IMPAIRED STUDENT

## Theoretical and Practical Considerations



Gary Owen Bunch, Ed.D.

*York University*
*Toronto, Ontario*



A College-Hill Publication

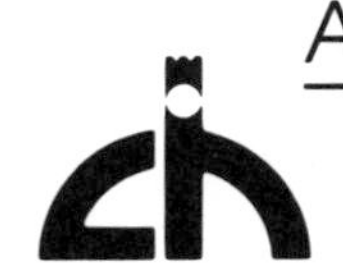

*Little, Brown and Company*
*Boston/Toronto/San Diego*

College-Hill Press
A Division of
Little, Brown and Company (Inc.)
34 Beacon Street
Boston, Massachusetts 02108



**Library of Congress Cataloging in Publication Data**
Main entry under title:

Bunch, Gary Owen, 1938-
The curriculum and the hearing-impaired student.

Includes bibliographies and index.
1. Hearing-impaired children—Education—United States—Curricula. I. Title.
HV2440.B86 1987 371.91'2 87-12783

**ISBN 0-316-11482-0**

Printed in the United States of America

To Dr. Bryan R. Clarke
Teacher, Mentor, Friend

# CONTENTS

# CHAPTER 1

# *Curricula and Hearing Impairment: A Perspective*

The dual topic of curriculum development and curriculum revision is a recurring one among educators of the hearing impaired. To a significant degree, dissatisfaction with existing curricula (Cole & Mischook, 1985; Griffey, 1981; Hasenstab & McKenzie, 1981; Lang & Propp, 1982; LaSasso, 1978) has been expressed. In response to this dissatisfaction, most schools for the hearing impaired and many individual educators have turned their attention to both curriculum development and revision. The result has been an abundance of locally created curricula mixed with a number of commercially available curricula. No one curricular approach, with the possible exception of that offered by Ling (1976),however, has been accepted by the majority of programs.

The reasons for the lack of any general agreement on acceptable, effective curricula are many and varied. Easterbrooks and Massey (1980) suggested that those charged with curriculum selection seize on curricula reflecting new concepts of learning, but abandon them when they fail to meet preconceived expectations, or "persist with a particular manageable approach which may be based upon outdated research in the face of current empirical and social evidence." Bunch (1978) suggested that the simple answer may be that the educational challenges centered about language acquisition are so great that no generally effective curriculum can be written at this point. A complicating factor in this specialized field is that little interest in the broad and narrow curricular problems facing educators of the hearing impaired has been evidenced by "outside" curriculum experts. Special education curricula in general have not drawn the attention of such experts (Tomlinson, 1982). Even for the few with expressed interest in exceptional children, hearing impairment is felt to pose no particular curricular challenge. Wilson (cited by Brennan, 1985) grouped exceptional children by their curricular needs. The first grouping included:

> *Children with defects of hearing, vision, or mobility without serious intellectual or emotional problems.* These children must acquire special, additional skills to overcome their disability, learn to use special equipment for recording or mobility. *They are capable of following the normal school curriculum* (italics added), though the time required for the necessary additional learning may reduce the number of subjects with which they can be involved at any one time. That problem may be overcome by extending their time in school or arranging follow-on curriculum in further education.

In a fashion typical of individuals unfamiliar with hearing-impaired students, Brennan accepted this analysis and extended it noting, "Their problems are considered to be the easiest" among the special needs groups. Most educators of the hearing impaired would dispute this assertion. They view the curricular challenge posed by hearing impairment as profound and complex. However, even professionals working in the field of hearing impairment have little extensive knowledge of the state of the art in their own field. To a significant extent those charged with curriculum development have concentrated on creating new curricula or revising existing curricula to meet the needs of day-to-day teaching. They have not stepped back to view curricula for the hearing impaired against the backdrop of what is occurring in education at large.

## BACK TO BASICS

Alhough this treatment of curriculum is not meant to be a discussion of basic principles of curriculum development, certain fundamental points are worthy of mention. The following chapters, each of which deals with a particular area of curricular interest, must be viewed within the framework of questions guiding the design of educational curricula in general. Tyler (1949) posed four questions accepted as basic to curricular design:

1. What educational purposes should the school seek to attain?
2. What educational experiences can be provided that are likely to attain these purposes?
3. How can these educational purposes be effectively organized?
4. How can we determine whether these purposes are being attained?

No matter which model of curriculum design one follows, these questions must be answered. For educators of the hearing impaired, direct response is hampered by a history of separation from the mainstream of education, lack of sufficient expertise in curriculum design, lack of means to share existing curricula, too great a concern with the specific problems of hearing impairment, and the need to deal with a markedly heterogeneous population. To begin the task of appropriate curriculum development it is essential to respond to Tyler's first question: "What educational purposes should the school seek to attain?" Discussion related to questions two through four will be found throughout the following chapters.

## Educational Purposes

Educational purposes, objectives, or goals may be viewed on a macro- or microcosmic level. The level of view adopted by those charged with the responsibility of curricular design will determine if special curricula are prepared for hearing-impaired children, if regular curricula for "normal" children are adapted, or if regular curricula are used in unadapted form. Whatever position is taken, the first point of consideration is determination of the overall purposes or objectives of the curriculum (Sass-Lehrer, 1984).

If special curricula are prepared, then there must be something about hearing impairment that makes the hearing-impaired learner different. The purposes attached to curricula will reflect the differences implied by this "hearing impaired as deviant" perspective. Studies describing the modest academic achievement, the limited language development, the speech development difficulties, the use of sign language, and the closed community preferences of many hearing-impaired individuals are interpreted as defining a population with highly individual needs. Once a curriculum designer has determined that the population of interest has special needs, these needs must be worked into the curriculum. Brennan (1985) noted: "Special needs and curricula interact in complex manner. The interaction arises from the demands made upon curriculum by the range and level of special needs, by the multiplicity of special needs presented by some children, and by the help and assistance required if pupils are to be maintained in appropriate curricula and educated efficiently."

No professional would deny that certain characteristics of hearing impairment demand that specific curricula must be designed to meet special needs. The fact that many hearing-impaired children have insufficient hearing for the normal development of speech means that special speech curricula must be designed. The fact that many hearing-impaired children require special assistance to maximize their use of residual hearing means that aural habilitation curricula must be designed. Such curricula, in and of themselves, address characteristics and learning needs not shared in similar fashion by average learners or other groups of exceptional learners. Specific purposes guide the instructional methods employed, the support materials selected, and assessment systems. In a sense, however, such curricula exemplify a microcosmic view of curricula and hearing impairment. The hearing impaired as a group possess special learning characteristics that create educational needs not shared by society in general. Curricula designed for the hearing impaired are therefore necessary, because curricula created for the bulk of individuals in society will not meet the special learning needs of the hearing impaired adequately. Such a philosophy cannot be faulted with regard to the readily definable ways in which the needs of hearing-impaired children are different and special. It is when this philosophy extends to areas such as reading, mathematics, and vocational training that an argument ensues. That argument centers about the question "Do hearing-impaired children possess learning characteristics sufficiently different from other learners to create a need for unique curricula in all areas?" If the response is affirmative, special curricula with their own purposes and objectives are required. If a negative response is appropriate, a variety of curricula designed for "normal" learners may be used in adapted or unadapted form.

The typical response is that all children share the same general educational objectives, that normal children and exceptional children, including the hearing impaired, are similar. This position exemplifies the macrocosmic approach in curriculum development. However, as soon as this is said, qualifications are introduced. While most agree that the process of curriculum planning and goal selection is the same for all children (Brennan, 1985; Lowell, 1967; Saif & Thiel, 1983), many argue that actual expectations must be different. Tudyman (cited in Lowell, 1967) noted that the subject matter presented to regular children will be appropriate for few deaf children. Brennan (1985) advanced the idea that the traditional hierarchical division of instructional priorities (and by implication, objectives) of (1) what *must* be learned; (2) what *should* be learned, and (3) what *could* be learned may not be appropriate for exceptional learners. Brill, Merrill, and Frisina (1973) suggested that curricula for hearing-impaired children should be coordinated with, but not be identical to, curricula for normally hearing children.

This "yes-no" response pattern in the area of educational purposes in curricula for hearing-impaired children is typical of the field. Most authorities recognize and support the position that macrocosmic curricular objectives must be similar for all learners. Experience, on the other hand, dictates that modification of these objectives to meet the learning styles and capacities of hearing impaired children is necessary.

The primary determiner of the extent of modification is degree of hearing loss. As Bess and McConnell (1981) stressed, "Curricular approaches for hearing-impaired children cannot be discussed without some attention to the various categories of impairments based on the severity of the hearing loss." Often schools educating severely and profoundly hearing-impaired individuals have written curricula specifically for the needs of their students. These curricula may reflect state or provincial curricula but actual functional objectives vary. A danger in locally created curricula is that the products of such creation may be narrow in scope (Department of Education and Science, 1978). However, many professionals believe that deaf students cannot cope with the full curricula of normally hearing students and, therefore, the objectives of such curricula must be modified. An additional factor to be considered is the presence or absence of multiple handicaps. Is the deaf-retarded learner different in needs than the deaf-blind or deaf-learning disabled or deaf-gifted learner? Are special curricula or special adaptations to curricula required for these learners?

Positions and questions such as these must be considered and answered in the determination of curricular purposes or objectives. While the macrocosmic concept of a common core curriculum across all learners is attractive, it is evident that many educators of the hearing impaired hold significant reservations regarding the "amount" of commonality possible. Whatever the view, it is acknowledged that firm purposes must be defined before the actual laying out of the curriculum is possible.

## SPECIAL NEEDS OF HEARING-IMPAIRED STUDENTS

The reservations of many eductors are rooted in the perception that hearing-impaired learners have special needs. These needs are interpreted as indicating that some hearing-impaired learners are unable to learn in the same fashion and to the same degree as normally hearing learners. Abel and Baker (1981) are among those who present this position. In their discussion on infusion of skills and content into the curricula of the Maryland School for the Deaf they concluded, "After a list of student needs was made, it became increasingly apparent that a traditionally designed curriculum would not best meet these needs."

If, indeed, hearing-impaired learners have special needs, these needs must be noted and examined. Implications for education must be considered and reflected in curricula. Among the special needs of hearing-impaired learners, thc following have been identified:

1. Special language instruction
2. Special speech instruction
3. Aural habilitation instruction
4. Instruction through manual methods
5. A visual emphasis in instruction
6. Differentiated curricula from different groups
7. Specially created support materials

## Language

Language development is the central concern of educators of the hearing impaired. No matter what the degree of hearing loss, that loss appears to disrupt normal language development for the majority of those affected. The greater the loss, the greater the disruption. The pervasive nature of special language need has been such that all other instruction, traditionally, has taken second place to language instruction. Various authorities have taken the position that all curricula must be viewed as presenting opportunities for the expansion of language. They reason that without a solid language base, content of other subjects cannot be learned. A number of highly specific language curricula have been written with the majority bearing little resemblance to those prepared for normally hearing learners. It is only in the case of integrated students that regular curricula have been used extensively and, even then, it is considered necessary that most students receive specialized assistance in language from a teacher of the hearing impaired. Curricula in other areas have been written and adapted to allow for the limited language ability of many hearing-impaired learners. The result has been a tendency to restrict the level of instruction until sufficient language ability is developed to cope with such texts as science and social studies, or to rewrite these texts in simplified language. The language handicap occasioned by hearing impairment has been, and continues to be, a major concern of those involved with any area of education of this population.

## Speech and Aural Habilitation

The need for special speech and aural habilitation curricula is recognized by the vast majority of professionals dealing with hearing-impaired individuals. In recent years aural habilitation has received increasing attention, as teachers, speech and language pathologists, and other professionals have discovered that even minimal residual hearing is useful to most hearing-impaired individuals. Contemporary curricula emphasize stress on hearing for speech use much more than did older curricula. With the advent of the newer curricular approach, or perhaps in some ways leading to it, has been a simultaneous significant improvement in hearing aids and other assistive devices. Curricula in this most important area must take into consideration the functional use of such devices.

Speech and aural habilitation are grouped for the purpose of this short discussion though each is given its own chapter in this text. The grouping here is due to the fact that to a greater degree than ever before the values of intertwining instruction in speech and aural habilitation is being recognized. While each may be examined separately, and may be presented in distinct curriculum packages, as they are in many schools and clinics, the present trend is to regard these two special needs areas as one.

Within this unity of vision it must be recognized that one major variable affects both learning to speak intelligibly and learning to use residual hearing effectively. That variable is the degree of hearing loss involved. Degree of loss dictates to no small degree, the individual's spontaneous development of speech skills and the type of hearing aid recommended. The greater the loss, the less spontaneous the development of speech in the majority of individuals. The greater the loss, the less residual hearing to work with, and the more powerful the hearing aid necessary for maximum stimulation. Careful consideration must be given to the curricular implications of greater or lesser hearing loss. While there are always individual exceptions to any rule, degree of loss, for the majority, is a major determinant of progress in both speech and aural ability. This fact must be realized in curricula in these two allied areas.

### Manual Methods

Over the years a continuing controversy has focussed on the relative merits of oral, aural, and manual methods of instruction. It is not the purpose here to add to that particular discussion except as it relates to curricular design. Recent years have witnessed a decline of emphasis on purely oral and aural instruction and the growth of a methodology known as total communication. Total communication theoretically combines speech, aural habilitation, speech reading, finger spelling, writing, and sign in a fashion designed to best meet the needs of hearing-impaired individuals. The movement to use of total communication has been documented by Jordan, Gustason, and Rosen (1979). Their survey of 1,051 programs in hearing impairment elicited 642 responses. There were 537 programs employing total communication as the major communication mode, and only 6 programs employed an oral and aural method as their primary communication system. This was almost the reverse of the situation 10 years earlier.

This movement has not been accompanied by the development of total communication curricula. Of the nine communications curricula described in *Curriculum Guide Bank* (1982), only one mentions manual methods. The balance focus on speech and aural skills. Curricula in both total communication methods and manual methods are not mentioned with any frequency in the resources reviewed for this text. It would appear that most professionals regard skill in finger spelling and sign as skills that hearing-impaired individuals will "pickup" as normally hearing individuals pickup speech and listening skills. It is assumed that it is not necessary to prepare curricula for total communication, but that curricula may be delivered by means of total communication.

Such an assumption is open to question. If a specific communication system is to become the common means of instruction, that system must be examined and assessed in terms of increased efficiency in instruction. Systems such as speech, aural habilitation and auditory training, finger spelling, and sign have individually been studied for effect on academic achievement. To date there is little hard evidence that total communication is superior to the use of other systems.

One of the characteristics of education of the hearing impaired over the years has been swings of emphasis from one communication mode to another. Changing philosophy rather than new evidence is often the effective agent in choice of communication method for emphasis. Popham's (1969) comment on means in instruction has relevance here: "Frequently the means are never justified in terms of whether they produce increasingly effective attainment of ends; it is considered sufficient that the means are acceptable."

The above discussion should not be taken as argument in favor of or against any particular communication system. As the author has said elsewhere (Bunch, 1979), such an argument is less than productive. The consideration of total communication as a means of instruction, however, is pertinent. If curricula for many hearing-impaired individuals are to be delivered through total communication, the writers of those curricula must note its use and effect on instruction.

## Visual Emphasis

It is commonly held that the auditory limitation of hearing impairment may be attenuated partially through the increased and deliberate use of visual aids. One major avenue of visual endeavor has been the use of sign, finger spelling, and speech reading as compensatory systems. The use of manual systems was discussed previously. Speech reading is also considered of major benefit to many hearing-impaired individuals. The extent of this interest may be seen in the various curricula in speech reading, (Berger, 1972; Fisher, 1977; Jeffers & Barley, 1979; Ordman & Ralli, 1976) and in suggestions to enhance speech reading in the literature, (Bess & McConnell, 1981; Erber, 1977).

The use of illustrations, films, slides, television and captioning has also been a focus of attention (Brennan, 1985). The suggestion that hearing-impaired individuals appear to employ specific visual strategies in learning is mentioned in a limited number of studies noting visual matching strategies (Bunch, 1979; King & Quigley, 1984; Scouten, 1980).

The logic of visual compensation for auditory limitation, the conventional emphasis on visually oriented instruction in education of the hearing impaired, and the few studies indicating specific visual strategies among the hearing impaired have led to a contemporary focus on media to assist in instruction of that population. These include captioned films (Gough, 1963; Parlato, 1982), television (Callace, 1970; Moore, 1955), slides (Schragle, 1982; Scott, 1932), and computers (Rathe, 1969; Stuckless, 1983). While such technical materials are not curricula in and of themselves, their role in education of the hearing impaired must receive consideration.

### Different Groupings Among the Hearing Impaired

The statement that the population of hearing-impaired individuals is far from homogeneous can be made for most populations, but it takes on special meaning in hearing impairment. There appear to be at least three distinct educational groups of hearing-impaired students: severely to profoundly impaired; mildly to moderately impaired; and the multi-handicapped (Bunch, in press).

The severely to profoundly deaf group is characterized by minimal spontaneous development of speech, significant need for specialized teaching of language and reading, and placement in segregated educational situations. Among this group are a number who make sufficient academic progress for eventual admission to post-secondary programs that provide special considerations for hearing-impaired students. Although making some academic progress, a larger group encounters significant difficulty, particulary in language and reading and does not proceed to post-secondary levels.

The mildly to moderately impaired group is characterized roughly by spontaneous, but noticeably imperfect, development of speech and language and placement in integrated settings with specialized support. This group is expected to make progress comparable to that of their normally hearing peers in the subjects in which they are integrated. Depending on degree of loss and ability, individuals within this group may require considerable assistance from a resource person in subjects such as speech, language, and reading.

The third grouping is that of the multi-handicapped, the numbers of which are considerable, with up to 60 percent of deaf children reported to have at least one handicap in addition to that of deafness (Brennan, 1985). This group is characterized by labored academic progress, a need for highly specialized instruction, and placement in segregated classes even within already segregated programs.

It is not the purpose of this discussion to examine the differences and similarities, or the numbers in each of these general groupings. That will remain for those involved in assessment and placement. However, the groupings are of concern to curriculum writers. Is it necessary to design unique curricula for each group? Will one curricula, with some alteration, be suitable for all these groupings? Are curricula used with normally hearing learners appropriate with specific modifications? Questions such as these must be posed and answered if all groups of hearing-impaired children are to receive the most appropriate education.

## SPECIALLY CREATED SUPPORT MATERIALS

Much effort in hearing impairment has been expended in the preparation of special curricular support materials. This effort has followed two paths: one has been that leading to the development of materials to support specialized areas such as speech and aural habilitation. In some sense one might not consider these specially created as much as created from a normal need for materials in curricular areas unique to hearing impairment. The other path, however, does lead to the creation of special materials to support study in areas of study shared by the hearing impaired and the normally hearing alike. Among these areas are language, reading, science, and social studies.

The primary motivation for the creation of such materials has been the impoverished language ability of many hearing-impaired individuals. This impoverishment has given rise to two distinct types of what might be termed "special linguistic" materials. The first is that which is controlled linguistically to assist the hearing-impaired individual to master language and reading independently. These materials begin with relatively simple linguistic demands and proceed developmentally through increasingly complex linguistic structures. King and Quigley (1985), in their review of special reading materials, note "The use of linguistic controls in these materials is seen as a vehicle for reducing the load on the beginning reader so that attention can be directed to "learning to read." Typical of this type of curricular resource material are *Apple Tree* (Anderson, Boren, Caniglia, Howard, & Krohn, 1980) and the *TSA Syntax Program* (Quigley & Power, 1979) in language, *Reading Milestones* (Quigley & King, 1981, 1982, 1983, 1984) and *The Language of Directions* (Rush, 1977) in reading.

The second type of material is that which is semantically, lexically, and conceptually controlled. This material is designed as support for content areas. To enable the hearing-impaired student to follow the conceptual progression of content, linguistic structures and vocabulary are controlled. As a result of controlled language, the student is not faced with the dual task of handling unknown language and unknown content. Typical of such material is the *Controlled Language Science Series* (Fleury, 1979, 1982) and *People Changing: The Irish Come to America* (Simon-Olsen, 1982). An allied type of controlled language, content area material may be found in captioned films and videotapes.

Not all educators accept the need for specially created curricular materials. Those who do argue that the language limitations of the population in question demand unique support materials. Theirs is a philosophy that has much in common with deficit-centered models in other areas of special education. Conversely, others argue for what might be termed a natural model in which the individual is exposed to the normal wealth of language in the environment. This text does not argue for one approach or the other. The undoubtedly severe linguistic handicap of the hearing impaired must be taken into consideration in the design of curricula. It must be realized, however, that the choice of support materials has much to do with how a subject is taught. Logically there must be a direct relationship between the philosophy apparent in a particular educational approach and those support materials chosen to enact it.

## THE REDUCTIONIST PITFALL

The preceding material presents brief discussions of major problems to be considered by those engaged in designing curricula for hearing-impaired students. The balance of the text is similarly concerned with such problems and the actual use of curricula. The natural result is a close examination of the tools of instruction—their limitations, and their strengths. Subjects are broken down into teaching units. Students are discussed in impersonal terms. The tools take on an apparent dominant role with only one aspect being considered of a student, the ability to learn, and only one aspect of the teacher, the ability to design and deliver effective curricula. This is an additional problem for curriculum developers.

Although concern with the effective delivery of instruction is laudable, it should not result in a mechanistic approach to the hearing-impaired individual. The subject to be taught is not more important than the learner in any educational situation. As the following chapters will make clear, many hearing-impaired individuals encounter overwhelming challenges in their attempt to conquer language and other subjects. This situation should never result in lack of consideration of the individual as both an individual and a person with many abilities not directly related to the problems of hearing impairment. Any topic of instruction or curriculum, is subservient to the totality of the individual. To be most appropriate, curricula will be designed to blend with the multiplicity of needs and abilities of the individual as a member of society. While many activities of curriculum design may be reductionist in nature, the total effort must address the whole and avoid becoming entangled in contemplation of the parts.

## SUMMARY

Hearing-impaired students are an unusually difficult group to teach. This difficulty arises, not from lack of interest, lack of potential, or inappropriate behavioral characteristics, but, from the incapacitating effect of being cutoff from normal auditory appreciation of the sounds of the world. One reflection of the depth of this general problem is the annoying problem of preparing instructional curricula that adequately take into consideration the manifold effects of hearing loss. At this point in time, educators of the hearing impaired have not succeeded in educating the average hearing impaired individual to the level of normally hearing peers in any area of study. This situation exists despite the fact that teachers of the hearing impaired are well trained, administrators are competent, and often imaginative, and considerable effort has been expended in small-group instruction.

One field that requires continued attention is that of curriculum design. Due to the traditional educational isolation of the hearing impaired from regular education, little assistance in this area has come from those researching and writing mainstream curricula. This situation has been so pronounced that even those examining the curricular needs of special populations incorrectly consider the needs of the hearing impaired to be minimal. The result of this isolation, and of society's warped view of the challenge of teaching hearing-impaired students, has been an insufficient and sporadic study of the curricular needs of this group. While individual educators and schools have struggled with curriculum design, revision, and implementation, minimal widespread action has been evident.

Educators in hearing impairment would be well-advised to concentrate efforts on a review of their basic purposes in educating hearing-impaired students. They must determine if their objectives are the same as those for normally hearing students, and, if so, whether they are achievable. They must determine whether regular curricula can be used without change, can be used in modified form, or whether specially designed curricula are necessary.

The following chapters have been written to assist those involved with hearing-impaired students in examining past and contemporary curricular practices in various areas of study. It is necessary to know which factors have influenced curricula across time and which factors are pointing to the future. The information in the balance of this text will assist in the comparative analysis of curricula and in the determination of curricular strengths, weaknesses, and needs.

## REFERENCES

Abel, S.K., & Baker, S.C. (1983). The infusion process of skills and content in curriculum development. In F. Solano, J. Egelston-Dodd, & E. Costello (Eds.), *Focus on infusion* (Vol. II). Silver Spring, MD: Convention of American Instructors of the Deaf, pp. 57-63.

Anderson, M., Boren, N., Caniglia, J., Howard, W., & Krohn, E. (1980). *Apple tree.* Beaverton, OR: Dormac.

Berger, K.W. (1972). *Speech reading principles and methods.* Baltimore: National Educational Press.

Bess, F.H., & McConnell, F.E. (1981). *Audiology, education and the hearing impaired child.* St. Louis: C.V. Mosby.

Brennan, W.K. (1985). *Curriculum for special needs.* Philadelphia: Open University Press.

Brill, R.G., Merrill, E., & Frisina, D.R. (1973). *Recommended organizational policies in education of the deaf.* Washington, DC: Conference of Executives of American Schools for the Deaf.

Bunch, G.O. (1978). Language without thinking. *ACEHI Journal, 4,* 39-41.

Bunch, G.O. (1979). Degree and manner of acquisition of written English rules by the deaf. *American Annals of the Deaf, 124,* 10-15.

Bunch, G.O. (in press). Teacher preparation in hearing impairment: A proposal. *Canadian Journal of Education.*

Callace, C. (1970). Basic principles for instructional television. *American Annals of the Deaf, 115*, 587-591.

Cole, E., & Mischook, M. (1985). Survey and annotated bibliography of curricula used by oral preschool programs. *Volta Review, 87*, 139-154.

*Curriculum Guide Bank*. (1982). Washington, DC: Gallaudet College Press.

Department of Education and Science. (1978). *Special educational needs* (Warnock Report). London: HMSO.

Easterbrooks, S.R., & Massey, C.B. (1980). Evaluation and continued assessment of the life cycle of curricula for the hearing impaired. *Volta Review, 82*, 393-398.

Erber, N.P. (1977). Developing materials for lipreading evaluation and instruction. *Volta Review, 79*, 35-42.

Fisher, M. (1977). *Lipreading for a more active life*. Washington, DC: A.G. Bell Association.

Fleury, P. (1979; 1982). *Controlled language science series*. Beaverton, OR: Dormac.

Gough, J.A. (1963). Captioned films for the deaf. *Volta Review, 65*, 24-25, 50.

Griffey, M.N., Sr. (1981). A survey of present methods of developing language in deaf children. In A.M. Mulholland (Ed.), *Oral education today and tomorrow*, Washington, DC: A.G. Bell Association, pp. 119-131.

Hasenstab, M.S., & McKenzie, L.D. (1981). A survey of reading programs used with hearing impaired students. *Volta Review, 83*, 383-388.

Jeffers, J., & Barley, M. (1979). *Look, now hear this*. Springfield, IL: Charles C. Thomas.

Jordon, I.K., Gustason, G., & Rosen, R. (1979). An update on communication trends at programs for the deaf. *Volta Review, 124*, 350-357.

King, C., & Quigley, S. (1984). *Reading milestones placement test battery*. Beaverton, OR: Dormac.

King, C.M., & Quigley, S.P. (1985). Reading and deafness. San Diego: College-Hill Press.

Lang, H.G., & Propp, G. (1982). Science education for hearing impaired students: State-of-the-art. *American Annals of the Deaf, 127*, 860-869.

LaSasso, C. (1978). National survey of materials and procedures used to teach reading to hearing impaired children. *American Annals of the Deaf, 123*, 22-30.

Ling, D. (1976). *Speech and the hearing impaired child: Theory and practice*. Washington, DC: A.G. Bell Association.

Lowell, E.L. (Ed.). (1967). *Report of special study institute: Curriculum planning for the deaf*. Los Angeles: John Tracey Institute.

Moore, L. (1955). Television as a medium for teaching speech reading and speech. *Volta Review, 57*, 263-264.

Ordman, K.A., & Ralli, M.P. (1976). *What people say*. Washington, DC: A.G. Bell Association.

Parlato, S. (1982). Educational captioned films and field evaluation: Broadening the base. In F. Solano, J. Egelston-Dodd, & E. Costello (Eds.), *Focus on infusion* (Vol. 1). Silver Spring, MD: Convention of American Instructors of the Deaf. pp. 168-171.

Popham, W.J. (1969). Objectives and instruction. *American Educational Research Association Monograph Series on Curriculum Evaluation, 25*, 32-64.

Quigley, S.P., & Power, D. (Eds.). (1979). *TSA syntax program*. Beaverton, OR: Dormac.

Quigley, S.P., & King, C. (Eds.). (1981, 1982, 1983, 1984). *Reading milestones*. Beaverton, OR: Dormac.

Rathe, G.H. (1969). Computer assisted instruction and its potential for teaching deaf students. *American Annals of the Deaf, 114*, 880-883.

Rush, N. (1977). *The language of directions*. Washington, DC: A.G. Bell Association.

Saif, P.S., & Thiel, L. (1983, June). *Application of a model of curriculum development and evaluation to content areas for hearing impaired students.* Paper presented at the joint meeting of the Association of Canadian Educators of the Hearing Impaired and the Convention of American Instructors of the Deaf, Winnipeg, Manitoba.

Sass-Lehrer, M. (1984). Curriculum revision: A step-by-step approach. *Perspectives, 2*, 10-12.

Schragle, P. (1982). Preparing captioned slides for classroom use. In F. Solano, J. Eglelston-Dodd, & E. Costello (Eds.). *Focus on infusion* (Vol. 1). Silver Spring, MD: Convention of American Instructors of the Deaf, pp. 177-179.

Scott, E.V. (1932). The use of slides in primary classes. *Volta Review, 34*, 56-58.

Scouten, E. (1980). An instructional strategy to combat the wordmatching tendencies in prelingually deaf students. *American Annals of the Deaf, 125*, 1057-1059.

Simon-Olsen, B. (1982). *People changing: The Irish come to America.* Providence, RI: Corliss Park Press.

Stuckless, R. (1983). The microcomputer in the instruction of hearing impaired students. Tool or distraction? *American Annals of the Deaf, 128*, 515-520.

Tyler, R.W. (1949). *Basic principles of curriculum and instruction.* Chicago: University of Chicago Press.

Tomlinson, S. (1982). *A sociology of special education.* London: Routledge & Kegan Paul.

# CHAPTER 2

# *Language Curricula*

The ultimate aim of every teacher responsible for developing the language of a hearing-impaired child is that the child will develop normal language ability. Some teachers have no doubt that, if certain methods are followed, the majority of hearing-impaired children can obtain language abilities similar to those of their hearing peers. They exhort teachers to follow their ideas closely to achieve success. We thus find the following statements in the literature (Fitzgerald, 1949):

> We have proved to our satisfaction that classification of words and thoughts (under key-words and the few symbols that we use) and the understanding that follows hasten, to say the least, the child's grasp of and spontaneous use of English.

and (Van Uden, 1977):

> The purely oral way remains the ideal for prelingually deaf children: more deaf children can be brought to the full culture of language, and this can be done on the average, better and sooner than by other means, provided the right methods are followed by qualified teachers.

and (Groht, 1958):

> Teachers who do not believe that normal deaf children can acquire the use of language as it is used by people who can hear, lack faith in the abilities and possibilities of the deaf.

Such statements fly in the face of research findings regarding the language achievement levels of hearing-impaired individuals. Researchers consistently have documented the inability of the average severely to profoundly hearing-impaired person to achieve a normal range of vocabulary and comprehension in language. Heider and Heider (1941), Templin (1950), Myklebust (1960), MacGinitie (1964), Brannon (1968), Nunnally and Blanton (1966), Garber (1967), Schmitt (1970), Di Francesca, Trybus, and Buchanan (1971), Quigley, Wilbur, and Montanelli (1974), Sarachan-Deily and Love (1974), Brennen (1977), Bunch (1978) and Moores (1981) are among those who have examined, in one way or another, the language development of hearing-impaired children. All agree that the average hearing-impaired youngster does not enjoy the ability to use language with the same facility as his hearing peers, or even that of much younger hearing children. There can be no doubt that some hearing-impaired individuals do achieve well and possess age-commensurate language abilities. Among them are many individuals with mild-to-moderate hearing loss and a significantly lesser number of individuals with severe to profound loss. There can be no doubt that past and present curricular methods in language have not been equal to the task of establishing acceptable standards of language ability in the hearing-impaired population in general.

The present text does not detail research into language achievement levels. The reader is referred to studies and works referenced, and to others, for supportive detail. One study is noted here to indicate typical findings in this area. Gentile and Di Francesca (1969) surveyed results on the Stanford Achievement Test across 21,447 children aged 7- to 17-years plus (see Table 2-1).

The low levels of achievement across the various categories noted give rise to little feeling of accomplishment among educators of the hearing impaired. Moores (1970) was not incorrect in stating that hearing-impaired children are "significantly inferior (to hearing children) in all aspects of language development and facility." Little evidence that older or newer curricula have altered the above facts or tempered such views is available.

## GENERAL CURRICULAR APPROACHES

Two general varieties of language curricula have been developed for hearing-impaired children. Both find their roots in the accumulated knowledge of classroom teachers. Both evolved slowly and demonstrate the melding of large portions of conventional wisdom and practice and modest portions of contemporary research. These two, the analytic (formal, structural, grammatical, constructionalist, scientific, systematic) and the natural (informal, synthetic, mother's method), or some combination or form of them are used throughout the English-speaking world today (Bunch, 1975; Griffey, 1981; Moores, 1982).

King (1983) found that four primary approaches were employed in the United States. The first three were the structural, the natural, and the combined, (i.e., melded aspects of the structural and the natural). These terms were used when a particular method was employed throughout a school or school division. King used a fourth term, "eclectic," for those instances in which

**Table 2-1.** Percent of Hearing-Impaired Subjects Scoring Above Specified Grade Levels by Age on Stanford Test of Achievement Language Items

| | Percent of subjects scoring at or above grade level noted | | | | | |
|---|---|---|---|---|---|---|
| **Age/grade level** | **Word meaning** | **Paragraph meaning** | **Vocabulary** | **Language** | **Word study** | **Reading** |
| Age 7* Grade 2.0 | 16.9 | 9.8 | 2.0 | | 11.3 | 10.7 |
| Age 8* Grade 3.0 | 3.5 | 2.3 | 1.8 | | 5.6 | 2.5 |
| Age 9* Grade 3.0 | 2.1 | 1.8 | 1.6 | | 4.9 | 2.0 |
| Age 10† Grade 4.5 | 0.2 | 0.4 | | 7.9 | 7.0 | 0.2 |
| Age 11† Grade 4.5 | 0.0 | 1.1 | | 11.5 | 5.4 | 0.0 |
| Age 12‡ Grade 5.5 | 3.3 | 3.7 | | 4.5 | 5.5 | 2.9 |
| Age 13‡ Grade 5.5 | 1.0 | 3.5 | | 5.4 | 7.3 | 2.9 |
| Age 14** Grade 7.5 | 0.7 | 2.1 | | 4.5 | | 1.1 |
| Age 15** Grade 7.5 | 0.4 | 2.5 | | 5.1 | | 0.4 |
| Age 16** Grade 7.5 | 0.3 | 0.7 | | 2.4 | | 0.7 |
| Age 17** Grade 7.5 | 0.4 | 0.4 | | 2.5 | | 0.4 |

Note: Data adapted from Gentile, G., and DiFrancesca, S. (1969).

* Primary I battery
† Primary II battery
‡ Intermediate I battery
** Intermediate II battery

individual teachers chose which of the three methods they would use. A fifth category, "others," indicated methods that did not fit comfortably under any of the above four. The responses from 233 participating systems are summarized in Table 2-2. The structural or analytic and natural approaches are obviously the choice of the great majority of educational programs. These two basic systems are discussed in detail below.

**Table 2-2.** Language Instruction Approaches Used with Hearing-Impaired Students by Percent

| Approach | Preschool | Primary | Intermediate | Jr. High | High |
|---|---|---|---|---|---|
| Structural | 5.2 | 7.4 | 9.9 | 10.9 | 8.7 |
| Natural | 34.1 | 6.2 | 4.9 | 1.5 | 4.4 |
| Combined | 36.3 | 58.0 | 55.9 | 48.8 | 47.1 |
| Eclectic | 23.0 | 27.3 | 29.1 | 38.6 | 39.4 |
| Other | 1.4 | 1.1 | .1 | .1 | .1 |

Adapted from King, C.M. (June 1983). *Survey of language methods and materials used with hearing impaired students in the United States.* Winnipeg: Joint Convention of ACEHI, CAID and CEASD.

## The Analytic Method

Proponents of the analytic method consider that language principles and structures must be presented in a planned, coherent fashion. Certain patterns characterize language and, if the hearing impaired child is to master language, he must learn the basic patterns and then extend them into more and more complex patterns. In general the analytic systems have been used more widely with students with greater than lesser hearing losses.

The essentials of present analytic systems may be found in the work of Heinicke (1729–1784), who followed a grammatical approach to language teaching. Heinicke formed various word types (nouns, prepositions, adjectives, adverbs, and verbs) into lists and then placed them artificially in basic sentence forms. Activities promoting memorization of these forms were devised for student practice. Eventually the analytic method crossed the Atlantic to the United States with Laurent Clerc in the form of Sicard's theory of ciphers. This theory of ciphers had grown from the work of de l'Epée, a contemporary of Heinicke. Like Heinicke, de l'Epée considered that words could fit into place in a sentence form according to a grammatical system. For some time the basic approach in many North American schools was to divide a sentence into component parts (nominative case, verb, objective case, preposition, and object of preposition) and interchange appropriate words as required (Clerc 1851; Moores, 1982). The basic analytic approach has undergone a variety of changes and continues to do so today.

Among these changing forms were systems such as the Wing Symbols (Wing, 1887) and the Barry Five-Slate System (Barry, 1899). The Wing Symbol system consists of letters, numbers and other symbols placed over written language to explain the form and function of the parts of a sentence. The main aspect of the Wing system is a series of eight symbols:

S = subject;

V = verb;

V‾‾‾‾‾ = transitive verb;

V‾‾‾‾‾Ↄ = intransitive verb;

‾‾‾‾‾V = passive verb;

O = object;

AC = adjective complement;

N = noun or pronoun complement.

The Barry Five-Slate System consisted originally of five divisions of a basic sentence. These divisions (subject, verb, object of the verb, preposition, object of the preposition) were used as fixed guides under which appropriate parts of a sentence were written. In group work these divisions were each on large separate slates. For individual work each child had a smaller slate appropriately divided. Eventually a sixth division or slate was added for time expressions. These systems were popular at the turn of the century. Though not in formal, generalized use at the present time, vestiges of these methods may yet be seen. Old ideas die hard, especially when newer ideas have not done away with earlier problems.

The Fitzgerald Key is the contemporary outgrowth of earlier analytic systems (Fitzgerald, 1949). This approach to language has been the most widely used among the structural systems (Quigley & Paul, 1984). The Key may be considered a generative system of language in that it provides the student with a set of rules from which to derive or generate a variety of sentences. From an initial emphasis on vocabulary acquisition under Key words (i.e., what; who; how many.) the teacher leads the children to the formulation of simple assertive sentence forms and then on to question forms and increasingly complex sentences. Stress is placed on correct syntactical order and gradual addition of sentence elements. A simplified form of the Key is found in many classrooms across North America. A typical display may appear as in Figure 2-1.

Though the majority of schools do not now use the Key in its full form, teaching aids and teaching methods reminiscent of the Key are common. King (1983) reported that 37.9 percent of programs responding to her study stated that they specifically used the symbol system associated with the Key. One school retaining essentials of the Key is Clarke School for the Deaf. Their language curriculum publications, *Language* (1972) and *English Curriculum: Upper School* (1978), clearly state that their formal or analytic approach is based on *Straight Language for the Deaf* by Fitzgerald (1949). "The Key is used in this method to establish the sentence pattern. It is built-up for the children

| Who: | What: | | |
|---|---|---|---|
| What:________ | Whom: | Where: | When: |

**Figure 2-1.** A sample of Fitzgerald Key headings.

step-by-step as new constructions are introduced. This pattern helps the child visualize the relationships of words, phrases, and clauses in the normal sequence" (Clarke School for the Deaf, 1972).

It is useful in attempting to understand the Key to read Fitzgerald's preface to *Straight Language for the Deaf*. It is clear that the method presented was designed to assist the child in cognitive development. "Back of the title, Straight Language, there lies the assumption that straight *language* implies straight *thinking*." It is clear as well that Fitzgerald considered her method to be a "natural" one. She eschewed "unnatural, mechanical language" and "mechanical ways of acquiring it." Finally it is of interest to note that Fitzgerald did not mean to set out a curriculum, or course of study. She specifically denied it, stating that attempting to lay down a course of study would take many books. However, the Key has been taken by many as a curriculum guide and the system has been molded by some into an unnatural, mechanistic method.

Over the years, the Key has led to the explication of a number of curricula. One of the earliest of these may be found in the two books comprising Buell's *Outline of Language for Deaf Children* (1952a, 1952b). Detailed schema for language instruction over a six year period are presented. More latterly are the Clarke School publication *Language* (1972) outlining the school's language approach for children up to 13 years of age, and *English Curriculum: Upper School* (1978) that focusses on the 13- to 17-year age range. Continued interest in the Key is apparent also in both Hudson (1979), in which the language program at the Kansas School for the Deaf is outlined, and in survey reports such as that by King (1983).

The Key, as the contemporary representative of traditional analytic approaches, has been criticized for a number of reasons. As Moores (1982) noted, the Key produces "essentially linear, left to right strings and cannot illustrate some logical relations between utterances which would be intuitively obvious to a native user of language." Griffey (1981) commented on the emphasis of vocabulary lists intrinsic to the Key and other analytic methods and deplored the apparent lack of understanding of the needs and lives of children. Similarly, but in a more general sense, Streng, Kretschmer, and Kretschmer (1978) observed that despite Fitzgerald's obvious brilliance of concept, many of those who subsequently used the Key did not possess her vision and grasp of language and reduced her method to mechanistic teaching. Their statement that "when the Key serves only as an end rather than as the means to straight language, it loses its value" is certainly valid. However, this type of statement is not to be associated with analytic methods only. It is a comment on the quality of training and instruction of teachers, rather than a comment on the viability of any one curricular approach. Perhaps the most telling comment is that analytic systems do not appear to give most hearing-impaired individuals the ability to internalize language rules.

While some traditional systems possess a generative aspect, they have been limited by inflexibility. Contemporary curricula have reduced this inflexibility to a greater or lesser degree. In general, recent curricular approaches have embraced a transformational-generative theme. Beginning with Chomsky (1957), linguists moved away from traditional, structural grammar theories to an emphasis on the syntactic relationship of words, phrases, and sentences. The child was seen more as an active and creative participant in the language development process and less as a relatively passive responder to stimuli. Language was viewed as having two levels: one, the deep or underlying rule level, where true understanding of language relationships existed, and two, a surface or performance level in which these understandings reached expression mediated by memory, fatigue, level of attention, and other factors. Between these levels operated rules or transformations that translated "internalized" knowledge into utterances. Educators of the hearing impaired, excited and enthused by this new view of language, and frustrated by lack of success with traditional methods, seized on generative-transformational concepts and produced new curricular approaches.

One of the earliest of these was *A Patterned Program of Linguistic Expansion Through Reinforced Experiences and Evaluations* (Apple Tree), (Caniglia, Cole, Howard, Krohn, & Rice, 1972), the most popular of contemporary analytical systems (King, 1983). Other early transformational curricula were *Lessons in Syntax* (McCarr, 1973) and, even earlier, *The Language Curriculum: Rhode Island School for the Deaf* (Blackwell & Hamel, 1971). These curricula accepted a relatively simplistic view of generative-transformational grammar and replaced the Key approach of building up basic to complex sentence forms with an approach based on a limited number of sentence forms. These were to be mastered and then manipulated or transformed through application of selected rules into other sentence forms. These early transformational grammar curricula were replete with new terminology and teaching ideas. However, they had leaped too quickly onto the generative-transformational bandwagon. Most linguists would not have agreed in the late 60s and early 70s that the theory was sufficiently far advanced to be translated successfully into practice. Certainly the concept of predictable sentence structures and basic rules that operated across large numbers of structures was appealing. As King (1983) reported 57.5 percent of programs used all of or part of the symbol systems associated with Apple Tree, 19.7 percent used Rhode Island, 19.3 percent used names of transformations, and other systems totaled 20.6 percent. The difficulty lay in an incomplete understanding of the theory being used, the fact that the field of linguistics itself only paused for a period of emphasis on syntactic relationships, and a rather cautious inclusion of some more traditional "crutches," such as a continuing dependence on vocabulary lists and a restricted set of basic sentence patterns. As Blackwell, Engen, Fischgrund, and Zarcadoolas (1978) noted, the introduction of these new curricula did not make any real difference in the internalization of syntactic rules and the emphasis on simple sentence formation continued to emphasize " 'straight language' rather than complex language." In many respects these early transformational grammar curricula were simply old methods in new clothing (see Table 2-3).

**Table 2-3.** Type Language Curricula and Systems Employed with Hearing-Impaired Children

| Developer | System | Characteristics |
|---|---|---|
| Heinicke (Germany, 1700's) | Grammatical approach | Word lists, basic sentence forms, artificial manipulation, stress on writing |
| Sicard (France, 1700's) | Theory of ciphers | Word lists, division of sentence into five parts, artificial manipulation, stress on writing |
| Wing (U.S., 1887) | Wing symbols | Division of sentence by functions of elements, sentence analysis through symbols, word categories |
| Barry (U.S., 1899) | Five-slate system | Division of sentence into five parts (later six), artificial manipulation, word lists |
| Fitzgerald (U.S., 1929) | Straight Language | Systematic build-up of sentences, word lists, no mechanical drill, key words, generative |
| Caniglia et al. (U.S., 1972) | Apple Tree | Basic sentence forms, stress on vocabulary, artificial manipulation, generative, transformational terminology, consistent evaluation, part of a program only |
| McCarr (U.S., 1973) | Lessons in syntax | Extended sentence forms, considerable language ability required, artificial manipulation, generative, transformational terminology, consistent evaluation, part of a program only |
| Blackwell et al. (U.S., 1978) | Sentences and other systems | Basic sentence patterns, cognitive emphasis, semantic emphasis, spiral curriculum evaluative methods, psycholinguistic model |
| Streng et al. (U.S., 1978) | Integrated language arts | Basic sentence patterns, cognitive/experiential approach, minimal grammar, psycholinguistic model |

Updated versions of transformational grammars have appeared. Among these are *Sentences and Other Systems* (Blackwell et al., 1978), which is a reworking of the Rhode Island Curriculum, and the experience-based integrated approach suggested by Streng, Kretschmer, and Kretschmer (1978). In some ways these approaches may not be considered truly analytic since they make use of natural method philosophy to a considerable degree. However, they do continue to accept such aspects as a limited set of sentence forms and a stress on vocabulary and structure.

These latter approaches attempted to move ahead with linguistic study and included some emphasis on semantics and pragmatics. They endeavored to integrate the concepts of current linguistic theory and the principles of Piagetian developmental psychology. Language development was not viewed as something separate from other developmental aspects of the hearing-impaired child. Integrated as well were principles of contemporary curricular design. Blackwell and associates (1978) stressed the contributions of Bruner and the concept of the spiral curriculum, while Streng and colleagues (1978) emphasized the need to plan experiences from which to derive language in an integrated language-arts model.

These more recent analytic approaches represent a positive movement in language work with hearing-impaired individuals. The emerging theories of linguistics provide a base for major curricular advances. Newer analytic curricula should prove superior to existing traditional approaches. Limitations continue to plague analytic methods, however. These are basically teaching methods and do not affect the whole child as a linguistic environment affects the whole normally hearing child. A movement in the direction of ecological curricula is apparent but it is not yet a reality. Most analytic approaches caution that they are not sufficient unto themselves to accomplish the task of adequate language development. A basic problem is that we do not fully understand how the "user" of language acquires his or her skills. Until we bring sufficient knowledge of "user" and "developmental schema" together, our attempts will be incomplete.

## The Natural Method

Though analytic methods were the choice of most early North American educators of the hearing impaired, a number opposed what they perceived as an inflexible, grammatical approach that did not require much more of the students than memorization. Among these was Greenberger (1879) who espoused a system of teaching grammatical principles and necessary vocabulary in the context of natural situations. Language was to rise from the needs of the child with teaching focussed on an exploitation of opportunities arising in daily activities. With Greenberger, the Lexington School began a long history of adherence to "natural" methods of teaching language to the hearing impaired, a history that continues to the present day. Essentially Greenberger, and others after him, put forth the curricular position that if children are taught language in an artificial fashion from a predetermined sequence of principles, they will use it in an artificial fashion, never translating it into a fluent, normal receptive, and expressive system. They consider that a natural language approach provides the best opportunity to avoid these weaknesses. The natural method has been used with students who have a wide range of hearing losses.

At approximately the same time as Greenberger developed his views, Alexander Graham Bell (1883) pursued and published information regarding a natural method of teaching language. Working with a 5-year-old child, Bell seized on daily play activities as a basis for teaching words and language in the immediate environment. The language of any situation was recorded on a chalkboard. Phrases were grouped together and the intonation patterns of speech represented by such devices as altering the size of the print to indicate emphasis.

The curricular views of such figures as Greenberger and Bell clashed with those of most earlier educators and considerable controversy resulted. This argument continues. Two recent educators who reject analytic methods completely and espouse natural language approaches are Groht (1958) and Van Uden (1977).

Groht emerged from the Lexington system as a firm proponent of the natural method. She believed beyond doubt that "the way to make it possible for the deaf child to gain this mastery (of language) is not by altering the language itself but by making it alive and desirable for him and by seeing that it meets his needs." Though Groht did not claim to have provided a curriculum in language, her book sketched the types of language activities she considered appropriate from preschool to the secondary level. Her ideas have been accepted as the basis for a curriculum by many. Schmitt (1966) outlined the basic principles of Groht's approach as:

1. Language and vocabulary must be supplied according to the child's needs rather than to rigid word lists and principle listings.
2. Natural language is acquired by repetition in meaningful situations rather than by drill and textbook exercises.
3. Language use is best taught through conversation and discussion, written compositions of all kinds, and through academic and skill areas of the curriculum.
4. When language principles need to be taught they should be introduced incidentally in natural situations, then explained by the teacher in a real situation, then practiced by the children through use of games, questions, stories, pictures and conversations (p. 94).

With these as a guide, and with the many teaching ideas supplied by Groht, teachers have felt able to teach hearing-impaired children of all ages and to do so successfully. They have not felt the need for a predetermined listing of sequentially arranged language principles.

Van Uden (1977) has continued the work by such as Groht and is among the most prolific of advocates of a natural instructional approach to language. He further developed the concepts of earlier educators and evolved a "maternal reflective method" in which he compared the influence of a teacher using this method to "the parents of hearing children, i.e., those who educate them through and in their mother tongue." Van Uden is convinced that modern psycholinguistic theory has provided sufficient insight into language development for the educator of the hearing-impaired child to succeed in teaching that child the mother tongue as a first language. He does not deny that the actual teaching may not be as informal as with a normally hearing child, but it can be similar.

Van Uden developed a "conversational" approach to spoken and written language. Intertwining theory, models and practical suggestions in a sometimes confusing fashion, he laid out his curricular approach. In doing so he noted continually that his method and an oral approach are mutually dependent, that the maternal reflective approach yields a cultural language base, that analytic (constructionalist) methods are limited and limiting, and that few hearing-impaired children would ever require assistance through manual communication.

### Summary of Analytical and Natural Approaches

Despite the claims of the advocates for one method or another, and the barbs of detractors, neither the analytic nor the natural approach has produced desirable levels of language ability across the general hearing-impaired population. The methods tend to produce admirable (and enviable) results in the hands of individual practitioners. There can be no doubt that Bell, Fitzgerald, Groht, Buell, and Van Uden made their systems succeed to their satisfaction. There can be no doubt, either, that these methods appear to be person-dependent. In the hands of one individual they are excellent; in the hands of many others, they yield mediocre results. The Key, for instance, was a brilliantly devised system and, when used appropriately, children learned English well. Unfortunately, in the hands of too many others, the Key was employed in a mechanistic fashion, feeding on the artificial drill activities deplored by Fitzgerald. A similar fate befell practitioners of the natural method as outlined by Groht. Without extensive knowledge of language, and without Groht's sensitivity to the method, many "were often left floundering in a sea of unstructured language problems" (Streng, Kretschmer, & Kretschmer, 1978, p. 128).

Over the years a variety of criticisms have been levelled at various methods. Lenneberg (1967) questioned whether the meta-language methodologies available for language instruction of the hearing impaired coupled with the deficiency in model examples occasioned by hearing impairment, would ever result in normal language ability for the hearing-impaired population. Garber (1967) criticized teaching methods for the hearing impaired for not exposing the hearing-impaired child to the extensive language experiences enjoyed by normally hearing children. Lowenbraun (1969) viewed language teaching methods for the deaf as deviating from the language acquisition patterns of other children. Doctor (1950) and Streng (1964) found a weakness in traditional methodologies with their strong tendency towards overwhelming teacher involvement and minimal child involvement. Moores (1981) regarded proponents of the analytic approach as "wedded to a deficiency or pathology model" that was unrewarding. Perhaps most telling are comments such as that by Griffey (1981). After viewing the field and the controversy between major curricular approaches she stated "sides are taken, and very often the welfare of the deaf child is lost sight of, in the controversy that ensues, because a particular method has become more important than the pupil." Bunch (1978) has suggested that this problem may have arisen because educators of the hearing impaired have been faced with a problem beyond their resources. When faced with a monumental task and offered competing resources, it is not unusual for the individual to seize on one of these resources, invest it with appropriate power, and wield it diligently and faithfully to the exclusion of other systems. It is a type of "true believer syndrome" that eases frustrations and acts as a security system.

## CONTEMPORARY CURRICULAR CONCERNS

Since the 1960s educators of the hearing impaired have been grappling with a new way of looking at language development, discussed briefly previously as transformational-generative language theory. In essence, language development is viewed as a result of the child interacting with an environment replete with auditory language. As children interact with their language environment, they test the language they hear, absorb or receive it, and integrate or internalize it into an emerging set of rules for expression. Eventually these internalized rules are tested on others in the environment and constantly modified and extended until an acceptably normal language corpus is developed. The child, equipped with an innate propensity for learning language (Lenneberg, 1967), demonstrates basic mastery of the majority of oral-language structures by the time he is ready to enter school. He is in command of the syntactic, semantic, and phonologic bases of his language and is ready to extend this oral command into the graphic sphere, in forms of reading and writing, to learn those few remaining language rules not yet mastered, and to continue in the development of discourse abilities.

Educators of the hearing impaired have been grappling with this new knowledge because it does not fit traditional curricular reasoning in language development for the hearing impaired. Past curricula are based on the assumption that language may be taught and taught successfully. Under analytic methods, a curriculum consisting of a designated sequence of language principles and suggestions for teaching procedures was laid out. The teacher taught through the sequence carefully, testing mastery as she went, and completed the curriculum by the end of a stated number of years. The number of years was raised and some of the higher level principles dropped for hearing-impaired children with multiple handicaps. Under the natural methods the teacher responded to the language needs of the child, divining needed principles from daily activities and teaching them. Over the years the child would demonstrate the need for all the usual principles of English and these principles would be taught in nonmechanistic fashion. A major problem with all of this, under both major curricular variants, was that it took place after the child passed the critical stage for language learning and had entered formal education. The child did not test his own emerging language rules and form his own decisions. The finished rules were taught to him either from a predetermined list, or because he appeared to need to use the principle in question. Flexible amounts of time for reception and internalization of rules were not given. Expression, close on the heels of the first exposure to the "rule," was the order of the day. Teaching procedures under both methods were similar (Bunch, 1975) and were developed on stimulus-response, direct imitation models.

Over the same period educators of the hearing impaired realized that language and thought are inextricably linked and no language curriculum is complete without an emphasis on cognitive growth. This recognition grew primarily from the work of Furth (1966) and others during the 1960s and is embodied at present in a number of language curricula (Blackwell et al., 1978; Streng et al., 1978). Contemporary curricula that do not stress cognitive development based on the work of theorists such as Piaget (1955) and Vygotsky (1962) lack a much needed dimension.

It would appear that much has occurred to make challenging the life of the curriculum developer of language for the hearing impaired. Concurrent with a change in language theory, and the emergence of cognition as a major factor in language curricula, came a push for integration. This did not mean only integration of hearing-impaired children, but also of teachers of the hearing impaired, and curriculum development linked with the mainstream of education. Prior to the 1960s the educator of the hearing impaired was able to evolve language schema that reflected experientially derived needs and did not draw heavily on curriculum development theory common to regular education. To a significant degree, curricula were developed in-house by experienced teachers of the hearing impaired and with little recognition of need for input from outsiders. This, too, has changed. There is a growing realization that concepts of curriculum development common in mainstream education must become common in both special education and in education of the hearing impaired. One of the early innovators in this regard was Grammatico who brought concepts from Taba to preschool curricula (Grammatico & Miller, 1974). Carrying this concept forward are Blackwell and associates (1978) who wove Bruner's concepts of the spiral curriculum throughout their work, teachers like Cole

(1980) who are attempting to base curricula on active involvement, deduction, induction, and exploration, and supervisors like Stone (1980) who are developing cognitive teaching styles in their teachers.

If the above points are drawn together a number of guidelines for the design of language curricula for the hearing impaired emerge. Not all these are unique to the area of hearing impairment though they do form a unique package. These guidelines are:

1. Provision of curricula appropriate for use during the critical stage of language acquisition.
2. Utilization of information gained in studies of normal language development.
3. Ensuring of receptive and expressive periods of sufficient duration to promote internalization of language rules.
4. Development of cognitive abilities and linguistic abilities simultaneously.
5. Alignment of curricula for the hearing impaired closer to the design of curricula for mainstream education.
6. Application of contemporary curricular theory in the development of language curricula for the hearing impaired.

## Critical Stage of Normal Language Acquisition

Children pass through a critical stage for language acquisiton. This stage begins at birth and is completed by age 4 or 5 years (Bryen, 1980; Hammill, Bartel, & Bunch, 1984; Hopper & Naremore, 1973). The brain is innately programmed for the acquisition of language and if this innate system is influenced by a normal language environment, language is acquired rapidly and according to a routine pattern (Dale, 1976; Lenneberg, 1967). If the language environment is severely disrupted, or if the innate system is damaged or incompletely developed, language acquisition is delayed or fails to occur. Moores (1970a, 1982) presents the possibility that "any language program that is initiated after age five—no matter what methods are used—is doomed to failure for the majority of deaf children." Though Moore's comment has not received wide attention within the field of hearing impairment, it posesses the weight of logic. If the human neurological system is designed to facilitate the acquisition of language, if neural pathways are set up and ready to go, lack of stimulation over a period of time may result in the deterioration of such pathways. A type of atrophy may set in as it does with other human systems that are inactive over lengthy periods. If such is the case, curriculum developers must be concerned with the early years, for this is the time when the system is still in condition to perform the task for which it was designed.

To a surprising degree, this is not yet the case. Few curricula have been developed for the preschool period. Two that have been developed are by Harris (1971), *Language for the Preschool Deaf Child*, and Northcott's *Curriculum Guide: Hearing Impaired Children (0-3 years) and Their Parents* (1977). It is difficult to find other curricula that, like these, emphasize language development and aim at a development parallel to that of the normally hearing child. The fact that both of these are not new indicates that some curricula developers realized the importance of the early years before the spate of present studies and articles excited interest. On the other hand, it is indicative of relative lack of activity in this area, in which one finds few contemporary curricula focussed on this area.

This is not to suggest that no activity is taking place. Indeed, there is a high level of interest in the implications of normal acquisitional patterns for the education of the hearing impaired. Sitnick, Rushmer, and Arpan (1977) developed an interesting *Parent-Infant Communication* curriculum for the years from birth to age 4. Within this curriculum is a clear realization that the parent and not the educator of the hearing-impaired child is the responsible person in early language development. In fact, two separate but interdependent curricula are offered; one for hearing-impaired preschoolers, and one for the parents of hearing-impaired preschoolers. Holmes and Holmes (1981) developed a language programming approach that follows a normal language acquisitional model. They stressed the importance of social discourse between the hearing-impaired child and mother. Research was cited indicating that there does appear to be a discernible stage-based developmental schema in the language acquisition of the hearing impaired. They went on to link lack of early exposure to sign language and a resultant inadequate linguistic environment to delays in language development. It is certainly a stretching of the literature to suggest, as these authors appear to do, that a curriculum based on early transmission of language through sign, as against oral methods, is warranted by available studies. It would not be a stretching of any point to suggest that manual communication or oral communication can be used to further linguistic aims and to stimulate early communication. Unfortunately, Holmes and Holmes did not develop this latter thrust in any detail.

Hasenstab (1983) also developed curricular ideas for young hearing-impaired children. She stressed the role of pragmatics as central to the habilitative process. Within the general topic of pragmatiacs, she developed the importance of the context in which language occurs, the idea of communicative intent, and the concept of discourse rules that govern interaction. In her short article, Hasenstab did not have room to do more than suggest these as focal areas of interest and to provide a few examples of how they might be understood and utilized. She did, however, succeed in drawing the importance of such areas of language development to the attention of those concerned with the design of early language curricula.

A theoretical model for language development based on research in normal language acquisition was offered by Knight (1979). He accepted the position that "hearing impaired children appear to go through similar developmental stages of English language as hearing children, though at a slower rate." His model was based on this questionable assumption. In developing the model Knight took into consideration a number of basic problems. Among these were (1) the doubtfulness of most family situations for hearing-impaired children developing a sophisticated sign language communication atmosphere, despite any advantages for ASL as a medium of communication; (2) the difficulty in providing full and unambiguous access to English as a native tongue for the hearing-impaired child in most family situations; and (3) the physical limitations of the visual system in transmitting a language evolved on the basis of an auditory environment and the relatively more efficient auditory system. It is not the purpose of the present discussion to detail Knight's model. Interested readers will find this presentation elsewhere. It is important, though, for those interested in language curriculum development to be aware of the types of problems Knight raises. These, and perhaps others, possess significant implications for curricula of general use across the critical preschool period of language acquisition.

The present text is also not the place to review what is known of normal language development. It is accepted that language development in the hearing impaired should follow the pattern seen in normally hearing children for the best results in language. Therefore, a number of basic points may be made for curriculum developers. These are:

1. Language curricula for the hearing impaired should reflect developmental patterns known to exist among normally hearing children.
2. Language curricula must be ecological in nature. They must deal with all aspects of the child's environment.
3. Language curricula must be designed for implementation at the earliest possible stage.
4. Ways must be found and detailed to involve parents and others in providing a linguistic environment for the hearing-impaired child from birth, through the critical stage of language acquisition, as well as later.

## Internalization or Memorization

An individual who has easy use of the mother tongue has developed a set of internalized rules for dealing with linguistic situations and producing appropriate language. Following a sufficient period of language reception the normally hearing person begins attempts at expressing language knowledge. This expression begins with single words at approximately 1 year of age and passes gradually through two-word and three-word stages and on to complete sentence forms. Other words are added to early nouns and verbs, such as adjectives, pronouns, and articles in a relatively predictable schedule. As expressive experimentation continues, endings appear on words and regular and irregular verb forms are used with increasing accuracy. It is important to emphasize that receptive opportunities in various situations must be provided the child before he is able to attempt his first expressions. In general, if not universally, these first expressive attempts are approximations of correct syntactic strings, of needed phonologic components and of semantic intentions. Little by little, however, the child assembles his linguistic world and internalizes language rules that will find currency at the expressive performance level.

This is the pattern desired for hearing-impaired children as well. Unfortunately, a number of dynamics interfere with the establishment of a routine linguistic environment and the hearing-impaired child's internalization of linguistic rules. The curriculum developer must be aware of these dynamics and create curricula that will allow for them. These dynamics include:

1. Late identification of hearing loss and subsequent lack of early, specific, and sustained attention to input.
2. Parental shock and confusion following identification of hearing loss and a subsequent drop in communicative interaction.
3. Tardiness in provision of appropriate amplification.
4. Decline in communicative attempts by those other than parents in routine or occasional contact with the child.
5. A desire to teach the older child a language principle and have him express it immediately without attention to the required receptive, integrative period.

At this point in language programming most hearing impaired students do not receive a solid, sustained linguistic experience from birth. Few receive such an experience even following identification. The rule is for hearing-impaired children to experience an impoverished linguistic environment to and past the point of school entry. They do not receive the type of constantly stimulating receptive linguistic experience necessary for establishment of a set of internalized rules that will produce acceptable linguistic expression. It is not clear whether a limited corpus of normal rules is established or if a mixture of normal and deviant rules is established. Evidence of the latter is available for the older hearing-impaired child (Brennen, 1977; Bunch, 1978; DiFrancesca, Trybus, & Buchanan, 1971; Wilbur & Quigley, 1974). Bunch (1979) extended this problem further than most in suggesting that some students may be attempting to memorize language rather than internalizing even the simplest rules successfully. He pointed out that much of the teaching style in schools and classes for the hearing impaired promotes memorization, and the wide and inconsistent pattern of responses is reminiscent of attempted memorization of too large and too intricate a body of material.

Language curricula must be designed to take these points into consideration. Those developed for use with young children must allow for receptive opportunity and expressive opportunity similar to that experienced by normally hearing children. If this is not possible, the curricula must emphasize that whatever the age of the child, reception, and a considerable amount of it, must precede expression. Too precipitous an attempt to force expression may well result in the child attempting to memorize language and, as we know too well, language is too complex for memorization. Following sufficient receptive opportunity, there must be allowance for expressive experimentation. The normally hearing child does not produce accurate expression at the first trial; A series of successive approximations is the norm. If this experimental period is denied or severely cut off, the child is forced to use forms determined by an outside agent and not by his developing an internalized set of linguistic rules. All too often educators of the hearing impaired violate these basic guidelines.

## Cognitive and Linguistic Abilities

Considerable interest has been focussed on the interaction of cognitive and linguistic abilities in the hearing-impaired population. If we go back to the 1920s and 1930s, we can see that individuals such as Fitzgerald were concerned with the interplay of cognitive and linguistic abilities as language is developed. In the 1960s considerable attention was turned in this direction with the publication of Furth's *Thinking Without Language* (1966). Furth put forward the Piagetian viewpoint that intelligence is not dependent on language acquisition. Hearing-impaired individuals could develop cognitively despite severe linguistic impoverishment given appropriate stimulation. Furth outlined appropriate stimulation through detailed curricular activities designed to minimize language need and maximize cognitive development (Furth, 1969, 1970, 1971). He argued that experience in real situations develops cognitive abilities. Language is important for the developed mind but experience is the teacher to that stage. Various aspects of Furth's conceptualizations may be criticized (Moores, 1982), especially his tendency to present empirically untested hypotheses as fact. However, he moved educators and others from their traditional focus on deficiencies of the hearing impaired, to appreciation of and capitalization on strengths. Moores (1982) summed-up well present views on hearing impairment and cognition:

> The available evidence suggests that the condition of deafness imposes no limitations on the cognitive abilities of individuals. In addition, no evidence suggests that deaf persons think in more "concrete" ways than the hearing or that their intellectual functioning is in any way less sophisticated. . . .
>
> Given the present state of knowledge, the most parsimonious approach would be that the evidence suggests that deaf and hearing children are similar across a wide range of areas traditionally related to the study of cognitive and intellectual abilities. The great difficulty encountered by deaf children in academic subject matter is not caused

by cognitive deficiencies. In fact, it is safe to say that educators of the deaf have not capitalized on the cognitive strengths of deaf children in the academic environment.

The Piagetian position is not the single one of interest regarding the education of hearing-impaired children or education in general. The work of Bloom and his associates (1956) is important in establishing the need for a cognitive dimension in curricula. Vygotsky (1962) presented an alternate view on the relationship of language and thought to Piaget and Furth. Bruner (1962, 1966) presented still different views, melding and adding to those of earlier theorists. The key point is that these views exist. They should form part of the background knowledge of the curriculum developer and form part of the warp and woof of the fabric of curricula. Even if thought may develop without language, it must be communicated through language.

To date language curricula for the hearing impaired have paid only token acknowledgement to the need to deliberately consider and include cognitive activities. The majority of curricular approaches reviewed in this chapter recognize that language and cognition are in some way related. Most, though, go little further. One exception is *Sentences and Other Systems* (Blackwell et al., 1978), in which the need to consider topics on a conceptual basis has been recognized and acted on. As the authors state:

> If the hearing impaired student is to become a successful member of technological society, then that student will have to develop the appropriate cognitive style. And, it is only the symbolic representation of language that will enable the child to organize objects and events and modify perceptual representations in order to reach this goal (p. 10).

## Mainstream Curricula

A significant number of hearing-impaired children attend school in integrated settings. Karchmer and Trybus (1977) found that 19 percent of the almost 50,000 students in a national survey were integrated for substantial portions of their educational day. Some 10 percent received itinerant services, 6 percent were in part-time classes and 3 percent received resource room support. These children require specific curricular attention. A later chapter deals in depth with the needs of this population. The following short section provides a few remarks on language curricula specifically.

The most significant characteristic of hearing impairment is its effect on language functioning. Even with the benefit of considerable residual hearing, the child requires careful language management. For the integrated hearing-impaired child, this management is the responsibility of both the regular class teacher and the teacher of the hearing impaired. Since the child will need to understand the language of all subjects for which he is integrated, no curricular area may be ignored. The major difficulties facing mainstreamed hearing-impaired students are:

1. Keeping pace with new vocabulary
2. Integrating new language concepts
3. Reading texts prepared for normally hearing peers
4. Following and participating in classroom discussion
5. Acquiring free and easy use of social language

If a child is to be integrated successfully, each of these difficulties must receive attention.

Vocabulary is a major focus in any program. No vocabulary list meets the needs of the teacher nor of the child. A two-pronged team attack is recommended. The regular classroom teacher must find ways to present new material and its attendent vocabulary in clear fashion. Simultaneously the resource teacher must reinforce the new vocabulary of the classroom and be prepared to preteach a good part of it. The hearing-impaired child in the regular classroom must deal with the normal language of that classroom. If the child is unable to keep up, the meaning of new topics is lost and he falls further and further behind.

Much the same may be said with regard to the texts and readers normally used in the classroom. Together the two teachers are responsible for ensuring that the hearing-impaired child keeps moving with his peers. This often means that the resource teacher must accept responsibility for preteaching material directly from texts and for reading stories and novels through with the child either before or as they are read in the classroom.

The final two points above refer to language and much more. Adaptations to a teacher's instructional style may be necessary. Some alterations to the classroom may be considered. An appropriate auditory environment must be ensured. Interaction with normally hearing peers must be designed, encouraged, and monitored (Antia, 1982, 1985). While not directly curricular concerns, these points have much to do with the child's ability to participate in classroom routines and instruction and to benefit from them.

## SUMMARY

The development of language ability in the average student is the most challenging of the tasks facing educators of the hearing impaired. Recent years have witnessed no breakthroughs in this area and it remains an area of constant activity for curriculum writers.

Two general approaches have met with favorable reception. These are the natural—presently described best by Van Uden (1977)—and the analytic, detailed by such authorities as Blackwell and colleagues (1978), and Caniglia and associates (1972). The natural approach relies on a language instruction method based on the teacher's perception of a student's needs. Formal lessons on predetermined necessary language principles are rejected in favor of lessons and activities drawing on the student's emerging interests and needs. This curricular approach is especially demanding of the teacher. Analytic or formal methods rely on a schedule of sequentially laid-out language principles. Proponents of this system consider that the most productive approach is one that has analyzed basic language needs, and that provides sufficient instruction and practice in them. Teachers using this approach must be consistently aware of the need to make language real for the student and to relate it to the student's interests. In actual practice the majority of teachers make use of aspects of both the natural and analytic systems in an eclectic attack on language development in the hearing impaired.

Recent research in the language of normally hearing children has provided curriculum writers with new grist for their mill. As information emerges on how language evolves in the natural situation, teachers fit it into present curricula, set about revising existing curricula, or attempt to develop wholly new curricula. These efforts are to be encouraged if progress is to be made in this especially difficult area.

## TYPE LANGUAGE RESOURCES IN REVIEW

*Apple Tree* (Program) J. Caniglia, N.J. Cole, W. Howard, E. Krohn, and M. Rice (1972)

*Language, Learning and Deafness* (Text) A.H. Streng, R.R. Kretschmer, and L.W. Kretschmer (1978)

*Lessons in Syntax* (Program) J.E. McCarr (1973a, 1973b)

*Natural Language for Deaf Children* (Text) M.A. Groht (1958)

*Sentences and Other Systems* (Program/Text) P.M. Blackwell, E. Engen, J.E. Fischgrund, and C. Zarcadoolas (1978)

*Structured Tasks for English Practice* (Program) E. Costello (1975); E. Costello and S.D. Lopez (1975–1977); E. Costello and I.B. Pittle (1977); Lane (1979); Lopez and Lane (1978); Pittle (1980); Pittle and Melman (1981)

*TSA Syntax Program* (Program) S. Quigley, and D.J. Powers (1979)

## *APPLE TREE*

### J. Caniglia, N.J. Cole, W. Howard, E. Krohn, and M. Rice

*Publisher:*

Dormac, Inc.,
P.0. Box 752,
Beaverton, OR 97005

Dominie Press Limited,
345 Nugget Avenue, Unit 15,
Agincourt, Ontario MlS 4J4

*Skills taught:* Basic structures of the English language

Age/grade range: Deaf students, nonnative speakers of English

Group size: Class group; individual

**THEORY:** *Apple Tree* draws on the transformational grammar position in linguistics first outlined by Chomsky (1957). The major contribution of transformational grammar to the study of language is the conceptualization of a sentence as possessing two levels of constituent structure. The first is that known as surface structure, essentially a phrase-structure form of grammar. This approach, popular through most of the 20th century, accounted both for the individual's intuition of how words are grouped together, and for a variety of types of ambiguous utterances. The second, the strength of the transformational grammar theoretical position, is the deep structure (a.k.a. base structure, or underlying structure) level (Dale, 1976). These two levels are related but not identical. The deep structure is basic, with various transformations taking place to produce a surface structure. Caniglia and associates (1972) consider the transformational grammar approach to be valuable in that it exposes the regularities of the English language. *Apple Tree* attempted to capitalize on these regularities through use of selected transforms. The authors considered that correct use of syntax promoted understandable expression of thoughts and feelings.

Caniglia and associates stated that the symbols and patterns of language are mediated through the auditory channel and experiences. When one is disrupted, and the normal manner of language acquisition is not possible, alternate means leading to the internalization of language are necessary. The alternate means selected by the authors is that of determining 10 basic language structures, arranging them in a set-sequence, and teaching them through the spiraling curriculum method entwined about the 5 fundamental steps of teaching.

The 10 language structures are sequenced in a fashion that allows the child to proceed from the known to the unknown. Each step in the sequence depends on sufficient vocabulary background. Ideas for vocabulary development are given.

The program is considered only one part of classroom language. The deaf child or nonnative speaker of the English language requires constant immersion in language in the classroom. Caniglia et al. states: "When the stage of maturity is reached, or when the language structure is provided, this environmental language will become meaningful and useful to the child."

**DESCRIPTION:** *Apple Tree* depends on teaching, in a predetermined order, the following structures:

| | |
|---|---|
| 1. $N_1$ + V(be) + Adjective | The girl is happy. |
| 2. $N_1$ + V(be) + Where | The dogs are under the deck. |
| 3. $N_1$ + V(be) + $N_1$ | Rebecca was a princess. |
| 4. $N_1$ + V | The widow cried. |
| 5. $N_1$ + V + Where | Martin dashed across the squash court. |
| 6. $N_1$ + V + Where + When | An elephant fell in the ring last night. |
| 7. $N_1$ + V + $N_2$ | Monkeys eat bananas. |

| | |
|---|---|
| 8. $N_1$ + V + $N_2$ + Where | Children chase cats around and around. |
| 9. $N_1$ + V + $N_2$ + Where + When | Mary played soccer on the field this morning. |
| 10. $N_1$ + V + $N_3$ + $N_2$ | Matthew bought his friends some coffee. |

Terms used in the program ($N_1$; V(be), etc.) are defined for the teacher prior to lesson one.

The content of each lesson is laid out and a teaching pattern with suggested strategies is presented. The suggestions are quite detailed and simple to follow. All lessons utilize the following five steps considered fundamental to teaching.

1. *Comprehension*: the development of new vocabulary and new concepts and the review of old vocabulary and concepts. This step is considered to provide time for necessary internalization.
2. *Manipulation*: the direct handling of, and being involved with, lesson materials. Through manipulation the child "develops an awareness that certain words fit into specific slots or positions in a sentence," and develops a visual image of language structure.
3. *Substitution*: the variation of only one element in a sentence structure at a time (e.g., the subject or $N_1$). This step is considered to allow exploration from the known to the unknown and to provide security and success.
4. *Production*: spontaneous use of the structure following comprehension and internalization.
5. *Transformations*: rearrangements of the ten basic structures into a variety of forms.

Throughout all lessons, two levels of evaluation are employed. A behavioral objective is stated. Then specific concepts within structure development (concept evaluation) and ability to produce the structure in question (unit evaluation) are evaluated. A criterion level is suggested.

A number of constant techniques are built into the series of lessons. One of these is the use of controlled or pleasure stories with controlled vocabulary and language structure that allows the student to read for his own pleasure. These stories allow for reinforcement of structure and vocabulary as well. An example is:

A DOG

The dog is grey.

The dog is hairy.

The dog is long.

The dog is not tall.

The dog is friendly.

The dog is sleepy.

The dog is happy.

The dog is not angry.

A second technique is the use of illustrations to represent specific concepts. One of these is the use of the " 'I don't know' rabbit" used as a visual indication to the student that a response of some type is required. Others are use of a drawing of a parachute lowering the word "not" into a sentence to show the negative transform, and an illustration of a rabbit with accompanying box around a word and a directional line and arrow to explain linguistic principles.

A student workbook accompanies the teacher's manual.

**EVALUATION:** This program is highly reminiscent of earlier analytical methods of language instruction. It appears much like the Fitzgerald Key (Fitzgerald, 1949) in modern dress, and like *Lessons in Syntax* (McCarr, 1973a, 1973b), it employs a truncated view of transformational grammar to teach a limited set of language structures. The structured format and useful lesson suggestions will appeal to teachers who prefer a well-defined curriculum. Students who benefit from lessons built on familiar procedures will find security in the program. It may be especially appropriate for students experiencing difficulty producing syntactically correct strings of language under unstructured approaches to language instruction.

The use of visual illustrations will assist some children. It is questionable whether it is necessary to employ such methods for students beyond the first two or three years of school. The idea of visual assists is valuable though, and should not be abandoned for those benefitting from it.

The teacher's manual is clearly laid out. A large number of useful teaching ideas are presented.

The authors quite rightly note that *Apple Tree* is most suited to deaf children. In fact, as noted above, it may be best suited for a subset of deaf children. Personal experience suggests it is most useful for children who develop language ability slowly and with great effort. It may also be useful with nonnative speakers of English but it is probable that other less structured approaches are preferable.

## *LANGUAGE, LEARNING & DEAFNESS*

### A.H. Streng, R.R. Kretschmer, and L.W. Kretschmer

*Publisher:*

Grune and Stratton, Inc.,
111 Fifth Ave.,
New York, N.Y. 10003

Grune and Stratton, Inc.,
55 Barber Greene Road,
Don Mills, Ontario M3C 2A1

*Skills taught:* Theory, application and classroom management of language

*Age/grade range:* Preschool through high school

*Group size:* class group; individual

**THEORY:** Streng, Kretschmer, and Kretschmer (1978) have written a text that covers a great many aspects of language and education of hearing-impaired children. They draw heavily on current views of language acquisition in normally hearing children. Against this backdrop of emerging knowledge they plot what is known of language development in the hearing-impaired child. At issue, to some degree, in their discussion is whether the hearing-impaired and the normally hearing child develop language in the same manner. This issue is summarized thusly "It is still not clear whether deaf children generally learn language like normally hearing children, albeit at a slower rate, or whether they are different or even deviant in their developmental patterns."

The result of this indecision, certainly not unique to these authors, is a compromise in which theory is translated to practice. Streng and colleagues adopt the position that hearing-impaired children can learn language in a "normal" fashion given sufficient stimulation, but that "adjustments" are necessary. The primary adjustments suggested are reliance on a set of five basic sentence patterns and a limited grammar designed to maximize probability of success. Given these adjustments and a sound grounding in language and child development, the authors suggest that teachers of a wide range of hearing-impaired children in a variety of situations may anticipate acceptable levels of success.

**DESCRIPTION:** The text reviews a variety of topics before coming to grips with the language teaching curriculum for hearing-impaired children. Among these topics are a summary of the history of education of the hearing impaired in the United States, with an emphasis on Public Law 94-142—The Education of All Handicapped Children Act (1975) in Chapter 1, and a quick review of aspects of the learning process (behavioral learning, S-R theory, Piaget's periods of intellectual functioning, psycholinguistics and learning, etc.) in the second chapter. Chapters 3, 4, and 5 (Establishing and Maintaining Communication), Language—The Basic Tool, and The Learning Environment in the Classroom Setting, respectively) continue the examination of major topics in a summary format. All assist in sketching the position of the hearing-impaired child in these areas. Most discussion, though, is a review of basic knowledge in child development, language acquisition, and pedagogical basics.

One important point, from a curricular point of view, that comes from these chapters is the selection of Streng's (1972) five basic sentence patterns as a grounding for discussion of language development. These sentence patterns are:

1. NP + AUX + VI (Intransitive verb sentence).
2. NP + AUX + VT + NP (Transitive verb sentence).
3. NP + BE + NP (Predicate nominative sentence).
4. NP + BE + ADJ (Predicate adjective sentence).
5. NP + BE + ADV (Predicate adverb sentence).

They suggest the substance from which the authors' general approach grew. They built "an experience-based integrated language arts program" about developmental language theory as presented in transformational grammar. In so doing they pursued the concept of intensive, planned stimulation and language experience aimed at reception and expression within a limited English grammar. Within their framework they perceived no necessary limitation on conceptual development or semantic knowledge. In fact, they considered the limitations of their suggested grammar to be beneficial in some ways. Not failing the possibilities within the realm of their suggested grammar, the authors encouraged the teaching of more complex structures to those children capable of mastering them. A very few excellently presented examples of how this particular curricular approach may be put into practice are provided.

The final chapters deal with "Reading and Writing in the Curriculum," "Assessment and Planning for Language Growth," and multihandicapping conditions in "Beyond Deafness." The work on reading and writing is well-planned and discusses clearly how these aspects of education may be treated within a conceptually based, experience-oriented approach. Assessment and planning are given rather short shrift with almost no discussion of the possibilities of formal assessment. Useful guides for assessing and analyzing language samples are provided and do much to clarify interpretation using a transformational and limited sentence pattern approach.

The final chapter, "Beyond Deafness," mentions a variety of handicapping conditions in addition to hearing impairment. Discussions of these conditions are quite short and primarily definitional.

**EVALUATION:** *Language, Learning and Deafness* is one of a very few attempts to deal with language and hearing impairment in a comprehensive manner. It presents a curricular concept that many will find valuable, a blending of naturalistic methods of teaching and a predecided acquisition sequence of syntactic structures. The groundings of the approach within psycholinguistic theory are readily apparent. Theoretical discussion and practical general procedures are supported throughout the text with direct references to implications for hearing-impaired children and through selected examples.

The authors did not claim to present a full curriculum and they do not. An idea is presented and is fleshed out to a minor degree. The reader will, however, need to do considerable extending of the examples presented to conceive a functional curricular framework. In some ways, it is regrettable that time, space, and effort were spent on historical overviews and surveys of additional handicaps, rather than on language development and ideas directly.

One may question the concept of a limited grammar as exemplified by five basic sentence patterns. Many teachers will find the approach too restrictive. Others will find the direct translation of transformational theory to practice to be premature and the terminology awkward. Be that as it may, Streng and colleagues have provided a workable thesis and an interesting blending of experience-based and structured approaches to language development for the hearing-impaired student.

## *LESSONS IN SYNTAX*

**J.E. McCarr**

*Publisher:*

Dormac, Inc.,
P.O. Box 752,
Beaverton, Oregon 97005

Dominie Press Limited,
345 Nugget Avenue, Unit 15,
Agincourt, Ontario M1S 4J4

*Skills taught*: Syntax

*Audience*: Deaf, hearing-impaired or linguistically disadvantaged students with a limited use of language

*Group size:* class group; individual

**THEORY:** Transformational grammar theories underlie the structure of *Lessons in Syntax*. (See *Apple Tree* for a brief review of this theoretical position.)

**DESCRIPTION:** McCarr's program (1973a, 1973b) was designed to teach specific transforms in a highly structured fashion. It emphasized correct syntactical form as a requisite for accurately conveying thoughts and feelings but was not to be considered an exclusive method. Other methods of teaching language should be employed as deemed appropriate by the teacher in the effort "to produce creative, spontaneous, expressive language."

The transforms taught through *Lessons in Syntax* are:

1. Negative transform
2. Yes/no questions
3. Wh-questions
4. "Because" and "so"
5. Relative clause transform
6. Participle transform
7. Indirect discourse
8. Passive transform

Each transform is presented in a unit broken into a series of steps. Each unit contains (1) unit objectives: a description of the performance skills the students will have when the unit is completed; (2) sub-objectives: descriptions of the intermediary performance skills that the students must acquire to achieve the unit objective; (3) steps: procedures to be used to help the students acquire the skill described in the subobjective; (4) evaluation of subobjectives: a testing procedure to determine if the students have acquired the skills described in the subobjectives; and (5) a unit evaluation: a testing procedure to determine if the students have acquired the skill described in the unit objective.

Detailed instructions are provided in each Unit for each step suggested. Heavy reliance is placed on behavioral objective and stimulus-response methodology. The typical student response is in written form. McCarr stressed that immediate presentation of the correct response (confirmation) is necessary to reinforce correct student response or assist in student correction of an incorrect response. Routine use of an overhead projector and a game situation format is recommended. Teachers are encouraged to modify the examples given in the *Teacher's Manual* (1973b), but the syntactic form used must be retained.

Teachers work from the detailed *Teacher's Manual* and students work in the *Student Workbook* (1973a). A key is provided relating activities in the manual to exercises in the workbook. The workbook provides questions down the right-hand side of the page with the correct answer immediately across on the left-hand side. A cardboard "glider" is provided to cover the left-hand answers until each right-hand item is completed.

**EVALUATION:** *Lessons in Syntax* is a contemporary version of traditional analytical or structured systems for teaching language to deaf and other language-impaired children. It employs transformational terminology and instructional objective and stimulus-response methodology to teach a limited but valuable subset of language patterns. The highly structured format will be attractive to teachers wanting a preplanned language program and to students most comfortable in a system with regular rules and teaching methods.

As McCarr pointed out, *Lessons in Syntax* cannot stand by itself as an entire language teaching program. It must be supplemented by other systems. The responses required of the student in the workbook cannot be considered sufficient "to produce creative, spontaneous, expressive language." Unfortunately this reviewer has seen teachers using the system almost as their sole language program.

The program may be best viewed as a program for deaf, rather than hard-of-hearing students who are encountering difficulty with language acquisition. It could form part of the program for language-capable students, but, in that case, would be a supplement to another basic approach rather than the central language method.

## *NATURAL LANGUAGE for DEAF CHILDREN*

### M.A. Groht

*Publisher:*
Alexander Graham Bell Association,
3417 Volta Pl., N.W.,
Washington, D.C. 20007

*Skills taught:* English language in general

*Age/grade range:* Preschool to high school

*Group size:* class group; individual

**THEORY:** Groht (1958) did not present a strong explanation of her theoretical viewpoint. Clearly, though, her belief is that language instruction must be child-centered, and that it must grow from the needs and interests of the child. Language is a tool for the development of the deaf child's imagination and reasoning power and is a key to the emancipation of the deaf. The teacher must present language instruction in an interesting, creative fashion avoiding drill and stereotyped language that stifle true development.

Basic to the natural approach is the need for a teacher who is well-trained in language and hearing impairment. The teacher must be aware of the difficulties faced by the deaf child, but must not allow this awareness to result in analytical teaching. The teacher must "believe that the way to make it possible for the deaf child to gain this mastery (of language) is not by altering the language itself but by making it alive and desirable for him and by seeing that it meets his needs."

**DESCRIPTION:** *Natural Language for Deaf Children* provides a longitudinal overview of aspects of language development from nursery school through the high school years. Groht returns again and again to her themes of language development based on the interests of the child, and language development to improve thinking skills. The book is written in an informal matter. Theoretical discussion is mixed with teaching ideas in a disconcerting fashion. It is difficult to uncover her ideas at times but each chapter does contain a central theme.

Chapter 1 reviews aspects of language development in normally hearing children in a free-ranging, anecdotal fashion. The deaf child and the difficulties imposed by his hearing loss are viewed against this backdrop. The need for early language stimulation is emphasized. Chapter 2 outlines the need for a nursery school experience and the need to begin lipreading immediately and consistently is underlined. The concept of meaningful repetition is introduced along with the need for a conversational approach, natural vocabulary expansion, and imitative speech. Chapter 3 outlines the content of the preschool age (5 years). What to teach and how to teach are treated simultaneously with an introduction of stress on increased direct teaching. Ideas are given on the setup of the preschool classroom, the writing of news, the use of expressions, questioning, number work, and other topics. Basic to Chapter 4 is the entry of the child to "real school." Topics such as the postponement of writing, vocabulary needs, news-writing procedures, pronouns, verbs, stories, the use of pictures, and teacher planning are addressed. In Chapters 5-11 the child's career is traced through the school years, giving teaching ideas, and reinforcing the concept of natural language. Chapter 12, the final chapter, amplifies on Groht's faith in the natural method. She reviews her early teaching experiences and the advantages of the natural method over more analytical methods.

**EVALUATION:** Groht wrote the classic text describing the natural language method, a method with a checkered history over the past hundred years and more. Hers was a summary statement of a teaching philosophy held by many. As such it is really not a curriculum but more of a position statement supported by numerous examples. The reader may obtain a general view of the philosophy and some general curricular rules, but a reasoned treatment of the topic either as philosophy or curriculum is not available in this publication. The discussion bounces and bounds from major to minor points, and from topic to topic, in a rather disorganized fashion. The main themes underlying the natural method do, however, emerge.

## *SENTENCES AND OTHER SYSTEMS*

### P.M Blackwell, E. Engen, J.E. Fischgrund, and C. Zarcadoolas

*Publisher:*
Alexander Graham Bell Assoc.,
3417 Volta Place, N.W.,
Washington, D.C. 20007

*Skills taught*: Language development in general

*Age/grade range*: Preschool through high school

*Group size:* Class group; school/system wide

**THEORY:** Blackwell and colleagues (1978) drew heavily on the theory and emerging practice of the transformational-generative view of language development. Basic to this view is the concept that any utterance is a representation of two levels of language, the deep structure of a person's language, and his surface structure. Deep structure refers generally to the set of linguistic principles learned by the individual to be a speaker of the language. These underlying linguistic structures are closely related to desired meaning or the semantic aspect of an utterance. The actual utterance is the surface structure. It is the person's transformation of underlying knowledge of linguistic principles into some perceptible language form. Both deep and surface structures are related through application of a set of rules or transformations that begin at the underlying or deep level and progressively act on knowledge generated at that level until an utterance is made. The authors regard transformational-generative theory as providing the theoretical base allowing for a creative view of curriculum development, a system geared to individual ability and "a system for producing and understanding sentences."

Other theoretical orientations support and interact with the transformational-generative view of language development fundamental to the curricular approach of Blackwell and associates. On the cognitive side, they appreciate Bruner's synthesis of Piagetian and Vygotskian positions on the relationship of language and thought. Bruner suggests that three levels of representation with direct relevance for education may be hypothesized (Bruner, 1966). The first is enactive representation involving action; that is, direct physical response to situations. Second is iconic representation involving principles of perceptual organization, of completing and extending thought through perceptual imagery. Finally there is symbolic representation through words in various forms. These three levels must be worked into a curriculum if it is to possess a sound cognitive foundation.

The general theories discussed are woven about a view of curriculum design with roots in Bruner's three basic curriculum processes, the acquisition, transformation, and evaluation of information. These are regarded as best utilized within the spiral curriculum model.

**DESCRIPTION:** The text outlining the general curricular approach of the Rhode Island School for the Deaf begins with three chapters presenting the theoretical positions adopted by the authors. These positions are discussed in brief in the earlier section on theory. Chapter 3, "The Process of Curriculum Design," forms a bridge between theoretical discussion and curriculum explication, and as such, it is an important pivotal chapter. Among other things, it defines and describes the four steps forming the framework for the developmental language program suggested, which are:

1. Exposure: the provision of a system of language stimulation in the classroom with an appreciation of the fact that not all words and structures must be familiar to the student. Exposure to unknown forms is normal and needed.
2. Recognition: awareness that language forms (e.g., print, questions) possess meaning including different meanings and that these can be interpreted, even if not perfectly.
3. Comprehension: understanding of given language structures.
4. Writing: use of written symbols to indicate language ability and to use them at different levels for different purposes.

These steps are reiterated throughout subsequent chapters as organizational tools for discussion of ideas and methods.

Central to the language-development ideas of Blackwell and associates is the sentence pattern approach, the use of a limited number of sentence types to form a base on which language may be developed. Such an approach is not new in hearing impairment. The authors, though, state that transformational-generative theory has provided a new way of using this approach, and that a pattern of interrelatedness of the sentences, not apparent previously, is now apparent. Using this new way of looking at language development big sentences can be made from little sentences in a more successful fashion. Their five basic sentence patterns are:

1. The girl laughs.<br>NP V
2. The girl plays baseball.<br>$NP_1$ V $NP_2$
3. The girl is happy.<br>NP LV Adjective
4. The girl is a football player.<br>NP LV NP

5. The girl is on the ball field.
   NP LV Adverbial

The balance of the text is a presentation of ideas for teaching, sentence analysis, and the development of more complex and abstract language. Some emphasis is given to the planning process, the need to actively develop cognitive skills, and to language assessment. In assessment the authors subscribe to the concept that language development is a continuum, and a prerequisite for instruction is to determine where the hearing impaired child falls on the continuum. A language sampling approach is advanced with a focus on linguistic readiness, oral skills, and written language. Also discussed is the use of tests, such as the Assessment of Children's Language Comprehension (ACLC), the Illinois Test of Psycholinguistic Abilities (ITPA), Carrow's Test of Language Comprehension (TACL), and the Peabody Picture Vocabulary Test (PPVT).

**EVALUATION:** *Sentences and Other Systems* presents an eclectic view of language development in hearing-impaired children. It applies views of cognition, linguistics, and curriculum development to education of the hearing impaired in a positive fashion. Andrews (1981) refers to "its imaginative application to the education of deaf children, preschool through secondary school." It is refreshing to read discussions of Piaget, Vygotsky, Bruner, and others as they do apply to education in general and also how they might apply to language development in the hearing-impaired population. The discussions are sketchy but well-articulated and should spark professionals in hearing impairment to read more deeply into issues in curriculum development generally. The text is valuable on that basis alone.

The attempt to use a restricted set of basic sentence patterns using a transformational approach is not unique to *Sentences and Other Systems.* In common with a number of other curricula, also, is an unwarranted degree of optimism for the possibilities of the transformational–generative approach. Simply put, we do not yet know enough about language development in normally hearing children, let alone hearing-impaired children, to come up with a final solution, or anything approaching it, using a transformational–generative approach. Certainly, use of a restricted set of sentence forms is a curious twisting of the emerging theory of that approach. Despite the above commentary, the authors have done an admirable job and their exciting, incisive ideas and suggestions provide one of the most powerful present curriculum designs.

The section of the book most in need of strengthening is that on assessment. An interesting variety of points are made, but the reader does not obtain a real sense of how to assess language in the hearing impaired. The task of presenting a strong overview in this area is intimidating. However, the attempt to mingle language sampling techniques suitable for normally hearing children with a few tests of questionable validity for hearing-impaired children does not work. Surprisingly, the few tests standardized on the hearing-impaired population are not mentioned.

## *STRUCTURED TASKS FOR ENGLISH PRACTICE (STEP)*

**E. Costello, L.G. Lane, S.D. Lopez, C.S. Melman, and I.B. Pittle**

*Publisher*:
Gallaudet College,
Division of Public Services
Florida Ave. at 7th St. N.E.,
Washington, D.C. 20002

*Skills taught*:
Articles, nouns, verbs, pronouns, adjectives, linking verbs, prepositional phrases, adverb clauses, infinitives, gerunds, conjunctions, compound and complex sentences

*Age/grade range*: Adult (Grade three reading level minimum)

*Group size*: Individual

**THEORY:** No theoretical discussion is provided in these works. Analysis of the material indicates reliance on a traditional grammar approach. STEP employs nonrigorous versions of programmed instruction and instructional objective theory. Basic to this material is the belief that the adult deaf person will improve his or her English ability through sustained self-instruction and practice on a sequence of English principles.

**DESCRIPTION:** The STEP materials consist of a series of nine student workbooks and a bulky *Teacher's Resource Guide*. Topics of the individual workbooks are:

1. Articles (including some examples)
2. Nouns
3. Verbs: past, present, and future
4. Pronouns
5. Adjectives and linking verbs
6. Prepositional phrases
7. Adverb clauses
8. Infinitives and gerunds
9. Conjunctions, compound, and complex sentences
10. Writing sentences

Each workbook is organized on a similar basis. A statement or short explanatory discussion is provided to clarify the principle under consideration (e.g., *A, an, the* and *some* are called articles). Following immediately is an exercise based on the principle. Each exercise begins with an explicit direction accompanied by an example (e.g., "Draw a line under the articles in this story." Example: Do you have *an* interesting job?). The student works through the exercise and checks his responses with an answer section provided.

Student involvement and progress are monitored in a number of ways. The teacher is encouraged to administer a pretest and a post-test. The pretest determines whether the student requires work on the principle in question. The teacher is required to show the student how to read the directions, complete the exercises, and use the answer book. In addition, the teacher must be available to help with vocabulary and other matters as required and to teach beyond the exercises provided. The final monitoring system is in the form of an overall instructional objective and subobjectives. For articles these are:

### Objective

Given a picture stimulus, the student will write a paragraph of at least five sentences using *a, an, the,* and *some* correctly within those sentences at least 90% of the time.

### Subobjectives

**RECOGNIZING ARTICLES** —Given a short newspaper story, the student will underline articles within that story and circle the nouns to which each article refers.

**USING *A* and *AN***—Given sentences with the articles *a* and *an* omitted, the student will write *a* or *an* correctly in the blanks.

**USING *SOME*** —Given sentences with the articles *a, an* and *some* omitted, the student will correctly write *a, an* or *some* in the blanks.

**USING *THE*** —Given a story with all articles missing, the student will supply the correct articles.

**WRITING SENTENCES WITH ARTICLES** —Given a series of pictures, the student will write a paragraph of at least five sentences using the correct articles.

The *Teacher's Resource Guide* contains sections on all principles presented in the workbooks. Expanded discussion of the grammatical concepts associated with each principle is provided as well as ideas for fundamental understanding of the principle (Basic Activities), additional exercises (Practice Activities), and a few thoughts on further practice (Expansion Activities).

The Guide also contains a section on evaluation, a general diagnostic test designed to determine if the student needs work in the various areas of interest, and both pretests and post-tests for each workbook.

**EVALUATION:** STEP impresses by its sheer size. A great deal of work and thought has gone into the workbooks and teacher's guide. The result is a thorough examination of the principles under consideration. The exercises are clearly structured with logical progression from one exercise to another. The series should provide a good review for the deaf adult.

STEP should be considered a supplement to the teacher's instruction. There is insufficient explanation of each principle for the student to work from the workbooks independently unless the student already has a fairly firm grasp of the principles. The majority of deaf adults requiring work at the level presented in the workbooks would also require constant monitoring from a teacher. The programmed aspect of the series is not well developed. It is a simple linear system with inadequate self-checking or immediate reinforcement.

The series of principles comprising STEP was drawn from analysis of errors made frequently by deaf adults. It is wide-ranging but does not cover all grammatical principles necessary for a complete curriculum. It is not presented as such and should not form the entire program of language instruction. It is an aid, not the program. As such it could be used with adolescents as well as adults.

No technical data is provided for the various tests included in the package. Reliability and validity are unknown. Determination of principles to be stressed is based on a single error in any of the areas of interest. This use of a single error to determine practice need could lead to over-inclusion of students.

In summary, STEP is most useful as a supplement to class instruction for adolescents and adults with sufficient reading ability. It is a well-structured series of workbooks with adequate practice between the workbooks themselves and the additional ideas in the teacher's guide.

## *TSA SYNTAX PROGRAM*

### S. Quigley and D.J. Power (Editors)

*Publisher*:

Dormac, Inc.,
P.O. Box 752,
Beaverton, OR 97005

Dominie Press Limited,
345 Nugget Avenue, Unit 15,
Agincourt, Ontario M1S 4J4

*Skills taught*: Negation, conjunction, determiners, question formation, verb processes, pronominalization, relativization, complementation, and nominalization

*Age/grade range*: 10 years and older

*Group size*: Class group: individual

**THEORY:** Quigley and Power (1979) do not explicate the theoretical beliefs underlying the *TSA Syntax Program* to any extent. They clearly state that this program is but one phase in a multiphase "program of research and materials development in the structure of the language of deaf children and youth." (1979) It is not put forth as an entire curriculum of language development and teaching. However, it must serve as the best view of the authors' curriculum ideas until a fuller discussion of these is available.

Quigley and Power accept the position that a naturalistic approach to language development is the approach of choice for deaf children. This approach is not reviewed. Instead, the authors point out that the naturalistic approach is not successful in establishing more than a limited command of standard English syntax in many instances. They advance the *TSA Syntax Program* as a vehicle to assist with the development of syntax in these instances. The program is designed with "the limited objective of providing a set of activities and structured materials for aiding the development and remediation of English syntax." The choice of structures and their ordering has been determined by the design and ordering of the Test of Syntactic Abilities (TSA) and the research leading up to it.

**DESCRIPTION:** The *TSA Syntax Program* is composed of a series of 20 workbooks dealing with 9 major areas of interest and 9 accompanying teacher's guides. The major areas are:

1. Negation: guide and 1 workbook
2. Conjunction: guide and 2 workbooks
3. Determiners: guide and 1 workbook
4. Question formation: guide and 3 workbooks
5. Verb processes: guide and 3 workbooks
6. Pronominalization: guide and 4 workbooks
7. Relativization: guide and 3 workbooks
8. Complementation: guide and 2 workbooks
9. Nominalization: guide and 1 workbook

Each teacher's guide presents a discussion and explanation of the syntactic structure in question, with a review of research on the development of that structure in both normally hearing and deaf children. The balance of the guide provides behavioral objectives to be attained in working through the workbook, a pretest, post-test procedure based on administration and interpretation of relevant subtests of the TSA, some technical material, and sections focussed on teaching suggestions to supplement and expand workbook activities.

Workbooks are designed on a programmed learning format. Activity pages provide progressively more challenging tasks. Considerable use is made of explanatory illustrations. Vocabulary and concepts are considered to be at the upper elementary level for 10- to 18-year-old deaf children.

Teachers are required to monitor progress through each workbook. When necessary the teacher must intervene to explain vocabulary and concepts or be prepared to provide games and activities.

**EVALUATION:** The *TSA Syntax Program* provides a highly structured approach to the development and remediation of English syntax. It treats syntax independently of semantics with the rationale that, though the two are inextricably intertwined, there is sufficient evidence of syntactical difficulty for that aspect to be dealt with alone. The exercises are well-prepared, sufficient practice is provided for each objective, and useful supplementary games and activities are provided.

This program must be viewed as a limited assist within a larger instructional approach. This fact is stated and restated by the editors. They appear to fear that some teachers may embrace the *TSA Syntax Program* as a core for a language program. This implied fear is a very real one. Teachers, frustrated with the continued inability of many students to write syntactically correct English, may view the opportunity to use an extensive, largely student-operated, systematically arranged language program as a boon. An added appeal would be the apparent success as the student worked through each workbook. One cannot expect that students who have demonstrated difficulty during years of exposure to these structures will suddenly begin to use them correctly following completion of a series of workbooks. Typically, little revision of creative written English may be expected.

It would appear that the prepost testing system may spread too wide a net. As the editors note, few deaf students will attain pretest scores that would indicate that they need not enter the program.

The *TSA Syntax Program* is quite extensive. The result is that it is quite expensive. It is a moot point whether the instructional value of the program outweighs the cost.

## REFERENCES


Andrews, J. (1981). Sentences and other systems—A language and learning curriculum for hearing impaired children (Review). *American Annals of the Deaf, 126,* 391.

Antia, S. (1982). Social interaction of partially mainstreamed hearing impaired children. *American Annals of the Deaf, 127,* 18-25.

Antia, S. (1985). Social integration of hearing impaired children. *Volta Review, 87,* 279-289.

Barry, K. (1899). *The five-slate system. A system of objective language teaching.* Philadelphia, PA: Sherman and Co.

Bell, A.G. (1883). Upon a method of teaching language to a very young congenitally deaf child. *American Annals of the Deaf, 28,* 124-139.

Blackwell, P. and Hamel, C. (1971). *The language curriculum. Rhode Island School for the Deaf.* Providence, RI: Rhode Island School for the Deaf.

Blackwell, P.M., Engen, E., Fischgrund, J.E., & Zarcadoolas, C. (1978). *Sentences and other systems.* Washington, DC: Alexander Graham Bell Association.

Bloom, B.S. (1956). *Taxonomy of educational objectives. Handbook 1. Cognitive domain.* London: Longmans.

Brannon, J.B. (1968). Linguistic word classes in the spoken language of normal, hard-of-hearing and deaf children. *Journal of Speech and Hearing Research, 11,* 279-287.

Brennan, M. (1977, March). Can deaf children acquire language? *The Deaf Canadian,* pp. 8-13.

Bruner, J.S. (1962). *On knowing: Essays for the left hand.* Cambridge, MA: Harvard University Press.

Bruner, J.S. (1966). *Toward a theory of instruction.* Cambridge, MA: Harvard University Press.

Bryen, D.N. (1980). *Inquiries into child language.* Boston, MA: Allyn & Bacon.

Buell, E.M. (1952a). *Outline of language for deaf children. Book I* (Rev. ed.). Washington, DC: Volta Bureau.

Buell, E.M. (1952b). *Outline of language for deaf children. Book 2* (Rev. ed.). Washington, DC: Volta Bureau.

Bunch, G.O. (1975). *An evaluation of natural and formal language programmes with deaf children.* Unpublished doctoral dissertation, University of British Columbia, Vancouver.

Bunch, G.O. (1978). Language without thinking. *ACEHI Journal, 4,* 39-41.

Bunch, G.O. (1979). Degree and manner of acquisition of written English language rules by the deaf. *American Annals of the Deaf, 124,* 10-15.

Caniglia, J., Cole, N.J., Howard, W., Krohn, E., & Rice, M. (1972). *Apple tree.* Beaverton, OR: Dormac.

Chomsky, N. (1957). *Syntactic structures.* The Hague: Mouton.

Clarke School for the Deaf. (1978). *English curriculum: Upper school.* Northampton, MA: Author.

Clerc, L. (1851). Some hints to the teachers of the deaf and dumb. *Proceedings of the Second Convention of American Instructors of the Deaf and Dumb, 2,* 64-75.

The Clarke School for the Deaf. *Language.* (1972). Northampton, MA: Author.

Cole, J.R. (1980). Thinking and curriculum. *Volta Review, 82,* 337-344.

Costello, E. (1975). *Structured tasks for English practice: Articles.* Washington, DC: Gallaudet College.

Costello, E., & Lopez, S.D. (1975). *Structured tasks for English practice: Prepositional phrases.* Washington, DC: Gallaudet College.

Costello, E., & Lopez, S.D. (1975). *Structured tasks for English practice: Verbs.* Washington, DC: Gallaudet College.

Costello, E., & Lopez, S.D. (1976). *Structured tasks for English practice: Adjectives and linking verbs.* Washington, DC: Gallaudet College.

Costello, E., & Lopez, S.D. (1977). *Structured tasks for English practice: Infinitives and gerunds.* Washington, DC: Gallaudet College.

Costello, E., & Pittle, I.B. (1977). *Structured tasks for English practice: Pronouns.* Washington, DC: Gallaudet College.

Dale, P.S. (1976). *Language development* (2nd ed.). Hinsdale, IL: The Dryden Press.

DiFrancesca, S., Trybus, R., & Buchanan, C. (1971). *Studies in achievement testing, hearing impaired students: 1971* (Series D, Number 11). Washington, DC: Gallaudet College Office of Demographic Studies.

Doctor, P.V. (1950). On teaching the abstract to the deaf. *Volta Review, 52,* 568-572.

Fitzgerald, E. (1949). *Straight language for the deaf.* Washington, DC: Alexander Graham Bell Association.

Furth, H. (1966). *Thinking without language: Psychological implications of deafness.* New York: Free Press.

Furth, H. (1969). *A thinking laboratory for deaf children.* Washington, DC: Catholic University.

Furth, H. (1970). *Piaget for teachers.* Englewood Cliffs, NJ: Prentice-Hall.

Furth, H. (1971). Education for thinking. *Journal of Rehabilitation of the Deaf, 5,* 7-71.

Garber, G.E. (1967). *An analysis of English morphological abilities of deaf and hearing children. Dissertation Abstracts International, 28,* 2373A. (University Microfilms No. 67-16-279).

Gentile, G. and DiFrancesca, S. (1969). *Academic achievement test performance of hearing impaired students* (Series D, Number 1). Washington, DC: Office of Demographic Studies, Gallaudet College.

Grammatico, L.F., & Miller, S.D. (1974). Curriculum for the preschool deaf Child. *Volta Review, 76,* 280-289.

Greenberger, D. (1879). The natural method. *American Annals of the Deaf, 24,* 33-38.

Griffey, M.N., Sr. (1981). A survey of present methods of developing language in deaf children. In A.M. Mulholland (Ed.), *Oral education today and tomorrow,* Washington, DC: Alexander Graham Bell Association, pp. 119-131.

Groht, M.A. (1958). *Natural language for deaf children.* Washington, DC: Alexander Graham Bell Association.

Hammill, D.D., Bartel, N.R., & Bunch, G.0. (1984). *Teaching children with learning and behavior problems* (Canadian ed.). Boston: Allyn & Bacon.

Harris, G.M. (1971). *Language for the preschool deaf child* (3rd ed.). New York: Grune & Stratton.

Hasenstab, M.S. (1983). Child language studies: Impact on habilitation of hearing impaired infants and preschool children. *Volta Review, 85,* 88-100.

Heider, R., & Heider, G.M. (1941). Comparison of sentence structure of deaf and hearing children. *Volta Review, 43,* 364-630.

Holmes, K.M., & Holmes, D.W. (1981). Normal language acquisition: A model for language programming for the deaf. *American Annals of the Deaf, 126,* 23-31.

Hopper, R., & Naremore, R.C. (1973). *Children's speech.* New York: Harper & Row.

Hudson, P.L. (1979). Recommitment to the Fitzgerald Key. *American Annals of the Deaf, 124,* 397-399.

Karchmer, M.A., & Trybus, R.J. (1977). *Who are the deaf children in "mainstream" programs?* (Series R, No. 4). Washington, DC: Gallaudet College Office of Demographic Studies.

King, C.M. (1983, June). *Survey of language methods and materials used with hearing impaired students in the United States.* Paper presented at the joint meeting of the Canadian Association for Educators of the Hearing Impaired and the Convention of American Instructors of the Deaf, Winnipeg, Manitoba.

Knight, D.L. (1979). A general model of English language development in hearing impaired children. *Directions, 1,* 9-28.

Lane, L.G. (1979). *Structured tasks for English practice: Adverb clauses.* Washington, DC: Gallaudet College.

Lenneberg, E.H. (1967). *Biological foundations of language.* New York: John Wiley.

Lopez, S.D., & Lane, L.G. (1978). *Structured tasks for English practice: Conjunctions—compound and complex sentences.* Washington, DC: Gallaudet College.

Lowenbraun, S. (1969). An investigation of the syntactic competence of young deaf children. *Dissertation Abstracts International, 31,* 4147A. (University Microfilms No. 70-07025)

MacGinitie, W.H. (1964). Ability of deaf children to use different word classes. *Journal of Speech and Hearing Research, 7,* 141-150.

McCarr, J.E. (1973a). *Lessons in syntax: Student workbook.* Beaverton, OR: Dormac.

McCarr, J.E. (1973b). *Lessons in syntax: Teacher's manual.* Beaverton, OR: Dormac.

Moores, D.F. (1970a). *Education of the deaf in the United States* (Occasional paper #2). University of Minnesota, Project No. 332189, Grant No. OE-09-332189-4533(032). Washington, DC: Department of Health, Education and Welfare.

Moores, D.F. (1970b). Psycholinguistics and deafness. *American Annals of the Deaf, 115,* 37-48.

Moores, D.F. (1982). *Educating the deaf: Psychology, principles and practices* (2nd ed.). Boston, MA: Houghton Mifflin.

Myklebust, H.R. (1960). *Psychology of deafness.* New York: Grune & Stratton.

Northcott, W.H. (Ed.). (1977). *Curriculum guide: Hearing impaired children (0–3 years) and their parents* (Rev. ed.). Washington, DC: Alexander Graham Bell Association.

Nunnally, J.C., & Blanton, R.L. (1966). Patterns of word association in the deaf. *Psychological Reports, 18,* 87-92.

Piaget, J. (1955). *The language and thought of the child.* New York: Meridian.

Pittle, I.B. (1980). *Structured tasks for English practice: Teacher's resource guide.* Washington, DC: Gallaudet College.

Pittle, I.B., & Melman, C.S. (1981). *Structured tasks for English practice: Writing sentences.* Washington, DC: Gallaudet College.

Public Law 94-142. (1975). *Education of all handicapped children law.* 20 U.S.C. SS 1401-1420.

Quigley, S.P., & Paul, P.V. (1984). *Language and deafness.* San Diego, CA: College-Hill Press.

Quigley, S.P., & Power, D.J. (Eds.). (1979). *TSA syntax program.* Beaverton, OR: Dormac.

Quigley, S.P., Wilbur, R.B., & Montanelli, D.S. (1974). Question formation in the language of deaf students. *Journal of Speech and Hearing Research, 17,* 699-713.

Sarachan-Deily, A.B., & Love, R.J. (1974). Underlying grammatical role structure in the deaf. *Journal of Speech and Hearing Research, 17,* 689-698.

Schmitt, P.J. (1966). Language instruction for the deaf. *Volta Review, 68,* 85-105, 123.

Schmitt, P.J. (1970). Deaf children's comprehension and production of sentence transformations and verb tenses. *Dissertation Abstracts International, 30,* 936A. (University Microfilms No. 69-15371)

Sitnick, V., Rushmer, N., & Arpan, R. (1978). *Parent-infant communication* (Rev. ed.). Beaverton, OR: Dormac.

Stone, P. (1980). Developing thinking skills in young hearing impaired children. *Volta Review, 82,* 345-352.

Streng, A.H. (1964). *Reading for deaf children.* Washington, DC: Alexander Graham Bell Association.

Streng, A.H. (1972). *Syntax, speech and hearing.* New York, NY: Grune & Stratton.

Streng, A.H., Kretschmer, R.R., & Kretschmer, L.W. (1978). *Language, learning, and deafness.* New York: Grune & Stratton.

Templin, M.C. (1950). *The development of reasoning in children with normal and defective hearing.* Minneapolis, MN: University of Minnesota Press.

Van Uden, A. (1977). *A world of language for deaf children* (3rd ed.). Amsterdam: Swets & Zeitlinger.

Vygotsky, L.S. (1962). *Thought and language.* Cambridge, MA: MIT Press.

Wilbur, R.B., & Quigley, S.P. (1974). Syntactic structures in the written language of deaf children. *Volta Review, 77,* 194-203.

Wing, G. (1887). The theory and practice of grammatical methods. *American Annals of the Deaf, 32,* 84-92.

# CHAPTER 3

# *Reading Curricula*

Reading may be defined as the meaningful decoding of a graphic symbol system that is coded to represent language and cognitive structures already possessed by the reader. Simply put, the individual cannot read and make sense of what has not been already experienced and stored in the form of language. Although the act of reading can result in new learning, that new learning is essentially the result of orderly and, perhaps, new arrangement of ideas presented in the form of words, phrases, and sentences already known. It is self-evident that including too great a number of new words, phrases, or concepts interferes with the act of reading. The individual's language base cannot sustain reading in such a situation.

The point that reading depends on previous language development is made here for one fundamental reason. Hearing-impaired individuals, in general, encounter significant difficulty mastering what we call language. The extent of that difficulty and the methods through which educators attempt to overcome it are discussed in an earlier chapter. Suffice it to suggest here that the hearing-impaired population meets with enormous difficulty in learning to read with average competence largely due to impoverished language development. As Browns and Arnell (1981) noted "Hearing-impaired children are . . . . deficient in language when they enter school. Seldom do they attain the same level of linguistic maturity as their hearing peers." If this is true, the reader, teacher, administrator, parent, and researcher will be in a position to appreciate why the design of effective curricula and support materials in reading is a formidable task. The balance of this chapter will review methods developed, theories of reading development in the hearing-impaired school population, and problems to be considered in the future development of materials and curricula. Present curricular practice will first be reviewed.

## EXISTING CURRICULAR PRACTICE

Approaches in reading instruction for hearing-impaired children roughly parallel those for other children (King & Quigley, 1985). Reading curricular systems can be divided into varying categories for discussion. Gibson and Levine (1979), in their examination of reading from a psychological perspective, suggested two broad classes. One is an information processing model in which reading is viewed as a fixed series of stages or events extending over time. The other, currently enjoying considerable attention, is the analysis by synthesis model. Goodman's miscue analysis is perhaps the best known example based on the analysis by synthesis model. An alternative method of discussing reading is one focussed on phonic instruction. Armbruster, Echols, and Brown (1982), Browns and Arnell (1981), Clarke, Rogers, and Booth (1982), Ewoldt (1981), Hirsh-Pasek and Treiman (1982), and Truax (1978) discussed these models and others briefly in the context of hearing-impaired students.

Whatever model is favored, the theoretical framework must take on substance in the form of an instructional approach to be of practical value to teachers. By and large approaches to reading development and instruction can be reduced to four general methodologies: basal reader, language experience, individualization, and programming. They need not be discussed more than briefly in this chapter as they are well-detailed in the literature. Teachers have put their faith in one or more of these approaches, sometimes choosing and discarding them one after the other. It is easy to imagine the disruption to curricula and instruction as teachers implemented the latest, or most available, most logical, or last advocated approach. If this is too cynical a statement, consider the words of Clarke and associates (1982):

> In short, the current state of instructional methodology is one of confused eclecticism. Obviously there is no preferred approach, and the best advice is that, if one method does not succeed after it has been given a reasonable trial, then another approach should be tried. (p. 65)

La Sasso (1978) and Hasenstab and McKenzie (1981) reported in detail on reading methods and materials used in the United States in recent years. La Sasso (1978) surveyed programs for the hearing impaired in the United States, Puerto Rico, and Guam, obtaining usable questionnaire responses in 507 of 960 cases. Hasenstab and McKenzie (1981) had a somewhat lower return rate for a United States program survey but still received a creditable 201 responses to 550 questionnaires mailed. La Sasso's was the larger and more general survey and sought information across a variety of areas and methods. In an amplification and extension of one of La Sasso's categories, Hasenstab and McKenzie inquired specifically into reading series most frequently used. The following information presented is primarily from the wider La Sasso survey, with pertinent additions from Hasenstab and McKenzie.

Two instructional approaches standout as the most frequently used primary or supplementary systems: language experience and basal readers. Basal readers are more popular as a primary approach, and language experience as a supplemental approach. Both the individualized approach and the programmed approach were employed to an appreciable degree in supplemental roles and to a lesser degree in primary roles. Percentage of use is given in Table 3-1 for varying levels of instruction.

It is interesting to note that at junior high school level (ages 13-to-15 years) and senior high school level (ages 16-to-18 years), many programs did not appear to use any of the four basic approaches as a primary instructional method (34.5 percent and 52 percent respectively). However, at the primary level (ages 5-to-8 years), a number of programs used more than one main approach, depending on instructional needs of the different groups of children.

Certain basal reader series are obvious favorites, whereas others are used less frequently. Hasenstab and McKenzie (1981) indicate that 40 percent of the programs they studied used either Scott-Foresman Reading Systems or Open Highways, 12 percent used the Ginn 720 or 360 Series, 8 percent opted for Houghton-Mifflin readers, 7 percent for Bank Street readers, 6 percent for other Macmillan readers, and 5 percent for Edmark. La Sasso found the following distribution: Reading Systems—35 percent, Bank Street readers—18 percent, Ginn 360—16 percent, Design for Reading by Harper and Row—7 percent, Open Highways—5 percent, Basic Reading System by Holt, Rinehart, and Winston—4 percent, and Houghton-Mifflin readers—3 percent.

## BASAL READERS

There is little doubt that given the foregoing information, the curricular approach of choice depends heavily on basal readers. This is not surprising given the finding of Bockmiller and Coley (1981) that more teachers felt adequately prepared to use basal readers than other techniques in reading instruction. It is also apparent that no one set of readers is considered most appropriate by a majority of teachers at any instructional level. La Sasso (1978) set out a chart of most frequently used basal readers by primary, intermediate, junior high, and senior high school levels. Scott-Foresman's Reading Systems was the favored series at the primary level used 37.9 percent of the time; intermediate school was 34.6 percent; junior high school was 34.1 percent, and senior high school at 26.8 percent. The variety of series in use is reflected in La Sasso's report that 40 different series were in use and Hasenstab's and McKenzie's report of 36 in use. The reasons for choosing certain series and rejecting others are varied and not well-explored in the literature. Benefits and drawbacks are mentioned but there is little intensive or extensive analysis. Some general comments (Ling & Ling, 1978) follow:

**Table 3-1.** Percentage of Programs Using Various Instructional Approaches as Primary or Supplementary Methods to Teach Reading to Hearing-Impaired Children at the Different Levels of Instruction

| Level of instruction | Number of programs | Percentage of programs using the various instructional approaches | | | | | | | | | | | |
|---|---|---|---|---|---|---|---|---|---|---|---|---|---|
| | | Basal reader approach | | | Language experience approach | | | Individualized approach | | | Programmed approach | | |
| | | P | S | T | P | S | T | P | S | T | P | S | T |
| Primary level (ages 5-8) | 448 | 47.8 | 21.7 | 69.5 | 43.1 | 36.6 | 79.7 | 10.9 | 16.7 | 27.6 | 9.3 | 20.3 | 29.6 |
| Intermediate level (ages 9-12) | 434 | 58.1 | 19.8 | 77.9 | 19.1 | 58.1 | 77.2 | 10.4 | 26.0 | 36.4 | 6.2 | 25.8 | 32.0 |
| Junior high school level (ages 13-15) | 289 | 36.0 | 21.7 | 57.7 | 12.8 | 42.6 | 55.4 | 12.5 | 29.7 | 42.2 | 4.2 | 21.7 | 25.9 |
| Senior high school level (ages 16-18) | 250 | 15.2 | 17.6 | 32.8 | 12.8 | 31.2 | 44.0 | 16.8 | 26.8 | 43.6 | 3.2 | 16.0 | 19.2 |

From La Sasso, C. (1978). National survey of materials and procedures used to teach reading to hearing impaired children. *American Annals of the Deaf, 123*, 25. Reprinted by permission.

P = primary; S = supplementary; T = total.

> One of the major benefits of following a basal reading series is that the vocabulary is carefully controlled, ensuring that new words are repeated several times throughout the book and are included for review later in the series. Unfortunately, most current basal readers were prepared by persons unaware of recent psycholinguistic developments. The result is the inclusion of syntactic structures which are beyond the comprehension of the normal-hearing beginning reader, and consequently far beyond that of the hearing impaired child.

and (Clarke et al., 1982):

> Teachers of the hearing impaired, however, express discontent with these packaged materials, citing the use of uncontrolled vocabulary, inappropriate language levels, and the phonetic emphasis of some of the programs.

Browns and Arnell (1981), in their discussion of basal reading programs, stressed that teachers must be flexible in their use of basal series. Readers are not to be worked through from start to finish in a routine manner. Selections are to be analyzed by the teacher for appropriateness in building skill areas, in providing reading in areas of student interests, and in being within the experiential and linguistic ranges of any specific group of hearing-impaired children. Browns and Arnell were forthright in their support of basal reading programs but also warn teachers of the inappropriateness of much basal material.

Other general criticisms relate to the unfamiliarity of textual material (Gormley, 1981, 1982; Schnepel, 1980), the need to rewrite basal readers to accommodate lexical and grammatical limitations (Hammermeister & Israelite, 1983b), the lack of general applicability of basal series (Truax, 1978), and syntactic complexity (Quigley, 1982). Although these general points are covered in diverse sources, La Sasso (1978), Hasenstab and McKenzie (1981), and King and Quigley (1985) provided the most exhaustive analyses. It is worthwhile to note the positive and negative aspects highlighted in the first two surveys as they pinpoint functional considerations with which curricula designers must deal in their work. King and Quigley (1985) expanded these discussions in a wide-ranging, incisive review of text-based variables that influence text difficulty, including the text of basal readers.

Which features to include in basal readers for the hearing impaired is of considerable interest to those charged with curricular responsibility. Table 3-2 provides a short list of aspects to consider.

From the table it is evident that considerable variability resulted from the surveys by La Sasso and Hasenstab and McKenzie. A partial explanation for this is that La Sasso dictated categories to be checked or not checked whereas Hasenstab and McKenzie provided an open-ended response format. However, two points emerge. First, aspects of value in basal readers for use with hearing-impaired students do not differ all that much from aspects considered valuable

**Table 3-2.** Desirable Aspects of Basal Readers Employed with Hearing-Impaired Students

| Aspect | La Sasso (1978) | Hasenstab and McKenzie (1981) |
|---|---|---|
| High interest level | × | × |
| Appropriate conceptual load | × | |
| Helpful support materials | × | × |
| Can be modified for use | × | |
| Attractive format | | × |
| Controlled vocabulary | | × |
| Sequential skill development | | × |
| Appropriate language level | | × |
| Useful diagnostic tests | × | |

for normally hearing students. Second, desirable features are so general as to provide little in the way of specifically useful information. Of the nine aspects noted, none stands out as uniquely applicable to hearing-impaired students.

Browns and Arnell (1981) added three additional points to those offered by La Sasso and Hasenstab and McKenzie: (1) basal readers must stress oral language development and reading for meaning from the earliest stages; (2) whatever series is chosen must provide for flexible use; and (3) stories must use natural language forms. Again, these points are not restricted to applicability to hearing-impaired students alone.

Information is also available on particular weaknesses of existing basal reader series (see Table 3-3).

Both the La Sasso and the Hasenstab and McKenzie studies showed wide variability in responses for the Ginn Bank Street readers but a close association for the Scott-Foresman readers. It is difficult to explain this apparently wide difference in professional opinion for two of three reading series. Hasenstab and McKenzie made no mention of it although they referred to the earlier La Sasso survey. In the face of such conflicting feedback from studies, it is difficult to pinpoint actual weaknesses of basal reading series. It might be supposed that the appropriate policy would be to avoid readers with apparent weaknesses and depend on those with apparent strengths. The foregoing discussion suggests that it is not possible to do so with confidence on the basis of available surveys and mention in the literature. No one basal reader series stands out as head and shoulders above the others.

The generally bleak situation with regard to the appropriateness of basal readers for many hearing-impaired learners is ameliorated to some degree by

**Table 3-3.** Weaknesses of Selected Basal Reader Series Frequently Employed with Hearing-Impaired Students as Indicated by Users

| | Scott-Foresman % | | Ginn % | | Bank Street % | |
|---|---|---|---|---|---|---|
| **Weakness** | **La Sasso*** | **Hasenstab† & McKenzie** | **La Sasso** | **Hasenstab & McKenzie** | **La Sasso** | **Hasenstab & McKenzie** |
| Uncontrolled vocabulary | 41 | 50 | 52 | 8 | 34 | 3 |
| Insufficient repetition of vocabulary | 69 | 71 | 52 | 0 | 37 | 0 |
| Inappropriate language or syntax development | 47 | 50 | 56 | 8 | 51 | 3 |
| Heavy phonic emphasis | 41 | 46 | 48 | 12 | 39 | 4 |
| Low interest at higher levels | 26 | | | 4 | | 13 |
| For linguistically competent only | 33 | | 51 | | 32 | |
| Acceleration too rapid | | 39 | | 11 | | 11 |
| Idiomatic or figurative language | 56 | | 57 | | 38 | |

*1978

†1981

delineation of desirable aspects and weaknesses. It should not be concluded that, simply because basal readers do not solve the problem of teaching reading to hearing-impaired learners, basal readers should not form part of a curricular package. Rather, such points indicate that care must be taken in the selection of basal readers. They must be reviewed for their strengths and weaknesses and for the degree to which they suit various populations of hearing-impaired children.

A major response to this difficulty has been made by a number of writers who have attempted to write readers specifically for hearing-impaired students. These authors took into consideration to a greater or lesser degree the weaknesses associated with basal reader series prepared for normally hearing children. The result has been a limited amount of reading material with attention focussed on control of vocabulary and syntax (King & Quigley, 1985). Only one series of basal readers written specifically for the hearing-impaired population has been published, *Reading Milestones* by Quigley and King (1981), which is reviewed at the end of this chapter. While this series has been widely accepted, it contains a number of significant weaknesses, as do other materials written for the hearing impaired.

Browns and Arnell (1981) provided a valuable resource for those selecting basal reading programs for inclusion in reading curricula. Their detailed criteria for the evaluation of basal series will assist in ensuring that the best possible choices are made. These criteria are given below. Those selecting basal reader series would do well to review their possible choices in terms of the items noted by Browns and Arnell.*

### *Criteria for evaluating basal reading programs*

Who are the authors?
What is the program's instructional approach to reading?
Are the goals governing the development of the program clearly stated?
Are those goals clearly reflected in the materials? Are the children helped to perceive the goals toward which they are working?

### *Content and teaching strategies*

Is the program strong in the teaching of readiness skills? Is it systematic?

Does the program provide for the continuous development of oral language skills from the earliest levels?

Are beginning readers brought quickly to reading real books?

Does the subject matter appeal to a broad range of children's interests?

Can it widen pupils' interests and horizons? Is an appreciation of literature developed?

Is there a good balance of subject matter?

Are the selections well written? Do they include recognized children's authors?

Do the stories reflect the natural language patterns of children and adults or is the language stilted and non-fluent?

Are the vocabulary and syntax appropriate to the designated reading level of the material?

Are the pupils' readers attractive in appearance?

Is the size of print suitable to the reader's age and ability?

Are the illustrations appealing to children? Are they well drawn and well distributed? Do they help tell the story, clarify meaning, or enhance the text?

---

*From: Browns, F., and Arnell, D. *A guide to the selection and use of readinq instructional material.* Alexander Graham Bell Association for the Deaf, Washington, DC: Reproduced with permission.

Are the students encouraged to develop an interest in words and take independent responsibility for their vocabulary?

Does the program teach sound-symbol relationships? To what extent is this the mainstay of the program?

Does the program teach the multiple use of word-attack skills; sound-symbol relations, word structure clues, context clues, and use of dictionary?

Does the program emphasize reading for meaning from the earliest levels?

Does it teach critical and evaluative comprehension in addition to literal comprehension?

Is there a language arts strand that teaches creative and expository writing?

Are reference skills, particularly those of locating and organizing information, given attention?

Are comprehension and study skills applied to content material as well as narrative material?

Do the correlated workbooks provide effective practice on the skills developed in the program? Do they provide for application to new contexts?

Are the workbooks well organized and attractive?

How is the program paced? Are the levels realistic at which skills and concepts are introduced and mastered?

Does the program provide pupils with self-directing activities so they can begin to take responsibility for their own learning? Are the activities meaningful and interesting?

*Teacher's edition*

Are lesson plans for teachers easy to follow?

Do the lesson plans provide adequate guidance for helping the pupils read and interpret each selection?

Are alternate teaching strategies and activities provided for children who progress slowly? For children who acquire skills rapidly?

Can the reading materials be used flexibly?

Is the management system efficient, effective, and easy to use?

Are there suggested bibliographies for teachers and students?

Is there a scope and sequence chart? Is it easy to follow?

*Parental involvement*

Does the program contain material that parents can use with their children to foster the development of reading?

Is the material easy to use? Are adequate instructions provided?

A common compromise position adopted by those dissatisfied with basal reader series designed for normally hearing children and unable to write completely new readers is to rewrite existing material. Illustrations are used unchanged while the text is altered to meet what are considered to be the language levels of a particular group. A great many hours have been devoted to this task and some schools have extensive libraries of rewritten books. The practice has been extended to recreational reading materials as well as to reading series. King and Quigley (1985) provide a set of guiding principles for the preparation of reading materials. Educators wishing to re-write texts for inclusion in their curricula will find the King and Quigley guidelines of value.

From the above discussion on basal readers as a favored curricular approach in reading instruction, a number of central points emerge that were found in the writings of a number of authorities in the field. While absolute agreement on all points was not the case, the frequency of mention and extent of discussion make these points loom larger than others.

1. Vocabulary must be controlled in its introduction, repetition and extent (Browns & Arnell, 1981; Hart, 1978; Hasenstab & McKenzie, 1981; King & Quigley, 1985; Rompf, 1981; Truax, 1978; Walter, 1978).
2. The introduction and use of syntactic structures must be controlled (Hammermeister & Israelite, 1983a, 1983b; Hasenstab & McKenzie, 1981; King & Quigley, 1985; Ling & Ling, 1978; Quigley, 1982; Robbins & Hatcher, 1981).
3. Specific reading skills, e.g., sounding out, comprehension, and inference, must be developed (Browns & Arnell, 1981; Hart, 1978; Hasenstab & McKenzie, 1981; Ling & Ling, 1978).
4. Interest levels must be appropriate (Browns & Arnell, 1981; Hart, 1978; Hasenstab & McKenzie, 1981; King & Quigley, 1985; Ling & Ling, 1978; Truax, 1978).
5. Content must be familiar (Browns & Arnell, 1981; Gormley, 1981, 1982; Gormley & Franzen, 1978; King & Quigley, 1985; Pearson, 1982).

The aforementioned points reflect the concerns and opinions of many. They are simple to state but surprisingly difficult to meet. The reasons for the difficulty are many, and this is not the appropriate place for an extensive discussion. Some idea of the complexity of preparing basal readers and other reading materials will be given in a later section dealing with theoretical positions in reading instruction for the hearing impaired.

## LANGUAGE EXPERIENCE

In essence the language experience approach focusses on learning through the interrelationships of words and language as spoken, listened to, and written by oneself and others. Content is derived from the student's experiences as guided and developed by the teacher. Soon after reading what they write of their personal experiences, students move on to the writings of others. Language experience is considered a reading method useful in introducing reading, in introducing sight vocabulary, in developing beginning reading skills, and in middle grade reading programming (Alexander, 1979). The major strengths of the method are its relating of an individual's experiences, interests, and language to the act of reading and the integration of thinking, speaking, listening, writing, and reading. Its most serious limitation is the demand for a teacher able to blend experiences into a continually advancing reading program (McNeil, Donant, & Alkin, 1980).

As noted by La Sasso (1978), language experience is second only to basal readers as the approach chosen by teachers of the hearing impaired. This is true especially at the primary level. One reason for its favored use at this level may be the almost complete lack of appropriate published materials for hearing-impaired children. A second reason may be its wide-spread use with normally hearing children of a similar age. Although it is true as well at other instructional levels, the gap between those using a basal reader approach and those using a language experience approach widens, whereas the gap between those using a language experience approach and those using alternative approaches narrows. At these other levels, language experience is favored much more as a supplementary than a primary method of reading instruction.

King and Quigley (1985) noted that teachers of the hearing impaired have a variety of definitions for the language experience approach. For some it means child-dictated stories only, for others child-dictated stories and teacher modification as necessary, and for still others, child-dictated stories, teacher modification, and teacher-written chart stories. This point is important for curriculum developers in that child-dictated stories frequently contain multiple examples of nonstandard English. Teachers of hearing-impaired children often must correct the language to render it intelligible in terms of English syntax and semantics. In many cases such correction is considerable. The value of using child-dictated or child-created materials must be weighed against the intrusion of teacher language imposed to agree with standard English rules.

Despite La Sasso's survey research indicating that the language experience approach finds use in a multiplicity of programs, there is little evidence for its use as a primary method in the literature on teaching reading to the hearing impaired. When mentioned in any detail, language experience appears as one component of a many-faceted reading program. Hart (1978) recognized the need to tie experience and reading firmly together and encouraged the use of language experience activities throughout the school. However, teacher-made materials do not predominate (at least in number) in her listing of materials required to support a program focussed on making reading meaningful.

1. Library books of all kinds
2. Basal readers
3. Supplementary readers
4. Textbooks
5. Workbooks and skillbuilders
6. Reference dictionaries, atlases, etc.
7. Teacher-made materials
8. Audio visual aids
9. Functional materials (Hart, 1978)

Truax (1978), Ling and Ling (1978), and Browns and Arnell (1981) also encouraged the use of language experience techniques in concert with other approaches and materials. Language experience is used to differing degrees at different instructional levels. Reference to the more detailed analyses of selected reading curricula at the end of this chapter will examine the actual use of the method.

Teachers of hearing-impaired children appreciate that language experience draws on events and knowledge familiar to the child. Considerable effort has been expended routinely at preschool and primary levels to provide experiences in everyday situations to build a base on which to develop language and reading. One explanatory example of techniques employed in this endeavor may be found in a short article on preschool experiences and follow-up activities by Melnyk (1977). Although the benefits of reading activities based on familiar topics have long been recognized, it is only recently that substantial theoretical support has buttressed this conventional wisdom. The work of Gormley and Franzen (1978) and Gormley (1981, 1982) on familiarity, text comprehension, and recall, and of Pearson (1982) on schema theory as it may relate to the hearing impaired, may be considered especially pertinent to the efforts of those charged with curricular responsibilities for reading. The positions put forward by these authors will be reviewed later in this chapter.

Although language experience is a method favored by many educators of the hearing impaired, it is difficult to find any extended discussion of how to apply the method with hearing-impaired students. Even King & Quigley (1985) in their major publication on reading devote only two pages to the topic. It would appear that those who prepare curricula assume that teachers responsible for instruction in reading know the basics of language experience and are able to adapt the general procedure appropriately for hearing-impaired children. That this may not be a secure assumption is noted by Hammermeister and Israelite (1983a):

Although the language-experience reading approach is often useful for hearing-impaired children, its primary disadvantage is related to the fact that these children frequently have delayed language skills. The teacher of the deaf may find that too many language concepts and basic vocabulary items are lacking, and that the creation of natural reading materials is not possible.

Hammermeister and Israelite (1983a, 1983b) are among the few who discuss in any detail a method of employing this particular approach. They base their presentation on a project undertaken in Australia by Hart, Walker, and Gray (1977). This study, the Mount Gravatt Research Project, collected data on the language used naturally by $2\frac{1}{2}$-to $6\frac{1}{2}$-year-old normally hearing children, analyzed it for word sequences at various levels, for context in which used, and for intended meanings. In essence the researchers found that the language of basal readers does not capture the natural language of children. They devised a language and reading program based on their analysis of natural language. The components of this program are the following:

**ORAL LANGUAGE WORK.** This work is conducted within a pragmatic situation established by the teacher for student interaction and discussion. Teachers use children's own language strings as much as possible.

**LINKING ORAL UNITS WITH THEIR WRITTEN FORM.** The teacher prepares "signaling units" on cards. Following practice for recognition and extension, the children create their own cards.

**WORD ATTACK SKILLS.** Practice is given in phonics, although no particular method of word attack is mandated.

**PRESENTATION OF READING BOOKS.** The teacher creates reading books using the natural language of the children following sufficient time and effort in the first three steps.

Hammermeister and Israelite (1983a, 1983b) suggested an adaptation of Hart and associates' method (1977), which they consider useful for hearing-impaired children.

1. Teacher determines appropriate language from an actual situation. Students are involved in practice.
2. Teacher introduces the written form in signaling units from student utterances in the actual situation. Students use their own cards to form the sentence. Considerable practice in combining signaling units to create new sentences follows.
3. Teacher presents the reading story but only following successful practice in combining signaling units.

The authors suggest that this method would be useful because it employs the language structures of the children, refers to known situations and requires the teacher to converse and interrogate in language forms known to the children. Furthermore, it is an integrated language-reading program that combines and blends the skills of listening, communicating, writing, and reading.

Language experience is the method of choice chiefly at the primary level with hearing-impaired students. Its use at this level is possibly directly related to the availability of published materials of an appropriate nature for this population. At other levels, when language experience is used, it is employed in a supplementary fashion as one of a number of approaches. Throughout its use, it has in its favor the values of containing material familiar to the student and employing words and terms of the student's choosing. Conversely the language deficiences of the typical hearing-impaired child create a need for the teacher to impose standard English terms and syntax over the student's writing. Lack of resolution of this conflict has limited the generalizability of this technique.

## INDIVIDUALIZED INSTRUCTION

Individualized instruction in reading refers to an approach in which the child self-selects reading material according to interest and level, the child and teacher hold frequent conferences to keep check on reading progress and difficulties, and temporary groups may be formed on the basis of need in some particular skill or skills (Savage & Mooney, 1979). Spache and Spache (1977) noted that there are five major areas of concern related to this approach:

1. Organization of materials, extensive record-keeping, multiplicity of skills exercises required, and need for a conferencing system.
2. Complexity of the required conferencing system.
3. Need to devise, carry out, and monitor the skills development program.
4. Need for independence in student actions.
5. Need for appropriately detailed record-keeping.

Among the strengths of the individualized approach are the respect for the learner basic to its philosophy, use of self-motivation and self-actualization, and the opportunity for small-group skills instruction. No method is without its thorns, however. The tendency of some children to be narrow and inappropriate in their choice of reading materials, the difficulty of scheduling conferences, the need for high-level observational skills, and the demand for a wide-ranging knowledge of both individual children and children's literature all challenge the teacher (McNeil, Donant, & Alkin, 1980). The relative gains and difficulties associated with this approach for learners with special needs have led various authors to suggest that the individualized reading approach is inappropriate for other than average populations (Kirk, Kliebhan, & Lerner, 1978; Savage & Mooney, 1979).

The inappropriateness of this approach for educators of the hearing impaired may be reflected in its relatively low level of usage in North America. La Sasso (1978) reported that it is favored as a primary method or as a supplementary method by few teachers at the primary and intermediate (9-to-12 years) levels. It appeals to a greater number at junior high and is the primary method of choice at senior high (16-to-18 years). Even at the highest level, however, it is used only by 42 of 250 programs as a primary method and by 67 of 250 as a supplemental method. Materials of choice at the various levels are, in declining order, library books, newspapers, the SRA Reading Laboratories, and trade books.

It is difficult to determine why the individualized instruction approach is not generally used. The literature does not comment directly on this aspect beyond La Sasso's (1978) statement that teachers appeared to use the individualized approach when they could find no suitable reading material for their students, and King and Quigley's (1985) hypothesis that programs making this choice may be those that emphasize literature study. However, experience with hearing-impaired children suggests a number of reasons why this particular method would not be a primary curricular selection: language difficulties of so many hearing-impaired children, impoverished vocabulary, syntactic difficulties, and semantic problems. These would seriously restrict choice of reading material. Another reason may be a lack of understanding of the approach on the part of many teachers. Just as in so many other areas, reading requires specific study; not all teachers have sufficient skills in individualized instruction to implement it effectively. Lack of background in teaching reading is a problem noted by Coley and Bockmiller (1980) and Bockmiller and Coley (1981) in their writings on preparation as teachers of reading among teachers of the hearing impaired.

It should be noted, too, that the term "individualized" is used dissimilarly by many professionals. Truax (1978), for instance, spoke of an individualized program within an integrated communication curriculum. She went on to outline the reading branch of such a program, emphasizing the need to involve recreational, functional, and informational reading. A teacher not conversant with the essentials of various reading approaches may interpret that what Truax proposed is individualized reading. This, however, is not one of the central structures in Truax's proposal. Similarly, Hart (1978) included individual reading in her curriculum, but it is only part of a much larger eclectic whole.

One of the few discussions of an individualized program is that offered by McCarr (1973). McCarr described a program in effect at Oregon State School for the Deaf for grades 7 through 12. The program is not reviewed in detail, although examples of a fifth grade and an eighth grade program are provided. McCarr basically stated that the program was individualized and that students self-selected materials from among more than 75 available choices. Many of the materials were self-corrective, and students each had an individual file folder in which a record of material read was maintained. Project LIFE material (Pfau, 1963–1974a) was used to pinpoint reading needs, and the teachers directed students to appropriate materials to meet those needs. Intertwined with the reading program was an optional speech program. McCarr noted that all students opted for speech instruction. Speech instruction focussed in part on language and vocabulary from the individual's reading materials.

A unique component of the Oregon program was the deliberate revealing of reading test scores to students. As McCarr explained it, the students were routinely surprised by their low achievement levels and were motivated to improve. She noted that an average gain of 1 year and three months was realized in the period from September to May. This gain is a most substantial one at this age level. Unfortunately McCarr offered no substantial evidence that this gain was a result of individualized instruction. Other factors may have contributed to, or occasioned, the gain.

It appears that most curriculum writers in reading for the hearing impaired believe that individualized reading should be one component of a reading program. Conversely many teachers decline to use this approach and use it only when no other approach is available. The manifold language difficulties of the typical hearing-impaired student restrict its use. It is valuable to have students choose their own materials, but such a procedure is best related to recreational reading within an eclectic reading program.

## PROGRAMMED READING

Programmed instruction is based on operant conditioning principles. Characteristically the approach encompasses individual rate of progress, careful sequencing of instruction, and immediate feedback and reinforcement. Polloway, Payne, Patton, and Payne (1985) noted the approach can be effective for students who do not require direct and frequent teacher monitoring. Additionally, programmed materials have been found valuable with remedial readers when specific skills are in need of reinforcement (Alexander, 1979).

As in regular education, programmed reading has never become a major approach in reading instruction for hearing-impaired students. La Sasso (1978) noted that fewer than 10 percent of programs list the programmed reading approach as their primary method at any level of instruction. Approximately one in five list it as a supplementary method. The method appeals most at the primary level (9.3 percent), which is not surprising given the traditional emphasis on specific skill acquisition at this level.

The most ambitious effort in programmed instruction for the hearing impaired was that known as Project LIFE. An effort was made over a lengthy period to create materials for the hearing impaired based on the known principles of programmed instruction. Pfau (1970a) noted these principles to be the following:

1. Sequential presentation of learning events
2. Relatively small increments of difficulty
3. Overt responses
4. Immediate knowledge of results
5. Self-pacing
6. High probability of correct responses
7. Meaningful material
8. High interest level
9. Gradual fading of prompts
10. Reinforcement
11. Review

Pfau considered that these points, blended with the principles of behavioral objectives, would form the base for useful instructional programs. The teacher was to "view herself as an intrinsic segment of the system and as a manager of learning events."

Eventually a large number of materials, especially reading and writing materials, was produced (Pfau, 1963–1974a, 1963–1974b). Although considerable interest was aroused in these materials and they were distributed widely, they became supplementary materials rather than the core of an instructional approach. Among the reasons for their relatively low acceptance were cost, restricted variety, need for constant teacher monitoring, and difficulty of devising an appropriate design for hearing-impaired children. One example of the type of difficulty encountered was noted by Pfau (1970b) following a study of reinforcement methods: "Although simple knowledge of results is adequate motivation for most students, it may be that this means of reinforcement is inadequate for other target populations." Additionally, though great care was taken to set acceptably restricted incremental learning steps, the rate of progress expected was too great for many children. This was especially apparent in the initial readiness level programs. However, despite these limitations Project LIFE is the most frequently employed programmed material used in programs for the hearing impaired. Following Project LIFE in frequency of use are Sullivan Programmed Reading and the SRA Reading Laboratories (La Sasso, 1978).

In summary, the programmed reading approach has not made a significant contribution to curricula in reading. As Kretschmer and Kretschmer (1978) noted with reference to programmed approaches in a variety of areas, although initial results were promising, long-term results have not sustained early indications.

## THEORETICAL POSITIONS

It is well known that hearing-impaired individuals taken as a group achieve at quite low levels in comparison to normally hearing peers. One of the more widely known achievement level studies is that by Wrightstone, Aronow, and Moskowitz (1963). These investigators found an average reading level of grade 3.5 for hearing-impaired students aged 15 to 16 years. What is less well known is how to change this low level of reading ability, or how to make instruction more effective. If clear-cut methods were known, revised or new reading curricula and materials could be prepared. Unfortunately at present too little is understood. As Robbins and Hatcher (1981) stated, "Research on the reading ability of the hearing impaired leaves us at a loss to explain their low reading achievement."

One basic position is that hearing-impaired children do not read well as a result of a basic impoverishment in language ability. Truax (1978) recognized this position when she remarked that "Too often a hearing-impaired child is said to have a reading problem, when in fact the problem is really language based." Until the problem of language development has been resolved to a significant degree, many hearing-impaired children will be unable to read well because of lack of strength in lexicon, language patterns and rules, and the semantic relationships of language. Quigley and Kretschmer (1982) echoed this position stating:

> Not only the code (printed symbols), but also the language (standard English) are unfamiliar. Thus, the task of learning to read often becomes a language learning process at the same time. These children may be able to crack the code of the printed message and be able to identify each individual word, but without a solid language base, comprehension does not occur.

Walter (1978) questioned even the ability to identify individual words. He found in his investigation of the ability of the hearing-impaired child to deal effectively with English words in print "that previous estimates of vocabulary development in hearing-impaired subjects are spuriously high." Curriculum writers, according to this finding, must review even assumptions of vocabulary strength.

A number of options emerge from such a position. One of these is to stress language development and research in language prior to extensive study and effort in reading. Although a significant body of professionals appear to accept this position, others believe that much can be gained by a simultaneous attack on both language and reading.

Quigley is the main proponent of the view that syntactic deficiencies are a major contributor to the reading problems of the hearing impaired and that one method of combating these problems would be to create syntactically controlled reading materials (Quigley, Power, & Steinkamp, 1977). This position grew from a lengthy and detailed series of studies investigating the syntactic abilities of hearing-impaired students. These studies are reviewed briefly in the chapter on language. Although there is no doubt that major deficiencies exist in this area, it remains to be seen if controlling syntax will raise the reading ability of the hearing impaired. A number of controlled reading materials have been prepared. Among these are *Reading Milestones* (Quigley & King, 1981), a basal reader program, and the *Controlled Language Science Series* (Fleury, 1979). The former is reviewed in this chapter, whereas the latter is reviewed in Chapter 5. A listing of additional "controlled" materials may be found in King and Quigley (1985).

It is worthwhile to note that Quigley and his colleagues are not alone in isolating syntax as a major cause of reading difficulties among the hearing impaired. Robbins and Hatcher (1981) found in their study of sentence comprehension that syntax was outstanding among other variables as the most significant contributor to low reading scores. They concluded that "Comprehension difficulties of hearing-impaired children seem to be due primarily to syntactic rather than morphological or semantic deficit."

Bryans (1979) looked beyond the sentence level emphasis of those whose primary concern is syntax. She suggested that a partial explanation of the low reading achievement levels of hearing-impaired students may be inadequate control of the features of connected discourse. To support this position she cites Wilbur's (1977) finding that young deaf children encountered significantly greater difficulty with pronoun usage when antecedent referents were located in previous sentences than when they were located in the same sentences as the pronouns. Bryans' position was that increased deliberate attention to referents, lexical substitution, and summary words will lead to improved comprehension of continuous discourse. She provided a series of sample exercises to clarify her point.

Maxwell (1974), too, looked beyond the sentence level in an article in which she presented a modest proposal for improving reading, stating that teachers concentrate on the development of "thinking skills," not simply vocabulary and content. As she noted "A student may be able to define every word in an article and still not be able to interpret the whole." Maxwell put forth a concept of prediction, reading, and verification, and prediction drawn from Stauffer's (1970) work on reading. At a certain level this proposal is reminiscent of Furth's concern with the development of thinking skills (1966a, 1966b). At another level it ties in with Bryans' theories (1979) and the thesis that teachers are overly concerned with vocabulary, phrase, and sentence-level learning in reading.

This general position is not focussed, as is Quigley's work, on major modification in reading materials and processes. It deals with what might be termed "mini-theories," methods of changing instructional emphasis rather than instruction itself. Consequently, such ideas are not of major relevance to curriculum designers. They are worthy of consideration and inclusion in curricula but are not major factors. At present, however, no major factors that can be addressed directly are sufficiently understood to cause major curricular change. Even the work of Quigley and King (1981) in producing controlled syntax readers has no fundamental effect on curricula. The instructional process does not change radically simply with the introduction of a new set of basal readers.

Radical change is a natural outcome of the theoretical position of Gormley (1981, 1982), Gormley and Franzen (1978), and Gormley and Geoffrion (1981). These authors argued that the hearing-impaired individual is a uniquely different reader. There is no viable graphic symbol system for what many consider the hearing-impaired person's first language, the language of signs. Thus, there is a need to read in another, nonnative language system. This basic difference is offered as explanatory, in large part at least, for the reading difficulties experienced by this population. The various authors proposed that one viable method of ameliorating these difficulties would be to maximize the familiarity of what the student reads. In this connection Gormley (1982) stated "Readers are more likely to be able to comprehend a selection about a familiar topic than an unfamiliar one." Two studies investigating the effect of textual familiarity on comprehension of third-grade level material (Gormley 1981, 1982) are illustrative of the empirical support for this position. In the first study (Gormley, 1981), both students and materials were at a third-grade level. The findings indicated that familiarity was a salient feature in reading achievement. The second study (Gormley, 1982) involved third-grade level materials and second-grade level readers. Again textual familiarity was a significant factor. So strong was the effect that, in the investigator's opinion, it overrode the effect of syntactic complexity. Other researchers, however, caution against over-interpretation of the effect of using familiar material in reading with hearing-impaired children (King & Quigley, 1985).

The theoretical positions reviewed briefly in the foregoing deal with what appear to be fundamental issues: internalization of syntactic rules, lack of control of connected discourse, reading as thinking, and the need to promote familiarity to benefit from the individual's experiential and cognitive background. In actual fact, we do not know how to teach the average hearing-impaired student to read at a level commensurate with age and intellect. Each of the positions discussed shed some light on a dark subject. However, to date the result has been simply to illuminate only a few areas without revealing the shape or extent of the problem.

## SUMMARY

Those concerned with curricula for reading with hearing-impaired students are engaged in a most difficult arena. Reading is a field of study in and of itself and presents sufficient challenge to any teacher or researcher. Within the field of hearing impairment, however, the teaching of reading is intertwined with and confounded by the language deficiencies of the average student. None of the four traditional approaches to reading instruction nor any combination of them is successful in establishing acceptable levels of reading ability in the hearing-impaired population. Why this is so, unless we simply accept the position that sheer language lack is the limiting factor, is unknown. A number of individuals have attempted and are attempting to identify the salient language, or cognitive, or experiential abilities of hearing-impaired readers. In so doing these researchers provide an excellent example to others and set forth valuable issues for examination. To date, however, these issues are insufficiently clarified and too conflicting to provide a stable base on which to build curricula that would give promise of resolving, to any appreciable degree, the wide spread reading difficulties of the hearing-impaired population.

## TYPE READING RESOURCES IN REVIEW

*Reading* Clark School for the Deaf (1972)

*Reading Curriculum* Louisiana School for the Deaf (1985)

*Reading Milestones* S.P. Quigley and C.M. King (1981)

*Teaching Reading to Deaf Children* B.0. Hart (1978)

## *READING*

### The Clarke School for the Deaf

*Publisher*:
Clarke School for the Deaf Northampton, MA 01060

*Skills taught*: Various skills related to the development of reading ability at the levels of developmental, functional, and enrichment reading

*Age/grade range*: Lower, middle, and upper school or reading readiness through grade 9

*Group Size*: Class group

**THEORY:** The theoretical position of Clarke School staff with regard to reading is not reviewed in any detail. In general, reading is regarded as an "essential learning skill" that provides the means for accessing information about the world. Every teacher is a teacher of reading in the information-gathering task. Though it is realized that there is no one way to teach reading, certain central aspects of the Clarke approach are discernible. Since most children learn to read through use of audition and oral skills, instruction must emphasize parallel skills in the hearing-impaired student. Auditory, visual, and speaking skills are trained and emphasized throughout the reading process in the attempt to create a thinking reader. The reading process may be broken down into composite skills such as word attack, vocabulary building, comprehension, dictionary, and study. These are taught as necessary parts of a larger skill in a definite bottom-up theoretical orientation.

**DESCRIPTION:** The Clarke School curriculum guide in reading provides an overview of essential skills over three school divisions: lower, middle, and upper, covering prereading through grade 9. Three levels or types of reading are described. These are:

1. Developmental reading—systematic acquisition and improvement of reading skills.
2. Functional reading—use of the above skills in the acquisition, interpretation, and organization of information.
3. Enrichment reading—use of developmental and functional skills for reading appreciation and enjoyment.

Developmental reading is organized under a number of main topics which, in turn, are organized under minor topics as follows:

Reading readiness
- Auditory
- Visual
- Procedure

Word attack
- Word configurations
- Noting similarities and differences
- Phonetics
- Phonetic sight reading

Vocabulary building
- Categorizing words
- Use in context and practice
- Multiple meanings
- Antonyms, synonyms, and homonyms
- Expressions and idioms
- Everyday vocabulary
- Language and vocabulary for nonacademic areas
- Developing vocabulary through composition and language activities

Comprehension skills
- Recognizing the main idea
- Reading for details: facts and sequence
- Serving relationships
- Drawing conclusions: making inferences
- Forming opinions
- Other activities involving critical reading

Throughout the Developmental reading section teaching examples and procedures are given. Each major and minor topic is introduced with a short rationale.

Functional reading is organized along similar lines. The topics for this section are:

Dictionary skills
- Steps in developing dictionary skills

Study skills
- Rate of reading
- Following directions
- Basic vocabulary for following directions
- Note taking
- Outlining
- Summarizing
- Locating and using reference materials
- Form for a bibliography
- Development of ability to write reports and do research projects
- Background experiences and reference materials

Library skills

Oral skills related to reading
- Developing the child's ability to ask questions

Reading for enrichment is quite short relative to the other main reading types. It is divided into "For appreciation" ("Introduction to American Literature") and "For recreation."

Considerable space is devoted to the detailing of materials for each school division. Under lower school materials it is noted that teacher-made materials form the great majority of items used until some proficiency is achieved in oral and written language, at which point a basal reading series is introduced. Even then, teacher-made materials continue to be used. Additionally, use is made of a variety of supplementary reading materials. Samples of an experience topic, a paragraph story, a holiday topic, and teacher's news are given.

At the middle school level, ages 10-to-14 and grades 2 through 4 approximately are covered. Alternate basic reading series are suggested for each year, and supplementary materials to develop the skills laid out for middle school are noted including transparencies and filmstrips. Basic reading materials, alternate basic reading series, supplementary materials, and skills to receive special emphasis for each year of middle school are noted.

Materials for the six years of upper school are given, divided for two ability tracks: Track 1 covers ages 12 to 17 and grades 2.5 to 5 approximately, while Track 2 covers ages 12 to 16 and grades 4 through 9 approximately. Regular materials and supplementary materials are used for each year of each track.

The Clarke School guide closes with short sections on a number of topics. These are:

Descriptions of commonly used reading materials at Clarke School

Evaluation

Suggestions for teachers

Suggestions for teachers to give parents

**EVALUATION:** The Clarke School reading curriculum presents a useful, if traditional, approach to reading instruction for hearing-impaired students. Its emphasis on a skills acquisition, "bottom-up" concept of reading development is well-accepted in the field. It does not, however, reflect contemporary research findings to any significant degree.

Division of reading instruction into developmental, functional, and enrichment reading gives the curriculum some depth and utility. The weight of emphasis, however, falls on the developmental and functional areas with minimal attention to reading for appreciation and recreation. The delineation of teaching ideas in the first half of the curriculum will prove of value to many teachers. Unfortunately, discussion of theory is limited and teachers may not grasp the underlying principles for the ideas presented. The result may be difficulty in designing new teaching ideas to complement the examples given.

The support materials listed are wide-ranging but dated. To a significant degree any teacher using the Clarke School reading curriculum as a guide would need to investigate more recently published materials.

Provision for two tracks or ability levels in reading at the upper-school division recognizes the fact that not all hearing-impaired learners achieve well in reading. This is a necessary point to make in any curriculum. Unfortunately again, the resources noted are dated. The concluding sections on evaluation, suggestions for teachers, and suggestions for teachers to give parents are useful additions to the curriculum. The evaluation section is quite short and general.

## *READING CURRICULUM*

### Louisiana School for the Deaf

*Publisher*:
Louisiana School for the Deaf,
P.O. Box 3074
Baton Rouge, LA 70821

*Skills Taught*: Various skills related to reading: vocabulary acquisition, comprehension, appreciation

*Age/grade range*: Grade 9 to grade 12

*Group size*: Class group

**THEORY:** No theoretical discussion or indication of theoretical position is given in the secondary level *Reading Curriculum*. This curriculum is but part of a lengthier curricula that begins at the readiness level. Though earlier stages are not reviewed here, as they are currently undergoing revision, it is possible, through them and through the secondary curricula, to determine the general theoretical thrust of the Louisiana School.

The lack of auditory skill during the preschool years and the subsequent difficulty in acquiring spoken language results in lack of normal awareness of the relationship between the spoken word and written language. This lack of awareness must be overcome by specific teaching focussed on the visual, tactile, and kinesthetic senses as well as impaired auditory sense. Because many of the skills basic to reading are not readily established, a skills acquisition approach emphasizing vocabulary acquisition, comprehension, and appreciation is necessary. This bottom-up approach is followed at all levels in a context that also recognizes the need to develop reading through the student's interests and to motivate the student to read.

**DESCRIPTION:** The secondary level *Reading Curriculum* discussed here was developed specifically for the 1985–86 school year but follows the design of previous curricula for this level.

The Louisiana School secondary curriculum contains two major programs, academic and combined, each of which has three strands: easy, moderate, and difficult. Each of these levels, in turn, require that a student read at a particular grade level and accomplish all objectives of a specified academic or combined program grade level (see Table 3-4). Subject areas are noted for each grade. These are the same for all strands of both the academic and combined programs except for grade 9 as follows:

Grade 9 (academic) — Short stories and poetry.

Grade 9 (combined) — Short stories.

Grade 10 — American literature.

Grade 11 — English literature

Grade 12 — World literature

General and specific target goals are set for each strand of the academic and combined programs for grades 9, 10, 11, and 12. The specific target goals break down the global skill of the general target goals into indentifiable teaching points.

A general target goal for the grade 9 academic program is to "Develop various literal comprehension reading skills." The complementary specific goal

**Table 3-4.** Relationships of Programs, Grades, Program Strands, and Strand Prerequisites in *Reading Curriculum* of the Louisiana School for the Deaf

| Program | Grade | Strand | Prerequisites | |
|---|---|---|---|---|
| | | | Reading level | Achievement level |
| Academic | 9 | Easy | Grade 5.5 | Grade 8 academic (easy) |
| | | Moderate | Grade 6.0 | Grade 8 academic (moderate) |
| | | Difficult | Grade 6.5 | Grade 8 academic (difficult) |
| Academic | 12 | Easy | Grade 7.0 | Grade 11 academic (easy) |
| | | Moderate | Grade 7.5 | Grade 11 academic (moderate) |
| | | Difficult | Grade 8.0 | Grade 11 academic (difficult) |
| Combined | 9 | Easy | Grade 3.0 | Grade 8 combined (easy) |
| | | Moderate | Grade 3.5 | Grade 8 combined (moderate) |
| | | Difficult | Grade 4.0 | Grade 8 combined (difficult) |
| Combined | 12 | Easy | Grade 4.5 | Grade 11 combined (easy) |
| | | Moderate | Grade 5.0 | Grade 11 combined (moderate) |
| | | Difficult | Grade 5.5 | Grade 11 combined (difficult) |

is "(a) find main ideas; (b) establish mood, setting, plot and characterization; (c) locate facts and details; (d) follow directions; (e) establish sequence; and (f) summarize stories."

The final entry for each year and strand of the Louisiana *Reading Curriculum* is a listing of textbooks and supplementary materials.

**EVALUATION:** The secondary school *Reading Curriculum* is concise and specific. It states clearly what the general objectives for each year will be, and follows-up with detailed specific objectives. These specific objectives will assist the teacher in determining which topics to select for lessons. This will be a boon to the beginning reading teacher.

A strong point of the approach of the Louisiana School is the meticulous determination of ability levels of students. Goals and support materials are designed to meet the needs and abilities of students and to continue the study of reading in a logical, consistent fashion.

To some degree the *Reading Curriculum* suffers from brevity. This is particularly true with reference to affective goals. Most teachers will find it easier to understand and achieve cognitively oriented goals, such as "Write book reports", than affectively oriented ones such as "Develop enjoyment of recreational reading" (both grade 9). It would be of value to have a section of the curricula in which ideas for achieving goals were noted.

## *READING MILESTONES*

### S.P. Quigley and C.M. King

*Publisher*:

Dormac Inc.
P.O. Box 1699
Beaverton, OR
97075-1699

Dominie Press Limited
1361 Huntingwood Drive, Unit 7
Agincourt, Ontario
MlS 3Jl

*Skills Taught*: Reading in general with primary attention to syntactic structures and vocabulary and secondary attention to decoding skills, comprehension skills and cognitive skills

*Age/Grade Range*: Beginning reading to approximately grade 4

*Group size*: Class groups

**THEORY:** *Reading Milestones* grew from the extensive, longitudinal research program in the area of syntactic abilities of hearing-impaired children headed by Quigley. The basic finding of this research has been that hearing-impaired children encounter exceptional difficulty understanding and manipulating syntactic structures that are well understood and manipulated by much younger normally hearing children. Reading materials based on the expectation that the reader will be able to handle syntactic structures with relative ease and be able to focus on the actual reading task involved, pose difficulties for hearing-impaired children. Additionally, it is well known that hearing-impaired children have difficulty in acquiring an adequate vocabulary pool and that other aspects of language (e.g., metaphor, idiom) are particular problem areas. As a logical and planned extension of earlier research, *Reading Milestones* was designed as a set of readers with controlled syntax and controlled vocabulary.

**PROGRAM:** *Reading Milestones* consists of eight levels, each with ten readers, ten workbooks, and a teacher's guide. Levels are color-coded.

Level 1—Red books
Level 2—Blue books
Level 3—Yellow books
Level 4—Green books
Level 5—Brown books
Level 6—Orange books
Level 7—Tan books
Level 8—Purple books

Levels do not correspond to grade levels but the authors state that by the end of level 8, the majority of students should be capable of using grade 4 readers and other materials.

Readers are fairly small booklets ($5\frac{1}{2}'' \times 8\frac{1}{2}''$). Early readers introduce one new syntactic structure (red, blue, and yellow books) and a restricted set of vocabulary. Later levels continue with these early structures, expanding and reinforcing them. Vocabulary is introduced slowly with two to three new words in each red book story working up to four to five new words per story in the yellow books. While vocabulary continues to be controlled, words are introduced more rapidly in the remaining series. An introductory section in each reader states the syntactic rule to be introduced and new vocabulary. Each new vocabulary item and an accompanying illustration and sentence is presented at the end of each reader. Illustrations are brightly colored and generally pleasing. Due to the need to control syntax and vocabulary, stories, especially in the early levels, tend to be stilted and of relatively limited intrinsic interest compared to other readers.

Workbooks are related directly to reinforcement of syntactic structures and vocabulary learned. Teachers are advised to clarify instructions. Exercises are largely self-instructional. Behavioral objectives are given in each *Teacher's Guide* and short tests are available in the workbooks. Exercises are simple and clearly presented.

One combined *Teacher's Guide* is provided for red, blue, and yellow books with individual guides for other levels. Each guide has an introductory section in which the theoretical base for the series and general plan of the series, including discussions of the various skills, are stressed throughout. Specific discussion of the level or levels involved is given with clearly presented summaries of syntactic structures and vocabulary. A useful suggested lesson format with well-detailed ideas for activities is included.

**EVALUATION:** *Reading Milestones* is not a complete curriculum and should not be treated as such.

This basal reader series is the single published series designed specifically for hearing-impaired students. It reflects contemporary research findings and selected emerging theoretical positions. The basic position of Quigley and King is that syntax and vocabulary are central elements in reading for hearing-impaired readers and must be controlled. Less concern is shown for control of semantics, aspects of comprehension such as inference, and familiarity of content. Complete lists of syntactic structures, vocabulary, idioms, and inferences found in the readers are recorded in the Teacher's Guides.

*Reading Milestones* is a valuable resource in reading. It provides a base for programs and will serve as a needed resource for teachers uncertain of how to approach reading with hearing-impaired students.

## *TEACHING READING TO DEAF CHILDREN*

**B.O. Hart**

*Publisher*:
A.G. Bell Association, Inc.
3417 Volta Pl., N.W. 1
Washington, D.C. 20007

*Skills taught*: Various aspects of reading and development of reading skills from preschool to advanced levels

*Age/grade range*: 3 to 17 years and preschool to grade 8 approximately

*Group size*: Class groups

**THEORY:** Hart (1978) defined reading as "the process of getting thought from printed symbols by associating known meanings with these symbols". She considered auditory ability and oral skills to directly support this process. The hearing-impaired child, due to both difficulty converting the printed form into the spoken form and generally slow language growth, experiences significant struggle in learning to read. Despite this acknowledged struggle, Hart considers it possible for progress in reading to be achieved.

Hart emphasized that there is no one way to teach reading; therefore, reliance on one approach is questionable. Reading is more than acquisition of a structure composed of related skills. Students must be motivated to read, reading must be based on the students' interests and experiences, and reading must be a successful activity. Beneath this general philosophy, however, is clear reliance on a bottom-up approach to reading instruction. Reading is regarded as a structure of skills that must be mastered and assembled into the act of reading.

**DESCRIPTION:** Hart adapted materials and techniques designed for normally hearing children to the reading needs of hearing-impaired children. She has not developed a unique approach for the hearing impaired, but drawn on what she considered useful in reading curricula generally to sketch out a systematic sequence of activities from preschool to grade 8 in a program designed to cover approximately 14 years of instruction.

*Teaching Reading to Deaf Children* begins with a short, but clear, statement of philosophy underlining the need to motivate the child to read through use of material related to the child's interests and experiences. This approach is similar to experience-based top-down reading curricula used with many normally hearing children. Although this is true, there is a basic conflict between the usual global emphasis of the top-down approach and the skill-based emphasis of much of Hart's work.

Four types of reading are proposed by Hart. These are:

1. Developmental-guided reading lessons focussed on basal readers, control of vocabulary, and gradual, sequential progress.
2. Functional-reading directed to the achievement of a pleasurable or informative activity, such as learning street signs or baking.
3. Recreational-self-motivated reading with minimal adult intervention.
4. Remedial-planned, directed teaching of vocabulary and language to correct reading deficiences.

Aspects of these four types of reading are discussed in Chapters 3 through 6 that outline the curricula for preschool, primary, intermediate, and advanced levels.

Preschool includes ages 3 through 6 and is considered as a prereading or readiness period. Aims and goals are stated and the importance of creating an appropriate classroom atmosphere emphasized. The preschool program is described as one of play-type activities and experiences that lead eventually to language on which to build reading. Noted as appropriate teaching topics are: (1) specific reading skills; (2) visual discrimination; (3) auditory discrimination; (4) left-right orientation; (5) hand-eye coordination; (6) interest in stories and plots; (7) sequential memory; and (8) awareness of printed language. Sample activities are offered for these and special attention given to memory, classification, generalization, visual discrimination, and hand-eye coordination.

The primary grades cover ages 6 to 9 and grades 1 and 2, and is presented as that at which the child learns to read — the level of guided reading. Areas stressed are development of (1) concepts and verbal meanings through experiences; (2) sight vocabulary; (3) word recognition techniques; (4) reading in thought groupings; (5) ability to read longer groupings; (6) beginning dictionary skills; and (7) reading comprehension. A considerable number of ideas for developing word recognition and sight vocabulary is given. Over the primary grade years, a program including developmental, recreational, and remedial reading is carefully built. Suggestions for trips, activities, projects, dramatic play, news reporting, use of audio-visual materials, *My Weekly Reader*, basal readers, workbooks, dictionaries, and teacher-made exercises in pursuit of these are listed.

General goals, specific goals, and the special problems of the intermediate level, ages 9-to-12 years, or grades 3 through 5, are outlined. It is at this level that the commonly substantial reading gains of earlier years begin to plateau. Hart suggests that to counter this plateauing effect, allow regular daily periods of approximately 45 minutes for developmental reading. Opportunities for functional and recreational reading, as well as remedial reading when appropriate, must be planned into the timetable. Again, teaching ideas for these types of reading are sketched.

The advanced level, ages 12 to 17, or grades 6 through 8, is described as a time of "mature, independent, critical reading habits" for some students. Those experiencing difficulty advancing in reading are to "be allowed to progress at their own rate." Topics discussed in this concluding chapter are: developing good work-study skills, an appreciation of literature, critical reading, and reading as a permanent interest.

**EVALUATION:** *Teaching Reading to Deaf Children* has been a valuable resource to teachers of the hearing impaired for many years. It describes a traditional approach to reading instruction and combines this with a philosophy many contemporary educators would find acceptable. It remains a valued guide for many teachers.

To a considerable extent, however, this curriculum guide is dated. It focusses on a skills acquisition approach reminiscent of the perceptual training emphasis of early work in learning disabilities. There is a definite conflict between the philosophy espoused and the basic approach to actual teaching described. The sample activities are valuable but too starkly skill-oriented without sufficient discussion as to how to blend skills into the global act of reading.

Hart recognized that some hearing-impaired learners would encounter difficulty in reading from the earliest stages. Her sections on "remedial" reading are designed for these students. As such they are valuable, although they suffer, from brevity. At the advanced level, such learners are dismissed and the discussion provided focusses on capable readers only.

Teachers will find Hart's publication a valuable resource for ideas both for teaching and curriculum development. It will not serve as a complete curriculum guide due to its traditional emphasis and a lack of recent update that includes contemporary ideas on approaching reading for the hearing-impaired population.

## REFERENCES

Alexander, J.E. (Ed.). (1979). *Teaching reading*. Boston: Little, Brown.

Armbruster, B.B., Echols, C.H., & Brown, A.L. (1982). The role of metacognition in reading to learn: A developmental perspective. *Volta Review, 84,* 45-56.

Bockmiller, P., & Coley, J. (1981). A survey of methods, materials, and teacher preparation among teachers of reading to the hearing impaired. *Reading Teacher, 34,* 526-529.

Browns, F., & Arnell, D. (1981). *A guide to the selection and use of reading instructional materials.* Washington, DC: Alexander Graham Bell Association.

Bryans, B.N. (1979). Breaking the sentence barrier in language and reading instruction. *Volta Review, 81,* 421-430.

Clarke, B.R., Rogers, W.T., & Booth, J.A. (1982). How hearing-impaired children learn to read: Theoretical and practical issues. *Volta Review, 84,* 57-69.

Clarke School for the Deaf. (1972). *Reading*. Northampton, MA: Author.

Coley, J., & Bockmiller, P. (1980). Teaching reading to the deaf: An examination of teacher preparedness and practices. *American Annals of the Deaf, 125,* 909-915.

Ewoldt, C. (1981). New techniques for research and evaluation in the reading of the deaf. In G. Propp (Ed.), *1980's Schools . . . Portals to Century 21.* Silver Spring, MD: Convention of American Instructors of the Deaf, pp. 240-246.

Fleury, P (1979). *Controlled language science series.* Beaverton, OR: Dormac.

Furth, H. (1966a). *Thinking without language.* New York: The Free Press.

Furth, H. (1966b). Research with the deaf: Implications for language and cognition. *Volta Review, 68,* 34-56.

Gibson, E.J., & Levine, H. (1979). *The psychology of reading*. Cambridge, MA: MIT Press.

Gormley, K.A. (1981). On the influence of familiarity on deaf students' text recall. *American Annals of the Deaf, 126,* 1024-1030.

Gormley, K.A. (1982). The importance of familiarity in hearing-impaired readers' comprehension of text. *Volta Review, 84,* 71-80.

Gormley, K.A., & Franzen, A.M. (1978). Why can't the deaf read? Comments on asking the wrong question. *American Annals of the Deaf, 123,* 542-547.

Gormley, K.A., & Geoffrion, L. (1981). Another view of using language experience to teach reading to deaf and hearing-impaired children. *Reading Teacher, 34,* 519-525.

Hammermeister, F.K., & Israelite, N.K. (1983a). Reading instruction for the hearing impaired: An integrated language arts approach. *Volta Review, 85,* 136-148.

Hammermeister, F.K., & Israelite, N.K. (1983b). Language and reading: Putting it all together. In F. Solano, J. Egelston-Dodd, & E. Costello (Eds.), *Focus on Infusion* (Vol. II). Silver Spring, MD: Convention of American Instructors of the Deaf, pp. 116-121.

Hart, B.O. (1978). *Teaching reading to deaf children* (2nd ed.). Washington, DC: Alexander Graham Bell Association.

Hart, N.W.M., Walker, R.F., & Gray, G. (1977). *The language of children*. Reading MA: Addison-Wesley.

Hasenstab, M.S., & McKenzie, C.D. (1981). A survey of reading programs used with hearing-impaired students. *Volta Review, 83,* 383-388.

Hirsh-Pasek, K., & Treiman, R. (1982). Recoding in silent reading: Can the deaf child translate print into a more manageable form? *Volta Review, 8,* 71-82.

King, C.M., & Quigley, S.P. (1985). *Reading and deafness.* San Diego, CA: College-Hill Press.

Kirk, S.A., Kliebhan, J.M., & Lerner, J.W. (1978). *Teaching reading to slow and disabled learners.* Boston: Houghton, Mifflin.

Kretschmer, R.R., & Kretschmer, L.W. (1978). *Language development and intervention with the hearing impaired.* Baltimore: University Park Press.

La Sasso, C. (1978). National survey of materials and procedures used to teach reading to hearing-impaired children. *American Annals of the Deaf, 123,* 22-30.

Ling, D., & Ling, A.H. (1978). *Aural habilitation.* Washington, DC: Alexander Graham Bell Association.

Louisiana School for the Deaf. (1985). *Reading curriculum.* Baton Rouge, LA: Author.

Maxwell, M. (1974). Teaching reading as a problem-solving activity. *American Annals of the Deaf, 119,* 721-723.

McCarr, D. (1973). Individualized reading for junior and senior high school students. *American Annals of the Deaf, 118,* 488-495.

McNeil, J.D., Donant, L., & Alkin, M.C. (1980). *How to teach reading successfully.* Boston: Little, Brown.

Melnyk, T.L. (1977). Teaching community awareness to hearing-impaired preschoolers. *ACEHI Journal, 3,* 99-102.

Pearson, P.D. (1982). A primer for schema theory. *Volta Review, 84,* 25-33.

Pfau, G.S. (1963-1974a). *Reading–language series* (Project LIFE). Albany, NY: Instructional Industries.

Pfau, G.S. (1963-1974b). *Pre-reading series* (Project LIFE). Albany, NY: Instructional Industries.

Pfau, G.S. (1970a). The application of programmed instruction principles to classroom instruction. *Volta Review, 72,* 340-348.

Pfau, G.S. (1970b). Reinforcement and learning—some considerations with programmed instruction. *Volta Review, 72,* 408-411.

Polloway, E.A., Payne, J.S., Patton, J.R., & Payne, R.A. (1985). *Strategies for teaching retarded and special needs learners.* Columbus, OH: Merrill.

Quigley, S.P. (1982). Reading achievement and special reading materials. *Volta Review, 84,* 95-106.

Quigley, S.P., & King, C. (1981). *Reading milestones.* Beaverton, OR: Dormac.

Quigley, S.P., & Kretschmer, R.E. (1982). *The education of deaf children.* Baltimore: University Park Press.

Quigley, S.P., Power, D., & Steinkamp, M. (1977). The language structure of deaf children. *Volta Review, 79,* 73-84.

Robbins, N.L., & Hatcher, C.W. (1981). The effects of syntax on the reading comprehension of hearing-impaired children. *Volta Review, 83,* 105-115.

Rompf, J.A. (1981). Helping the deaf community college student improve his reading skills. *American Annals of the Deaf, 126,* 825-828.

Savage, J.F., & Mooney, J.F. (1979). *Teaching reading to children with special needs.* Boston: Allyn & Bacon.

Schnepel, J.R. (1980). Experiences and an approach to teaching reading to hearing-impaired children. *Volta Review, 82,* 236-241.

Spache, G.D., & Spache, E.B. (1977). *Reading in the elementary school.* Boston: Allyn & Bacon.

Staufer, R. (1970). *The language-experience approach to the teaching of reading.* New York: Harper & Row.

Truax, R.R. (1978). Reading and language. In R.R. Kretschmer & L.W. Kretschmer (Eds.), *Language development and intervention with the hearing impaired.* Baltimore: University Park Press, pp. 279-310.

Walter, G.G. (1978). Lexical abilities of hearing and hearing-impaired children. *American Annals of the Deaf, 123,* 976-982.

Wilbur, R.B. (1977). An explanation of deaf children's difficulty with certain syntactic structures in English, *Volta Review, 79,* 85-93.

Wrightstone, J., Aronow, M., & Moskowitz, S. (1963). *Development of reading test norms for deaf children* (P.N. 22-262). New York: Bureau of Educational Research, Board of Education.

# CHAPTER 4

# *Mathematics Curricula*

Educators throughout North America would readily support the notion that the development of mathematical abilities is one of the critical elements within an individual's school career; however, there is little evidence that this philosophy has had much impact on those responsible for mathematics curricular development, program design, or pedagogical strategies specifically related to the academic needs of the hearing impaired. A review of both past and current literature in deaf education quickly substantiates this belief.

During the 1984 and 1985 period, less than 2 percent of all reported research and demonstration projects in schools and classes for the deaf in the United States and Canada were designated as mathematics proposals. Of the doctoral dissertations written on deaf education for the same geographic area during 1983 and 1984, approximately 4 percent dealt with some aspect of mathematics concept or skill development. (American Annals of the Deaf, 1985)

The July 1986 edition of the *Journal for Research in Mathematics Education* (JRME), prepared by the National Council of Teachers of Mathematics (NCTM), listed research reported in approximately 65 educational or psychological journals or publications. Of the 565 entries describing research summaries, articles, and dissertations published in 1985 in Canada and the United States, not one was specifically related to mathematics education for the hearing impaired. Despite these observations, it should not be concluded that mathematics education for the hearing impaired is totally neglected. It simply appears that mathematics research and development within deaf education does not currently enjoy a high placement on the priority lists for professional investigation or additional funding to support research. There are, in fact, a number of educators and school programs that have attempted to research and develop specialized curricula and materials designed to meet the identified needs of the hearing-impaired school populations.

For several years, the Pre College Programs division of Gallaudet College has published *Perspectives For Teachers of the Hearing Impaired*, a magazine designed to give professionals in education of hearing-impaired students a forum to share teaching strategies, announce conferences and courses, and to describe nontechnical information regarding curriculum investigations and trends. *Perspectives* has included teacher-written articles concerning specific aspects of such mathematics curricula as geometry, consumer math education, and the use of computers in mathematics programming.

Traditionally, individuals or schools for the deaf have developed *in-house* mathematics curricula for their own populations; however, these programs are generally based on the curricula developed and mandated by the local boards of education for their regular school populations, or the guidelines rely to a great extent on a particular textbook series. A survey of both past and present mathematics curricula throughout North America suggests that these are common practices (Taylor, 1986). Mathematics curricula generated by teachers specifically for use with hearing-impaired students are not extensive. In spite of this, there have been several well-researched and designed documents that will be described later in this chapter.

Unfortunately, the endeavours of the individual educator or a school's curriculum committee rarely gain much widespread attention in comparison to the research findings and program innovations presented in the speech, audition, communication mode, or language and reading areas. This is not surprising since preservice and in-service training maintains the tenet that teachers of hearing impaired are primarily language teachers and that all other subjects, including mathematics, science, and social studies, do not require the same intensive teacher training because these areas simply require adaptations or modifications of the curricula presented in the general educational milieu. Modifications usually involve controlling the vocabulary and syntax used to present the material and an increased use of manipulative and visual aids. Although these adaptations or modifications are generally applied in programs for the deaf, few hearing-impaired individuals achieve the same level of academic understanding or success as do their hearing peers. It appears as though deaf educators have undervalued the importance of research in mathematics curricula and teaching strategies required by their special populations.

A comparison of the literature and sample curricula offerings currently available to those that existed historically in schools and classes for the deaf, reveals an amazing similarity. The only obvious differences appear to be in the areas of computer-assisted instruction and a stronger focus on consumer education and life skills, especially for the less intellectually able population.

## HISTORICAL PERSPECTIVES

For the most part, mathematics curricula and activities for the hearing impaired have followed the trends established in the regular educational systems.

### Early Traditions

Until the mid 1950s both types of school programs maintained a traditional approach to mathematics. They were text-based and discouraged the use of concrete manipulatives beyond the primary grades. Math teaching strategies emphasized a group teaching orientation with large does of mental arithmetic, rote memory activities for learning, and drilling basic facts and applications of arithmetic formula and geometric theorems along with step-based problem-solving approaches. Applications of the fundamentals focussed on the perceived needs of the time: e.g., interest and tax rates, calculating acreage, and farm production. Parents and teachers were comfortable because the "basics" had not changed significantly from their own school experiences. For the hearing impaired, this type of mathematics education posed many difficulties due to the reliance on memory, the rapid transition from concrete to abstract reasoning required, and the lack of manipulative materials. It is not surprising that in schools for the deaf, elementary programs emphasized the most basic of arithmetic operations and that a high percentage of high-school-aged students were channeled into vocational training classes. Statistical data for graduating students in this time period is unavailable; however, data to the late 1960s indicates that only few hearing-impaired individuals had, on standardized achievement tests in mathematics, attained beyond a sixth grade level.

### Curriculum Reform: "New Math"

In the mid 1950s the United States began a process of complete curriculum reform in the areas of mathematics and science education. Initially this reform was prompted by the technological competition that was developing between the United States and the Soviet Union. Scientists, educators, and the general public debated the issues related to improving the quality and depth of school mathematics programs, especially at the secondary and post secondary levels. Then in 1959, the College Entrance Exam Board (CEEB) published a report, *The Commission on Mathematics*, that suggested widespread changes within secondary school mathematics programs in order to encourage a more mathematically and scientifically knowledgeable population. These proposals placed strong emphases on the reorganization and integration of traditional math topics, utilizing a more deductive developmental approach with a greater focus on patterns and relationships. New topics, such as logic, probability, statistics, and modern algebra were also to be introduced. The CEEB's report initiated considerable curriculum revision within high school settings.

At the same time, the concepts of Bruner (1962) encouraged educators to examine more closely the levels of conceptual understanding required in mathematics and science. Bruner's work provided a basis for a psychological evaluation of traditional school programs as well as support for the evolving curriculum reforms and suggestions.

Added to these developments was the 1963 Cambridge conference report of the National Council of Teachers of Mathematics, *Goals For School Mathematics, grades K–12*, which indicated a need for research and curriculum revitalization across the school's mathematics continuum from primary to secondary grades.

The *Commission on Mathematics* and *Goals For School Mathematics, Grades K–12* reports, combined with the emerging psychological and educational research findings, prompted tremendous growth in mathematical research, curriculum innovations, model programs, teacher training, and materials development. This growth was well-supported through both public and private funding. Psychological issues such as readiness for learning, intuitive versus analytical thinking, and concrete experiences versus formal operations were examined. Experimental curricula and teaching strategies based on Bruner's philosophy and Piaget's theories of cognitive development quickly appeared. For most educators, the main thrust of the mathematics curriculum reform was to reduce the amount of rote learning and to replace it with psychologically appropriate content and methodologies for mathematics learning.

By the mid 1960s, "New Math" was the focus across both the United States and Canada. Two major projects that had some influence on the mathematics programs of the hearing impaired were established.

In Ontario, the *Nuffield Mathematics Teaching Project*, originating from Great Britain, along with the work of Biggs and MacLean in *Freedom to Learn* (1969) and the Ontario Ministry of Education's *Living and Learning* report (1968), changed the focus of many of the mathematics curricula across the province at all school levels. Educators for the hearing impaired involved in adapting regular school curricula for use with this population readily saw the advantages of new math with its emphases on manipulative materials and pschologically based learning progressions. Although the initial efforts at providing more appropriate curriculum content and teaching strategies for the hearing impaired evidenced some of the same problems that the regular educational programs experienced (e.g., the teaching of number bases and strong focus on set theory), the basic tenets of the new math philosophy that promoted increased understanding of math concepts and procedures, as well as a reduction in the levels of math anxiety, was evident. By the early 1970s the Ontario programs for the hearing impaired, at least at the primary and junior levels, had developed curricula and teaching strategies derived from the mathematics reform proposals. These improved students' conceptual and skill development in more areas of mathematics than in the past. Observant teachers of the deaf quickly distinguished between the beneficial and inappropriate aspects of new math for the hearing impaired.

It is difficult to ascertain the amount of curriculum revision for the deaf experienced in other provincial programs in Canada during the 1970s. Few materials in the mathematics areas were distributed or even informally discussed. A readily accessible national forum to do so did not exist at that time.

In the United States during the 1960s a multitude of experimental new math projects appeared especially in university programs with a teacher education component. The School Mathematics Study Group (SMSG), the University of Maryland Mathematics Project (UMMaP), the University of Illinois Committee on School Mathematics (UICSM) and the Minnesota Mathematics and Science Teaching Project (MINNEMAST) became synonymous with new math. A number of teachers and schools for the deaf in the United States readily seized opportunities to adapt or modify such projects for use in their mathematics programs. A lesser-known but extremely important project during the late 1960s was the Madison Project, an experimental curriculum and development project originating from Syracuse University and Webster College. During the summers of 1969 and 1970, Gallaudet College offered Summer Math Institutes on its campus to teachers of the deaf throughout the United States and Canada. Although the instructors for these courses were not teachers of the deaf, nor were they actually involved primarily in deaf education, they were presenting curricular content and teaching strategies appropriate for the hearing impaired that had evolved from the Madison Project. It is significant that Gallaudet College chose to host such summer programs on their campus. As a participant, this author had the opportunity to discuss and evaluate the fundamental philosophy and components proposed by the summer institutes with teachers of the deaf who worked with similar populations under the same constraints. In the author's opinion, these math institutes exemplified material a sound mathematical programming for hearing-impaired students from Kindergarten through grade 12 might include. Curriculum proposals were not bound to a text or to a predetermined set of learning objectives identified with a particular age or grade level. In fact, much of what was proposed at that time is strongly supported and suggested within the context of the current cognitive psychological research findings.

It would, however, be very misleading to suggest that programs for hearing impaired adopted the new math movement on a widescale basis. Very often classes and programs simply included new types of manipulative materials, as they became available, or began to use them more extensively beyond primary grade levels. In addition, a greater effort to introduce or expand nonoperational topics was seen (e.g., graphing, three-dimensional geometry, and probability). However, the concepts underlying contemporary approaches to mathematics education throughout regular education did not permeate deeply and extensively in mathematics curricula for hearing-impaired students.

## REACTION TO THE CURRICULUM REFORMS OF 1955 TO 1975

By 1975 many parents, educators and much of the general public had become disenchanted with the perceived results of new math. They felt that 20 years of revision and innovation had done little to improve the status of mathematical literacy in the United States. Longitudinal studies of achievement levels of students indicated minimal increases in some areas and decreases in others. Colleges and universities decried the lack of conceptual understanding and low basic-skill levels of their freshmen. Business and industry claimed that students lacked basic skills and the ability to apply mathematics to different situations. Parents believed too much time was spent playing with math and insufficient time spent on mastering simple facts and algorithms. These negative views of new math were not entirely justified. Critics tend to view the entire two decades from 1955 to 1975 as the "new math movement" when, in fact, several separate developments occurred during that period. During those 20 years, many different mathematics curricular ideas and teaching strategies surfaced, receded, and were abandoned, or resurfaced and were modified. It was a period in which vast amounts of time and money were spent on research and development. Considerable debate has arisen over the success or failure of this era in mathematics history. Those who viewed the revisions and innovations as failures claim that the curricula content cascaded downwards from their intended population targets to young children who had little need for it (National Council of Teachers of Mathematics, 1975). Most of the dissatisfaction really amounted to the following:

1. There was a lack of teacher training on a widespread basis.
2. There was a lack of public understanding for both content and methods being utilized.
3. Considerable funds were invested in research and demonstration projects but far less invested at the classroom level.
4. The necessary materials were not readily available.
5. Traditional approaches and beliefs are always extremely difficult to change.

An analysis of curriculum guidelines for that period also indicates that many of the concrete experiences suggested were not tied to practical applications of the concept with resultant minimal retention or transfer of knowledge and skills. Little attention was paid to *connections* required in mathematics so that particular activities were viewed in isolation from a larger goal. For example, many curricula samples included heavy emphasis on the study of other number bases but then did little to reinforce our own decimal system. Elementary students learned how to plot and draw equations on coordinate graphs without ever learning either the relationship between those activities or the later study of algebra and geometry at the secondary level.

However, the period between 1955 and 1975 provided many positive results. Compared to the traditional approaches in mathematics, rote memory was downplayed in favor of understanding; manipulation of concrete materials extended beyond primary grades; there was a continued assessment of teaching methods and curriculum content; further research was initiated in the areas of conceptual development and cognitive growth; and the realization grew that current technology could and should be employed in the educational setting.

To a minor extent, schools for the hearing impaired were involved in this debate. In those programs, in which the teachers had consciously selected appropriate curricular items and teaching strategies from the new math period considered to aid hearing-impaired students to more fully understand abstract concepts or for the teachers to break down complex mechanical operations into visual and sequential chunks, the controversy was largely ignored.

## BACK TO BASICS OR FORWARD WITH FUNDAMENTALS? (1975– )

Since 1975, in the United States and Canada, there has been a very strong movement to return to *the basics* in mathematics programs across the educational continuum. Fortunately, this has not meant a return to the traditional math of the first half of the century. In contrast to the New Math era, which was really an attempt to increase and enrich the mathematical knowledge levels of college-bound students and was directed, in the main, by university and scientific technical mathematicians, the current trends have been more realistic. Educators in both the mainstream and in special education settings are more cognizant of what constitutes practical needs for today's students.

Because of the research and curricular concerns that evolved from the previous decades, current leaders in the field of mathematics have encouraged the development of mathematics curricula that would more closely consolidate the *understanding* of mathematical patterns and structures simultaneously with *computational competence* and *realistic applications* in problem-solving.

A major trend in general education has been towards ensuring appropriateness and accountability of school programs. In the United States (Public Law 94-142, 1975) and Canada (Nova Scotia, 1969; Saskatchewan, 1971; Manitoba, 1976; Newfoundland, 1979; Quebec, 1979; Ontario, 1985), compulsory special education legislation has had a profound effect on all branches of education especially in programs for the hearing impaired. There has been a greater impetus in defining specific learning objectives, individualized educational programming, mastery learning approaches (precision learning), and computer-assisted instruction. With reference to mathematics education for the hearing impaired, there has been an increase in the use of programmed learning materials, implemented particularly in conjunction with individualized programs. Most commonly found kits in elementary hearing-impaired classrooms are:

SRA Math Lab (Scientific Research Associates)

ADLM Math Lab (Developmental Learning Materials)

PAL Math Program (Project Life)

Key Math Teach and Practice (American Guidance Service)

Key Math Early Steps (American Guidance Service)

Oregon Math Computation (Dormac)

Veri Tech (for Versa Tiles)

Within the past decade, computer-assisted learning programs in the areas of counting, number concepts, number recognition, sequencing, computation at all levels, geometry, logic, probability, statistics, and work problems have become prominent. Many programs for the hearing impaired have developed their own instructional discs that control syntax and vocabulary without sacrificing the original intent of the curricula. By generating their own computer programs in math, teachers of the hearing impaired have solved the language problems of many of the commercially prepared materials. In order to reduce duplication of effort, many teachers have begun computer program exchanges with other schools that encourages the extra benefit of providing a sharing of curricular ideas.

A third area of concern enunciated clearly in the National Council for Teachers of Mathematics' *An Agenda For Action* (1980) was:

> The higher order mental processes of logical reasoning, information processing and decision-making should be considered basic to the application of math curricula and teachers should set as objectives the development of logical processes, concepts and language, including the identification of likenesses and differences leading to classification (and) the precise use of such language as 'at least', 'at most', 'either-or', 'both-and' and 'if-then.'

Although these concepts are agreed upon by most mathematics teachers of the hearing impaired, few curricula guidelines are outlined in such a way as to ensure that higher order mental processes are developed internally. Many programs are designed in such a way that the teacher's higher order mental processes are imposed on their students. Perhaps as students are introduced to computers at an earlier age and allowed to experiment in designing computer programs independently we might see more student-generated applications to the logic- and statistical-type problems in the higher grades.

## CONTEMPORARY CURRICULA CONCERNS

Throughout the previous descriptions of mathematics education for the hearing impaired, it was quite obvious that the curricula and teaching methodologies over the years have remained unremarkable. Concerns described in the traditional mathematics era remain with us today in spite of improved technology, higher academic expectations, and an influx of research findings in educational psychology. The following is a brief description of areas which, in my opinion, deserve priority if mathematics curriculum development and delivery of programs are to improve in the near future.

### Achievement Levels in Mathematics for the Hearing Impaired

An examination of the results of the Stanford Achievement Tests for Hearing Impaired (SAT-HI, 1986) for most students in schools for the hearing impaired indicates that mathematics levels are much higher than for any other subject area. Computation scores are commonly two or more grade levels above the reading and language levels. This pattern of achievement in mathematics is consistent with research done by Di Francesca (1971) and Trybus and Karchmer (1977). As educators we have come to expect and accept this phenomena without giving notice to the fact that these mathematics levels are still much below those of our students' hearing peers.

A closer examination of the subtests and sections in the mathematics portion of SAT-HI will generally indicate strength in areas that typically require computation. Two concerns arise from these observations (Broadbent & Daniels, 1982):

1. Mathematics curricula and classroom programs at all levels must be evaluated in terms of what constitutes a well-rounded mathematics program, outside of computation skills.
2. Recent research indicates that there are no cognitive reasons for the average hearing-impaired student to lag behind his or her hearing peers in mathematics.

Preliminary observations of SAT-HI results, completed in Ontario, Canada, for mainstream hearing-impaired students, for the period of 1984 to 1986, show a different pattern of achievement. Results indicated that this population generally achieves higher scores in the language and reading areas than in the mathematics areas, although scores on the latter tests are sometimes above those of students in schools for the deaf. Interestingly, the subtests in mathematics for mainstreamed hearing impaired showed the same pattern of greater strength in areas requiring computation than in concepts or applications, as was demonstrated by students in schools for the deaf (Ontario Provincial Schools, SAT-HI Data 1985-1986).

Because there are increasing numbers of hearing-impaired students in mainstreamed programs, the different patterns in mathematics and language-reading achievement levels deserve investigation. Initial questions should address the grade placement, support services available, curricula content, and delivery of mathematics programs for the mainstreamed hearing impaired.

## Availability and Use of Current Technology

Because our society continues to have increasing access to efficient and less expensive forms of technology, mathematics educators and those responsible for establishing educational policies have repeatedly stated that all students of every age should have the opportunities to explore the use of calculators and computers.

It is suggested that the implementation of calculators begin in elementary grades and that they should be more readily used at any grade level by students who cannot compute basic arithmetic algorithms quickly and accurately, or that they be used when the computation involved is not the primary purpose of a mathematics activity. A typical statement found in a curriculum guideline (Ontario Ministry of Education, 1985) on the use of calculators is:

> The calculator has become an integral part of our way of life. In recognition of this fact, schools should ensure that students become proficient and discerning in the use of calculators. Estimation and mental calculation should be used to verify calculator results.

If mathematics curricula for hearing-impaired students incorporated this philosophy and policy, it is my opinion that the precious time currently used for excessive drill and practice on complex computations could be better utilized on other aspects of mathematics. Secondly, hearing-impaired students might be encouraged to remain in mathematics courses for more of their secondary school programs.

With the availability of computers in school programs there has been a tendency to use them for drill and practice systems. "Mathematics students are now able to use computers and programmable calculators as problem-solving tools, as well as in student-machine interaction, at a level beyond simple drill and practice" states the National Council of Teachers of Mathematics (NCTM) (1975).

In the NCTM's *An Agenda For Action* (1980) it is stated: ". . . take full advantage of the power of computers at all grade levels.

- computers should be used in imaginative ways for exploring, discovering and developing mathematical concepts and not merely for drill and practice.
- curriculum materials that integrate the use of the computer in diverse and imaginative ways should be developed and made available."

At the elementary level in mathematics programs for hearing-impaired students, it is a rare observation to witness computers being used as advocated by the NCTM. Computers are often the tool for delivery of individualized programs which can, depending on the mathematics curricula and preferred teaching methodologies, become a valuable or wasteful use of instructional time.

### Implications of Research in Cognition

Programs for the hearing impaired, especially those which are operated by state or provincial governments, are often very insulated from the mainstream of education. Frequently there is little awareness of what research is being done or how research findings might be applied to curricula or program delivery in programs for the hearing impaired. Within the past decade there has been considerable investigation in the area of cognition, by both psychological and educational researchers, that could have a positive effect on curriculum content in mathematics and teaching strategies used to deliver it. Most researchers agree that competence in mathematics involves two main areas–computational skill and conceptual understanding. Gagné (1985) has suggested that differences in conceptual understanding for mathematics arise because individuals organize knowledge differently. This organizational system, in turn, affects what information is attended to in problems, what is then recalled, and lastly how one actually solves problems. How hearing-impaired children process information and then retrieve it from memory has been an area of interest in deaf education for many years. Within the context of cognition, specifically in concept-attainment procedures, how new mathematical concepts and skills are presented to hearing-impaired children should be a major concern. Since differences in the organization of information will exist, educators need to more carefully consider how new concepts will be introduced, the rate of processing required to encode new information, types of rehearsal strategies that the hearing-impaired child might use to encourage retention of the material, and how *learning* of the concept can be fairly assessed. This approach suggests that complex and abstract aspects of mathematics could be presented more successfully.

### A Well-Rounded Mathematics Curricula

Most contemporary mathematics curricula for the hearing impaired, from junior grades through secondary, usually include the following areas: computation, estimation, measurement, geometry, graphing, and problem-solving. For mathematics in the 1980s additional curricula areas should include computer applications and consumer math relevant to the likely experiences for the ages of the students.

Although these areas appear in the curricula, there is evidence to suggest that actual classroom programs rely heavily on the computational areas. (Daniele, 1982). If recommendations by the NCTM and by various state and provincial school authorities were enacted, the use of calculators would reduce this tendency. Secondly, since SAT-HI results and classroom observations support each other, it appears as though in-service training for teachers should become a priority and teacher preparation programs should be revised in this area.

In my opinion, many teachers feel obligated to present items that can be tested objectively. Very often, teachers of the hearing impaired rely on evaluation of answers rather than on the cognitive processes involved, because the latter are far more difficult to assess. The development of assessment instruments for curriculum evaluation of noncomputational areas is a strong need at every grade level.

## Program Delivery for Mathematics Curricula

Regardless of how well designed a mathematics curricula is, there are several factors that inhibit achievement at all grade levels. Among them are: amount of the timetable devoted to mathematics instruction, time on task, use of visual-manipulative materials, level of abstract processing required, and the appropriateness of individualized activities.

In a study by Daniele (1982) involving intermediate and junior high school mathematics classes for the deaf, a number of these concerns were clearly substantiated on the basis of 14,000 observations of 76 students from 12 different classes in specialized schools for the deaf.

1. The correlation between the observed rates of academic engagement and mathematics achievement was $r = 0.49$ ($p = .001$).
2. Independent student seatwork accounted for 65 percent of all elapsed mathematics instruction time.
3. Twenty-six percent of all elapsed time was used for unrelated work, transition, and interruption.
4. The most popular general activity was seatwork (pencil-paper), which composed 39 percent of all class time.
5. Only 18 percent of the sessions were devoted to introduction and explanation of course content.
6. Visual aids and concrete materials were only used for 3 percent of the lessons.
7. Computer use and one-on-one adult-child work each made up about 6 percent of class time.

It is apparent that such concerns must be addressed by those designing and delivering mathematics curricula. Until they receive due consideration, program delivery in this important area of education will not be as efficient or as effective as is desirable.

## SUMMARY

Mathematics as a school subject for the hearing impaired maintains a special status in comparison to all the other aspects of their academic program. Teachers do not expect their students to compute complex operations if they have not demonstrated competence with basic facts. An analytic teacher is able to reduce topics to manageable steps and develop concepts and skills in an hierarchical fashion. Mastery of most areas of the mathematics program is more easily evaluated than is speech or reading comprehension or written composition. Due to the nature of the context, remediation and enrichment in mathematics should be relatively uncomplicated. On the surface, mathematics curricula should be the one area in which adaptations and modifications of the curricula used in regular educational programs should pose fewest difficulties. However comfortable an individual feels with these notions, mathematics education for the hearing impaired must become a greater concern if these students are to develop the type of mathematical foundation they require in today's technological society.

Contemporary concerns in mathematics education involve both the curricula content and the methodology used to present it. When educators in programs for the hearing impaired recognize the need for investigation and development in all areas of mathematics our students will be able to maximize their natural potential as current research suggests that they can.

## MATHEMATICS CURRICULA IN REVIEW

*Kendall Demonstration Elementary School Mathematics* (KDES) P. Mackall, I. Dayoub, R. Frye, and K. Cocoran-Horn, K. Mann, L. Long, and A. Baldini (1982)

*Mathematics Curriculum: Basic Level* N. Addison, C. Arkley, M. Buligan, B. Lalonde, R. Lavoie, D. MacDonald, N. McKenna, V. Taylor, and N. Wren (1985)

### *KDES MATHEMATICS*

**P. Mackall, I. Dayoub, R. Frye, K. Cocoran-Horn, K. Mann, L. Long, and A. Baldini.**

*Publisher*:
Pre College Programs
MSSD Box 114P
Gallaudet College
Washington, D.C. 20002

*Skills taught*: Meaning: sets, numbers, numeration;
Computation: operations and properties;
Applications: measurement and geometry relations, statistics and graphing problem-solving.

Age/grade range: Four strands designated as preschool, primary, elementary and middle school.

Group Size: Class and individual.

**THEORY:** The *KDES Mathematics* curriculum clearly states its two interwoven philosophies in its introduction. In relation to current mathematics theory, the curriculum aims at combining "meaning and drill and practice to develop computational skills; but with an emphasis on applying those computational skills in problem-solving situations." With respect to learning theory, it incorporated the developmental stages in learning suggested by the work of Piaget, Bruner, Diennes, and Galperin. The design of the units for each grade range suggests concept attainment strategies involving a hands-on approach. Follow-up activities incorporate specific textbook pages with related commercially prepared workbooks and games. The curriculum content and activities would appear to be appropriate for class, small group, and individual instruction.

**DESCRIPTION:** The *KDES Mathematics* program covers preschool (ages 2 to 5), primary (ages 5 to 9), elementary (ages 9 to 12), and middle school (ages 12 to 15). In the introduction, each grouping is given the typical intellectual stage markers: e.g., for primary and elementary, "Instruction should focus on using manipulatives as an introduction to concepts and skills, using visual imagery to further learn these concepts, and attempting symbolic functioning." A useful aspect attached to the objectives for goal areas is a suggested instructional level, which would enable a teacher to use the curriculum flexibility. For students who have not achieved mastery of an objective designed for their age grouping, the teacher could return to a previous level for reinforcement activities. This information is conveniently located in the Scope and Sequence Chart (Table 4-1) listing of objectives as A = Awareness, L = Learning, R = Review/Recycle: applying student's "knowledge of the concept with a higher level of materials/activities.")

The actual guideline is divided into four sections, with each section listing the objectives by number, a description of the objective, vocabulary required, activities, manipulatives, and a suggested evaluation process. The "Activities" section may include specific teaching strategies, a description of written seatwork to be prepared by the teacher and references to commercially prepared workbooks, and textbook references. The "Materials" section may list text references, manipulatives, and games. The suggestions for "Evaluation" include both informal and formal types of assessment and range from a simple task such as, "Ask student what happens when you add zero to a number" to "Paper Test *HM Mathematics 4*, Test 7 Part B." (The test series, *HM Mathematics*, is consistently referred to throughout the curriculum, although the lack of these texts would not cause difficulties for a teacher using this curriculum).

The KDES curriculum offers three appendices: Appendix A lists types of coded counting materials to be used in conjunction with the activities and materials for each objective; Appendix B is a general materials list including such items as cuisenaire rods, dice, and gameboards; Appendix C provides a 1-page Profile sheet (Figure 4-1) for each of the four age range sections.

**EVALUATION:** The *KDES Mathematics* curriculum authors have produced a comprehensive guideline incorporating sound psychological and mathematical theory for hearing-impaired students. It is a locally devised curriculum that is developmentally structured but flexible, enabling a school system to use it from preschool through intermediate grade levels for a broad range of intellectually functioning students. It is ideal for Individualized Educational Programs (IEP). Although it suggests specific text references with the objectives, it does not overly rely on the use of a textbook, a common problem of locally devised curricula that have been developed in programs for the hearing impaired. In comparison to other mathematics curricula for this particular population, it is well sequenced with a great deal of variety in both activities and suggested methods of evaluation. The inclusion of evaluation procedures *with* the

Table 4-1. KDES Scope and Sequence Chart

Operations and Properties (OP)

| Ojectives | | | PS | P | E | MS |
|---|---|---|---|---|---|---|
| OP | 01 | Demonstrate the meaning of the addition sign (+) as combining sets | A | L | | |
| OP | 02 | Add whole numbers: | | | | |
| | | OP 02.01 using one-digit addends with sums to 10 | A | L | | |
| | | OP 02.02 using basic facts | | L | | |
| | | OP 02.03 using a series of one-digit addends | | L | | |
| | | OP 02.04 using two numbers without regrouping | | L | | |
| | | OP 02.05 using multiples of 10 | | L | | |
| | | OP 02.06 using two numbers with regrouping | | L | R | |
| | | OP 02.07 using a series of numbers | | L | R | |
| OP | 03 | Memorize the basic addition facts (sums to 20) | | L | | |
| OP | 04 | Apply the identity element for addition | A | L | | |
| OP | 05 | Apply the commutative property of addition | | L | R | |
| OP | 06 | Apply the associative property of addition | | L | R | |
| OP | 07 | Demonstrate the meaning of the subtraction sign (−) as a removal of members of a set. | A | L | | |
| OP | 08 | Subtract whole numbers: | | | | |
| | | OP 08.01 using one-digit numbers. | A | L | | |
| | | OP 08.02 using basic facts. | | L | | |
| | | OP 08.03 using two numbers without regrouping. | | L | | |
| | | OP 08.04 using multiples of 10. | | L | | |
| | | OP 08.05 using two numbers with regrouping. | | L | R | |
| OP | 09 | Memorize the basic subtraction facts (sums to 20) | | L | | |
| OP | 10 | Apply the identity element for subtraction | A | L | | |
| OP | 11 | Demonstrate that addition and subtraction are inverse operations: | | | | |
| | | OP 11.01 by finding a missing minuend using addition | | L | R | |
| | | OP 11.02 by finding a missing addend using subtraction | | L | R | |
| | | OP 11.03 by using the inverse operation to check addition and subtraction computations | | L | R | |

| | | | |
|---|---|---|---|
| OP 12 | Demonstrate the meaning of the multiplication signs (×, •): | | |
| | OP 12.01 as repeated addition | L | |
| | OP 12.02 as forming arrays of objects in rows and columns | L | |
| | OP 12.03 as combining equivalent sets | L | |
| OP 13 | Multiply two whole numbers: | | |
| | OP 13.01 using basic facts | L | |
| | OP 13.02 using a one-digit multiplier and no regrouping | L | |
| | OP 13.03 using a one-digit multiplier and regrouping | L | R |
| | OP 13.04 using a two-digit multiplier | | L |
| | OP 13.05 using a multiple of 10 | | L |
| | OP 13.06 using a three-digit multiplier | | L |
| OP 14 | Memorize the multiplication facts | L | |
| OP 15 | Apply the commutative property of multiplication | L | R |
| OP 16 | Apply the associative property of multiplication | L | R |
| OP 17 | Apply the distributive property of multiplication over addition | | L |
| OP 18 | Demonstrate the meaning of the division signs (÷, $\sqrt{\ }$): | | |
| | OP 18.01 as repeated subtraction | L | |
| | OP 18.02 as separating a set into equivalent sets | L | |
| | OP 18.03 as separating a set into a given number of subsets | L | |
| OP 19 | Divide two whole numbers: | | |
| | OP 19.01 using basic facts | L | |
| | OP 19.02 using basic fact with remainders | L | |
| | OP 19.03 using a one-digit divisor | L | R |
| | OP 19.04 using a multiple of 10 | | L |
| | OP 19.05 using a two-digit divisor | | L |
| | OP 19.06 using a three-digit divisor | | L |
| OP 20 | Memorize the basic division facts | L | |
| OP 21 | Demonstrate that multiplication and division are inverse operations: | | |
| | OP 21.01 by finding a missing factor using division | L | R |
| | OP 21.02 by finding a missing dividend using multiplication | L | R |
| | OP 21.03 by using the inverse operation to check multiplication and division computations | L | R |

Kendall Demonstration Elementary School (1982), pp. 79-119, 255-261. Reprinted with permission.

Student ______________________________

Elementary Level

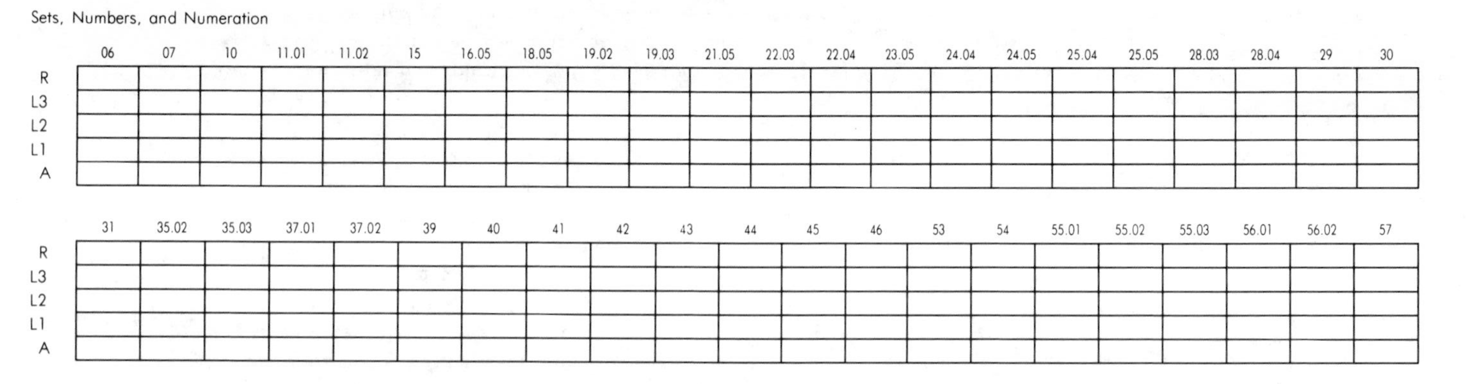

Sets, Numbers, and Numeration

| | 06 | 07 | 10 | 11.01 | 11.02 | 15 | 16.05 | 18.05 | 19.02 | 19.03 | 21.05 | 22.03 | 22.04 | 23.05 | 24.04 | 24.05 | 25.04 | 25.05 | 28.03 | 28.04 | 29 | 30 |
|---|---|---|---|---|---|---|---|---|---|---|---|---|---|---|---|---|---|---|---|---|---|---|
| R | | | | | | | | | | | | | | | | | | | | | | |
| L3 | | | | | | | | | | | | | | | | | | | | | | |
| L2 | | | | | | | | | | | | | | | | | | | | | | |
| L1 | | | | | | | | | | | | | | | | | | | | | | |
| A | | | | | | | | | | | | | | | | | | | | | | |

| | 31 | 35.02 | 35.03 | 37.01 | 37.02 | 39 | 40 | 41 | 42 | 43 | 44 | 45 | 46 | 53 | 54 | 55.01 | 55.02 | 55.03 | 56.01 | 56.02 | 57 |
|---|---|---|---|---|---|---|---|---|---|---|---|---|---|---|---|---|---|---|---|---|---|
| R | | | | | | | | | | | | | | | | | | | | | |
| L3 | | | | | | | | | | | | | | | | | | | | | |
| L2 | | | | | | | | | | | | | | | | | | | | | |
| L1 | | | | | | | | | | | | | | | | | | | | | |
| A | | | | | | | | | | | | | | | | | | | | | |

Operations and Properties

| | 13.04 | 13.05 | 13.06 | 17 | 19.04 | 19.05 | 19.06 | 22 | 24 | 25 | 26 | 27 | 28 | 29 | 30 | 32.01 | 32.02 | 32.03 | 32.04 | 32.05 | 32.06 | 32.07 | 32.08 | 32.09 | 32.10 | 33.01 | 33.02 | 33.03 | 33.04 |
|---|---|---|---|---|---|---|---|---|---|---|---|---|---|---|---|---|---|---|---|---|---|---|---|---|---|---|---|---|---|
| R | | | | | | | | | | | | | | | | | | | | | | | | | | | | | |
| L3 | | | | | | | | | | | | | | | | | | | | | | | | | | | | | |
| L2 | | | | | | | | | | | | | | | | | | | | | | | | | | | | | |
| L1 | | | | | | | | | | | | | | | | | | | | | | | | | | | | | |
| A | | | | | | | | | | | | | | | | | | | | | | | | | | | | | |

| | 33.05 | 33.06 | 33.07 | 33.08 | 33.09 | 34.01 | 34.02 | 34.03 | 34.04 | 34.05 | 34.06 | 34.07 | 34.08 | 34.09 | 35.01 | 35.02 | 35.03 | 35.04 | 35.05 | 35.06 | 35.07 | 35.08 | 36 | 37.03 | 37.04 | 37.05 | 38.03 | 38.04 |
|---|---|---|---|---|---|---|---|---|---|---|---|---|---|---|---|---|---|---|---|---|---|---|---|---|---|---|---|---|
| R | | | | | | | | | | | | | | | | | | | | | | | | | | | | |
| L3 | | | | | | | | | | | | | | | | | | | | | | | | | | | | |
| L2 | | | | | | | | | | | | | | | | | | | | | | | | | | | | |
| L1 | | | | | | | | | | | | | | | | | | | | | | | | | | | | |
| A | | | | | | | | | | | | | | | | | | | | | | | | | | | | |

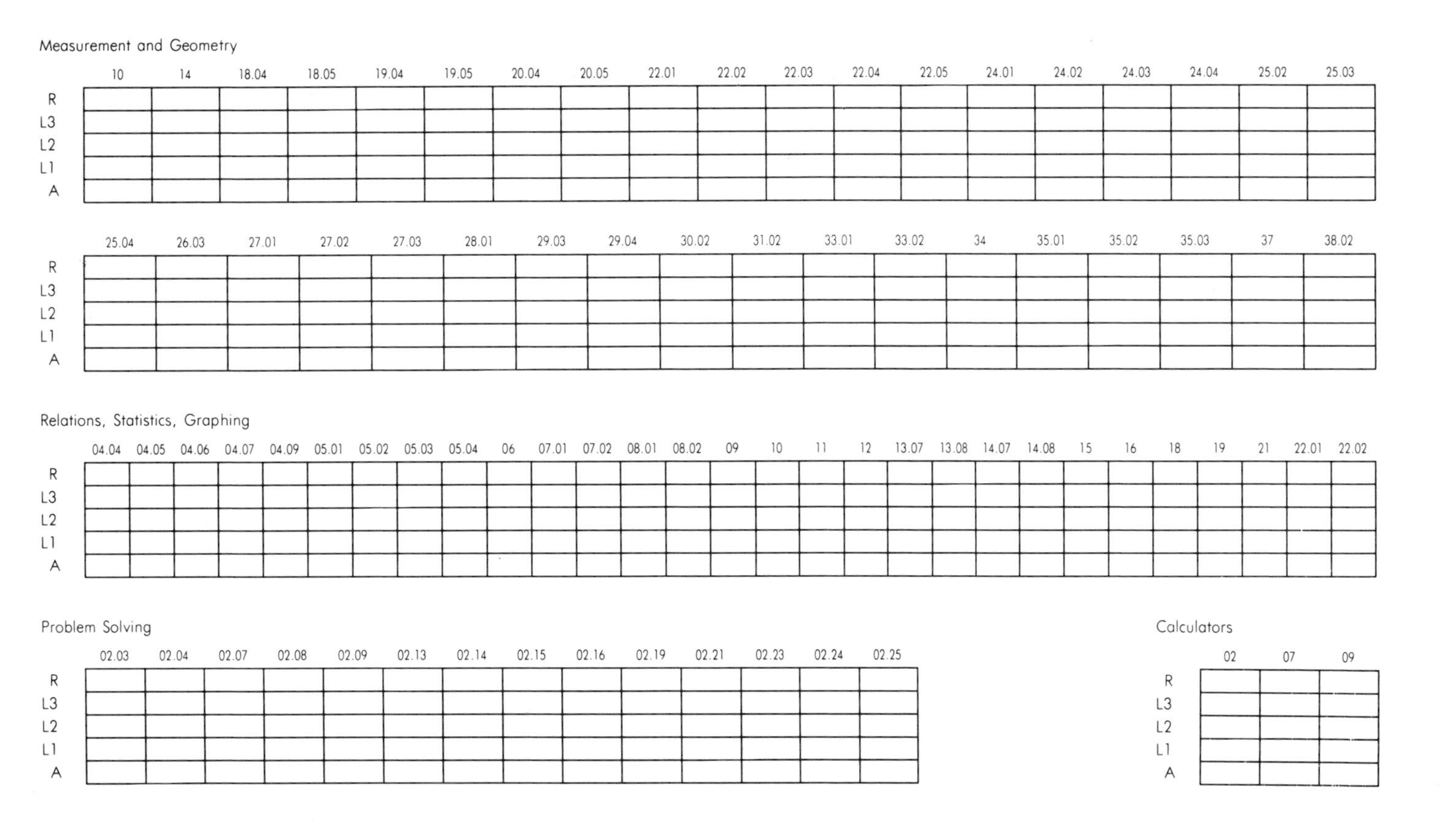

Measurement and Geometry

| | 10 | 14 | 18.04 | 18.05 | 19.04 | 19.05 | 20.04 | 20.05 | 22.01 | 22.02 | 22.03 | 22.04 | 22.05 | 24.01 | 24.02 | 24.03 | 24.04 | 25.02 | 25.03 |
|---|---|---|---|---|---|---|---|---|---|---|---|---|---|---|---|---|---|---|---|
| R | | | | | | | | | | | | | | | | | | | |
| L3 | | | | | | | | | | | | | | | | | | | |
| L2 | | | | | | | | | | | | | | | | | | | |
| L1 | | | | | | | | | | | | | | | | | | | |
| A | | | | | | | | | | | | | | | | | | | |

| | 25.04 | 26.03 | 27.01 | 27.02 | 27.03 | 28.01 | 29.03 | 29.04 | 30.02 | 31.02 | 33.01 | 33.02 | 34 | 35.01 | 35.02 | 35.03 | 37 | 38.02 |
|---|---|---|---|---|---|---|---|---|---|---|---|---|---|---|---|---|---|---|
| R | | | | | | | | | | | | | | | | | | |
| L3 | | | | | | | | | | | | | | | | | | |
| L2 | | | | | | | | | | | | | | | | | | |
| L1 | | | | | | | | | | | | | | | | | | |
| A | | | | | | | | | | | | | | | | | | |

Relations, Statistics, Graphing

| | 04.04 | 04.05 | 04.06 | 04.07 | 04.09 | 05.01 | 05.02 | 05.03 | 05.04 | 06 | 07.01 | 07.02 | 08.01 | 08.02 | 09 | 10 | 11 | 12 | 13.07 | 13.08 | 14.07 | 14.08 | 15 | 16 | 18 | 19 | 21 | 22.01 | 22.02 |
|---|---|---|---|---|---|---|---|---|---|---|---|---|---|---|---|---|---|---|---|---|---|---|---|---|---|---|---|---|---|
| R | | | | | | | | | | | | | | | | | | | | | | | | | | | | | |
| L3 | | | | | | | | | | | | | | | | | | | | | | | | | | | | | |
| L2 | | | | | | | | | | | | | | | | | | | | | | | | | | | | | |
| L1 | | | | | | | | | | | | | | | | | | | | | | | | | | | | | |
| A | | | | | | | | | | | | | | | | | | | | | | | | | | | | | |

Problem Solving

| | 02.03 | 02.04 | 02.07 | 02.08 | 02.09 | 02.13 | 02.14 | 02.15 | 02.16 | 02.19 | 02.21 | 02.23 | 02.24 | 02.25 |
|---|---|---|---|---|---|---|---|---|---|---|---|---|---|---|
| R | | | | | | | | | | | | | | |
| L3 | | | | | | | | | | | | | | |
| L2 | | | | | | | | | | | | | | |
| L1 | | | | | | | | | | | | | | |
| A | | | | | | | | | | | | | | |

Calculators

| | 02 | 07 | 09 |
|---|---|---|---|
| R | | | |
| L3 | | | |
| L2 | | | |
| L1 | | | |
| A | | | |

**Figure 4-1.** KDES Pupil Profile Summary Sheet. Reprinted with permission of Kendall Demonstration Elementary School (1982).

objective is unusual, but much needed, and emphasizes the use of alternative assessment strategies.

The *KDES Mathematics* curricula goes beyond the realm of most curricula because it encompasses an entire mathematics educational approach, not just a listing of content to be presented. The KDES curriculum is well-presented with cross referencing, color and number coding for the content, and related Scope and Sequence Charts and Pupil Profile Sheets. It is an excellent example of what a locally devised curriculum for hearing-impaired students could be if a curriculum committee were given access to expert advice, time to develop, field test and revise their efforts, and funding to support such a long term project.

## *MATHEMATICS CURRICULUM: BASIC LEVEL*

**N. Addison, C. Arkley, M Buligan, B. Lalonde, R. Lavoie, D. MacDonald, N. McKenna, V. Taylor, and N. Wren**

*Publisher:*
Ontario Provincial Schools for the Blind and Deaf
Mathematics Curriculum Development Committee
Ontario Ministry of Education, Provincial Schools Branch.

*Skills taught*: Basic mathematics skills essential to daily living: problem solving; sets, numerals, ordinals, place value; computation; measurement, fractions; decimals and percent; geometry.

*Age/grade range*: Grades 6 to 12 (limited intellectual ability).
*Group size*: Small group or individual instruction.

**THEORY:** The committee involved in the formulation of this curriculum chose to design a nongraded, developmentally sequenced program that would provide mathematics skills necessary for daily living. Effort was made to correlate curricula objectives to related life skills and vocational skills. The curriculum favors a concrete manipulative position focussing on meaningful related problems with an emphasis on the use of calculators to reduce disproportionate amounts of computation drill.

**DESCRIPTION:** The committee developed this curriculum with the view that classroom teachers or tutors unspecialized in the area of mathematics often have difficulty obtaining or choosing appropriate goals and relevant materials for students who have not grasped basic mathematics concepts or skills by age 12. Although the suggested objectives and activities are generally written with the young adolescents and low-functioning senior-grade students in mind, much of the curriculum would be appropriate for special education groups of all ages. The curriculum is composed of five sections: (1) Introduction; (2) a Scope and Sequence Chart; (3) Sequential Objectives; (4) Activities (coded to each objective); and (5) Appendices of suggested activities, references, and commercially prepared games.

A key feature of the Ontario Provincial Schools curriculum is its coordination of objectives and activities. The Scope and Sequence Chart (Fig. 4-2) has been divided into five developmental levels, with each level specifying the appropriate objectives for each of 14 skills areas. For example, in Level 1 on the Scope and Sequence Chart, students should master objectives 1 through 14 in addition.

The student will:

1. Perform addition facts to 5
2. Use the following symbols correctly; + and =
3. Find sums to 5 in vertical format
4. Find sums to 5 in horizontal format
5. Find sums to 5 with one addend being an empty set or zero
6. Find sums from 6 to 10
7. Find sums to 10 in vertical format
8. Find sums to 10 in horizontal format
9. Find sums to 10 with one addend being an empty set or zero
10. Add 3 numerals to produce a sum less than 10
11. Find sums to 20
12. Find sums to 20 in a vertical format
13. Find sums to 20 in a horizontal format
14. Find sums to 20 with one addend being an empty set or zero

A Skills Mastery Sheet, to be duplicated for each student and maintained in his record file, accompanies the Scope and Sequence Chart.

In the Activity Section of this curriculum, each activity is coded to a specific objective and very often a range of activities is described to appeal to the various ages and interests of the targeted population. The authors have borrowed heavily from activities developed for the *Kendall Demonstration Elementary School Mathematics Curriculum* (1982) but have also included activities, suggestions from teachers across the province, adaptations of activities from various journals and ideas gained at math conferences and workshops.

| | Level I | Level II | Level III | Level IV | Level V |
|---|---|---|---|---|---|
| Problem Solving | 1-10 | 1-12 | 1-18 | 1-23 | 1-29 |
| Sets | 1-16 | 0 | 0 | 0 | 0 |
| Numerals | 1-5 | 6-25 | 26-42 | 43-61 | 0 |
| Place Value | 1-5 | 6-11 | 12-21 | 22-26 | 0 |
| Ordinals | 1-3 | 4-7 | 0 | 0 | 0 |
| Addition | 1-14 | 15-16 | 17-24 | 0 | 0 |
| Subtraction | 1-4 | 5 | 6-8 | 9-13 | 0 |
| Multiplication | 0 | 1-2 | 3-8 | 9-18 | 0 |
| Division | 0 | 1-6 | 6-9 | 10-16 | 0 |
| Time | 1-12 | 13-24 | 0 | 25-30 | 0 |
| Length | 1-2 | 0 | 3-6 | 7-8 | 0 |
| Capacity | 1-2 | 0 | 3-4 | 5-6 | 0 |
| Mass | 1-2 | 0 | 3-5 | 6-7 | 0 |
| Temperature | 1-2 | 0 | 3-4 | 5-7 | 0 |
| Money | 1-2 | 3-6 | 7-13 | 14-16 | 16-38 |
| Fractions | 1-3 | 4.5 | 6-9 | 10-13 | 0 |
| Decimals and Percent | 0 | 0 | 1-7 | 8-9 | 10-11 |
| Geometry | 1-6 | 7-16 | 17-20 | 21-26 | 0 |

**Figure 4-2.** Scope and Sequence Chart. From Addison et al. (1985). Reprinted by permission.

**EVALUATION:** The Ontario Provincial Schools Branch has produced a comprehensive mathematics curriculum that would enable the most apprehensive teacher to present a viable program to a difficult population of hearing-impaired students. It is designed to ensure concept development in graduated steps with an avoidance of the usual computation-type follow-up activities. From this standpoint, it is excellent for use in developing Individualized Educational Plans (IEPs). Because of the design, students may enter the program at any grade level and continue at their own academic pace, or "graduate" from this program to a more difficult mathematics course. It would be especially useful for students entering from other school programs who require tutorials in specific areas of the mathematics curriculum. Students who successfully complete the program are eligible for a mathematics credit towards their secondary school diploma in Ontario.

Especially valuable is the variety of activities to be done in the context of games, individual or class projects, and the correlation to industrial arts, cooking, and sewing content.

Initial reading of the curriculum and an analysis of the specific objectives suggest that the content falls below that of a grade-3 mathematics textbook; however, this is indicative of needs of the target population. An uninformed parent might be disturbed by its reality.

Appropriate placement of a student in this type of developmentally sequenced program necessitates accurate evaluation of needs and achievements. Pretest and post-test instruments are essential. Information in this area is lacking but is in preparation.

From a cosmetic and user-friendly point of view, this curriculum could be improved with color-coded paper so that matching objectives and activity sections could be more easily accomplished.

Although a well-trained mathematics teacher might question the need for such an emphasis on activities, this curriculum should impress on every teacher that follow-up activities do not always need to be taken from texts or be uninteresting drill sheets.

## REFERENCES

Biggs, E.E., and MacLean, J.R. (1969). *Freedom to learn*. Canada: Addison Wesley Ltd.

Briars, D.J. (1983). An information-processing analysis of mathematical ability. In R.F. Dillon and R.R. Schmeck (Eds.), *Individual differences in cognition* (Volume 1). New York and London: Academic Press.

Broadbent, F., and Daniele, V. (1982). A review of research on mathematics and deafness. *Directions 1982* (pp. 1, 27-36). Washington, D.C.: Gallaudet College.

Bruner, J. (1962). *The process of education*. Cambridge, MA: Harvard University Press.

College Entrance Exam Board. (1959). *Commission on mathematics*. New York, NY: Program for College Preparatory Mathematics. Author.

Daniele, V.A. (1982). *A naturalistic study of Intermediate and junior high school level mathematics classes in schools for the deaf, with emphasis on time-on-task*. (Unpublished dissertation). Syracuse, NY: Syracuse University.

Di Francesca, S. (1971). *Academic achievement test results of a national testing program for hearing-impaired students, United States: Spring 1971*. Washington, D.C.: Gallaudet College.

Addison, N., Arkley, C., Buligan, M., Lalonde, B., Lavoie, R., MacDonald, D., McKenna, N., Taylor, V., and Wren, N. (1985). *Mathematics curriculum: Basic Level*. Ontario Ministry of Education. Toronto, Ont: Provincial Schools Branch.

Gagné, E. (1985). *The cognitive psychology of school learning*. Boston and Toronto: Little, Brown and Co.

MacKall, P., Dayoub, I., Frye, R., Cocoran-Horn, K., Mann, K., Long, L., and Baldini, A. (1982). *Kendall Demonstration Elementary School mathematics* (KDES). Washington, DC: Pre College Programs, Gallaudet College.

National Council of Teachers of Mathematics. (1963). *Goals for school mathematics: Cambridge Conference Report*. Reston, VA: Author.

National Council of Teachers of Mathematics. (1975). *Overview and analysis of school mathematics*. Reston, VA: Author.

National Council of Teachers of Mathematics. (1980). *An agenda for action: Recommendation for school mathematics of the 1980s*. Reston, VA: Author.

National Council of Teachers of Mathematics. (1986). *Journal for research in mathematics education*. Reston, VA: Author.

National Council of Teachers of Mathematics. (1975). *Overview and analysis of school mathematics grades K-12*. Reston, VA: Author.

Ontario Ministry of Education. (1968). *Living and learning*. Ontario, Canada: Author.

Ontario Ministry of Education. (1985). *Mathematics: Intermediate and senior divisions*. Ontario, Canada: Author.

Ontario Provincial Schools. (1985-86). *Stanford achievement tests for hearing impaired (SAT-HI), Ontario school board programs, Assessment scores for hearing-impaired students in programs supervised by Ontario school boards*. Toronto, Ont: Unpublished raw data. Author.

Pre College Programs, Gallaudet College. (1982). *KDES Mathematics*. Washington D.C.: Gallaudet College.

Taylor, V. (1986). *A review of mathematics curricula for hearing-impaired students*. Unpublished manuscript.

Trybus, R., and Karchmer, M. (1977). School achievement scores of hearing-impaired children: National data on achievement status and growth patterns. *American Annals of the Deaf 1977, 122,* (pp. 66-69).

## FOR FURTHER READING

Clarke School for the Deaf. (1970). *Mathematics curriculum.* Northampton, MA: Author.

Daniele, V.A. (1983). *Teaching arithmetic and mathematics to the hearing impaired: Priorities and basic skills for 1983 and beyond.* Paper presented at the 1983 North American Convention on the Education of the Hearing Impaired, Winnipeg, Manitoba.

Heddens, J.W. (1964). *Today's mathematics: A guide to concepts and methods in elementary school mathematics.* Chicago, IL: Science Research Associates.

Jensema, C. (1975). *The relationship between academic achievement and the demographic characteristics of hearing-impaired children and youth.* Series R, No. 2. Washington, DC: Office of Demographic Studies, Gallaudet College.

O'Neill, V. (1961). *Teaching arithmetic to deaf children.* Washington, DC: Alexander Graham Bell Association.

# CHAPTER 5

# *Science Curricula*

Science education has received scant attention over the years from educators of the hearing impaired. Surprisingly few articles and even fewer substantial works have been published in this area. The number of publications in the past quarter century dealing directly and extensively with science curricula may be counted on the fingers of two hands. This is not to say that science as a subject has been totally ignored in programs for the hearing impaired. However, science and the design of appropriate curricula have received little emphasis in programs that focus on language development and the basic task of establishing 2-way communication.

Within education as a whole the 1960s and the 1970s were a period of emphasis on science education. Sputnik was a major motivator for the creation of science curricula that would enable individuals and nations to better meet the needs of the space age. As Hedges (1968) noted, "The effect of science on contemporary life is becoming greater and more complex, and in its wake is raising new scientific, moral and theological problems." To meet these freshly perceived needs, a major switch from content-oriented science curricula to process-oriented curricula was considered necessary. In the United States the result has been major curricular publications, such as the *Science Curriculum Improvement Study* (ESS) and *Science—A Process Approach* (SAPA). These new curricula "placed emphasis on the process of science as inquiry and on an understanding of the broad framework of the respective branches of science, rather than on specific bodies of content. The facts of science are treated as outcomes of experimentation and discovery, rather than the basic ingredients of the learning experience."

An analogous major change has not permeated science education for the hearing impaired. Lang and Propp (1982) are among the few professionals concerned with substantial improvement in this area of the broad curriculum. They noted that "the dearth of literature in teaching science to hearing-impaired students at all levels of education may be indicative of the state-of-the-art of science teaching in contemporary school programs." Sunal (1984) lamented the lack of science curricula and support materials available for hearing-impaired students of all ages in both residential and mainstreamed environments. In his view many teachers consider science too difficult a subject for the hearing impaired. They cannot conceive of methods to effectively teach the concepts and material of science to this population.

Curricula for the hearing impaired have been developed, however; some of these are adaptations of curricula for normally hearing children and others are the result of extensive experience in dealing with hearing impairment and application of contemporary curricular approaches to the design of science programs specifically for the hearing impaired. Other individuals have studied the state-of-the-art in science education for the hearing impaired, contributed valuable insights on science, or suggested specific techniques for teaching science effectively. Battaglia, Scouten, and Hamil (1982) are among those who have no doubt as to the ability of hearing-impaired students to learn scientific concepts effectively. They stated "It is clear that hearing-impaired students can be successful science students when given all the necessary tools and some competent instruction."

## ADAPTED CURRICULA

A number of educators of the hearing impaired consider the approach of choice to be adaptation of existing curricula for normally hearing children. In their view the process of teaching children to think scientifically is the same whether a child is able to hear well or not. Contemporary curricula, with their focus on thinking skills and broad generalizations, as opposed to memorization, offer benefits to all children. This view fits in well with that of Hedges (1968) who defined science as, "a way of thinking and solving problems; it is the way in which discoveries are made, rather than the concepts discovered." This definition applies to all in the field of science, hearing impaired or not.

An added advantage is that contemporary process-oriented curricula were devised by experts in the field with more time and resources at their command than are normally available to those in programs for the hearing impaired. In the view of those supporting the adaptation model, the development of broadly conceptualized curricula with appropriate attention to national needs and movements yields more effective and efficient results than locally devised curricula. Sunal (1984) summed up the rationale for the adaptive approach in stating that the development of new programs requires considerable expenditure of time and money, whereas adapting existing programs allows the funneling of available resources into work on improving the chosen program to meet the specific requirements of hearing-impaired students. In Sunal's (1984) consideration, educators have the best of both worlds in opting for the adaptive approach.

Sunal and Sunal (1981a, 1981b, 1981c) have been among the major proponents of the adaptive approach. It is worthwhile to review the basic aspects of their model for the adaptation of science curricula. Fundamental to the approach used by Sunal and Sunal is the necessity of establishing general goals for a science program prior to selecting the program to be adapted (Sunal, 1984). The general goals for any adaptation should be the following:

1. Placing value on science
2. Encouraging the development of skills, interest and attitudes, including cognitive and language development
3. Making science an integral part of a student's life.

Furthermore any program considered for adaptation should demonstrate certain characteristics. Primary among these is that the goals of the selected program be appropriate for the hearing-impaired students who are to be taught. Any adaptation of the program should increase the probability that the curriculum will result in effective learning. This is an especially fundamental point given the wide range of functioning found among hearing-impaired students in any program. A second characteristic is that program goals are those that foster the hierarchical acquisition of skills. Sunal (1984) outlined these skills as observing-describing, investigating-manipulating, organizing-qualifying and generalizing-applying. In addition, any curriculum should focus on major conceptual themes, with each theme integrating the hierarchy of skills in a problem-solving manner. Sunal recommended the themes proposed by the Committee on Curriculum Studies of the National Science Teachers Association.

1. Structural patterns exist in all matter.
2. Order occurs in time and space.
3. Change and interaction are universal.
4. Living objects change and interact.

Once program goals are established, an instructional plan must be determined. Sunal specified a three-part sequence including introductory exploratory activities, a development phase for concretely based teaching of concepts, and a final double phase comprised of practical application by students and evaluation by the instructor.

In Sunal's analysis (1984) this three-part approach would lessen the problems hearing-impaired students experience in reading a regular text, and render learning more effective. He cautioned that the work and concepts presented not be at a level above the students' stage of development as judged by problem-solving abilities. Sunal also warned of six problem areas commonly found in traditional curricula. Any adaptation must deal with these areas, but, fortunately, he also suggested strategies that he considers effective in dealing with the problems. Any strategy may be used in more than one of the identified problem areas.

| *Problems* | *Strategies* |
|---|---|
| 1. Emphasis on facts and memorization versus skills and science processes | — Reorganization of material and effectiveness testing with students |
| 2. Activity with known results versus discovery and activity with unknown results | — Paraphrasing of language and activities |
| 3. Amount of independent reading versus active participation in meaningful activities | — Isolation of key words and phonics in a listing for each lesson |
| 4. Appropriate materials (for hearing-impaired students) | — Development of identification (name) tags and of language cards (individual cards bearing pertinent questions) |
| 5. Difficult terminology | — Development of enrichment activities |
| 6. Advanced level concepts | |

Considerable space has been devoted to the views of Sunal and Sunal for two reasons. One is that their appreciation of the difficulties involved in teaching science to hearing-impaired children is wide-ranging and penetrating. They present a cohesive, comprehensive overview of the adaptive approach. The second reason is quite pragmatic: No other individuals have contributed so widely to this topic in the recent past. The contributions of the Sunals and their colleagues form the most comprehensive body of contemporary work on the adaptation of existing science curricula for the hearing impaired (Sunal, 1984; Sunal & Burch, 1982; Sunal & Sunal, 1981a, 1981b, 1982). As such they are mandatory reading for those interested in the adaptive process.

Others have written either on very broad aspects of adapting curricula for the hearing impaired or on quite narrow topics focussing on one aspect of adaptation. Fitzgerald (1968), for instance, stressed the value of the behavioral objective model that she considered well-suited to contemporary problem-solving process-oriented curricula. DeWalt (1968) also encouraged the use of adapted approaches: She proposed a teaching model based on a resource teacher who develops science concepts in appropriate fashion for the instruction of hearing-impaired children. The classroom teacher provides backup language and communication method support. DeWalt went on to sketch certain adaptations. These include stress on the language problems of hearing-impaired children, with suggestions on how to compensate for the effect of these problems, and the gradual building-up of the scientific problem method from a simplified form in early grades to a more complex form in late elementary and early high school grades.

Battaglia and colleagues (1982) also discussed adaptations of the laboratory method. They stated that appropriate use of the laboratory report is uncommon in programs for the hearing impaired due to lack of instruction in the correct method of preparing laboratory reports. Their adaptations are based on the position that "a science teacher needs to help hearing-impaired subjects internalize facts and procedures, develop problem solving skills, sharpen laboratory skills, and acquire sufficient language competence to write laboratory reports that are acceptable in real work situations." They suggested that, at present, teachers use one of three basic, and basically flawed, strategies for instruction in laboratory procedures:

1. Demonstration by the teacher followed by imitation by students
2. Simplification and rewriting of language and vocabulary by the teacher followed by student reading and performance
3. Provision of unadapted manuals for students to struggle through

Battaglia and colleagues argued that the first method will not result in internalization of the procedure, the second will not prepare students for real work situations, and the third will result in frustration. They proposed an adaptation founded on the position that every teacher of science is also a teacher of language. Their adaptation incorporated suggestions put forward by Scouten (1979) in his presentation of an instructional model for the language needs of a laboratory report.

The method involves prereading of a particular experiment in a laboratory manual followed by the building-up of a "personalized plan of the work derived from the text." The personalized plan of work is developed by overhead-presented teacher questions such as, "What will you do first?" and written student responses such as, "I will heat the test tube in a hot water bath." Procedural steps are dealt with singly and in order. Technical language is dealt with as necessary. The student then performs the experiment following the plan. Four steps alter the personalized plan to acceptable laboratory report form. Given the sentence "I will heat the test tube in a bath of hot water," the steps would be:

1. Delete the subject "I," which is never used in laboratory reports.
2. Place the object, "the test tube," at the beginning of the sentence. It then becomes the subject: *The test tube*

3. Change the future-tense verb "will heat" to the past passive "was heated": The test tube *was heated.*
4. Add the adverbial phrase *"in a hot water bath"*: The test tube was heated *in a hot water bath.*

Use of the foregoing system with National Technical Institute for the Deaf biology students in 1979 and 1980 was evaluated for effectiveness through responses to an attitudinal questionnaire. Results indicated increased confidence, immediate improvement in report language, a positive change in the quality of student in-class questions, increased work in less time, and heightened independence in the laboratory.

A somewhat unusual use of an adapted curriculum is described by Grant, Rosenstein, and Knight (1973, 1975). These authors used a life science curriculum, *Me Now,* designed for educable mentally handicapped students with six Model Secondary School for the Deaf (MSSD) students. These students, aged 16 years and 7 months to 19 years and 8 months had restricted language and science skills as judged by Stanford Achievement Test (SAT) scores. The *Me Now* materials were considered worthy of use in a feasibility study given their low verbal content, high hands-on character, and high interest level. The materials were not adapted in any fashion. A four-month study was conducted. Although six students do not form an appreciable group, results were favorable. Substantial cognitive gains were noted, information retention was apparent, and positive affective change was found.

The positive aspects of adapted already-existing science curricula were discussed earlier. Although these values are undeniable, some authorities also see limitations. These are noted in point form as follows:

1. Curricula designed for regular classrooms do not meet the needs of all groups of hearing-impaired students (Clarke School for the Deaf, 1975; Hedges, 1968).
2. Curricula require extensive rewriting especially for younger hearing-impaired students. This rewriting may result in over-simplification of both process and content.
3. Many contemporary curricula continue to be to content oriented (Hedges, 1968; Lang & Propp, 1982).
4. It is not enough to consider curricula alone. Subject matter, teaching facilities, classroom design, class schedules, teaching assignments, and teaching load are important variables. These may well vary in the specialized educational setting from the regular education setting for which the curricula were devised (Fitzgerald, 1968; Lang & Propp, 1982; Leitman, 1968).
5. It is extremely difficult to judge the cognitive and problem-solving levels of hearing-impaired students. Curricula designed for normally hearing children may or may not be appropriate for hearing-impaired children when these basic parameters are considered (Hayden & Woodward, 1968; Sunal, 1984).

6. Most contemporary process-oriented curricula are designed for secondary levels of education; few are available for the levels at which the majority of hearing-impaired students function (Fitzgerald, 1968; Hedges, 1968).
7. Few teachers of the hearing impaired possess sufficient preparation in science to select curricula to adapt, to prepare appropriate adaptations, and to teach process-oriented curricula as they are designed to be taught (Lang & Propp, 1982).
8. Insufficient varieties of effective materials are available to support inquiry-based science curricula (Lang & Propp, 1982).

Those who opt to follow the adaptive model for science curricula must deal with the above limitations.

## CURRICULA DESIGNED FOR HEARING-IMPAIRED STUDENTS

A considerable number of professionals have chosen to design wholly new science curricula for hearing-impaired students. It is hoped that this decision was taken after careful consideration of the values and limitations of adopting and adapting curricula prepared for the broad range of average, normally hearing students. Be that as it may, the literature reflects concern with the limitations of adapted curricula noted earlier. These concerns and others have led to the development of special curricula. Evident in this development is an explicit acceptance that specially designed curricula, in common with regular curricula, must focus on process, problem solving, and activity.

Curricula written specifically for hearing-impaired students are found routinely in schools and special classes for the deaf (Sunal & Burch, 1982) where integration is not a primary consideration. Teachers in these situations deal only with hearing-impaired children and are intensely concerned with creating curricula that such children may master. The result often is the development of "*in-house*" curricula that reflect aspects of curricula being studied by normally hearing children, but which would not be considered simply adaptations of such curricula. The reasons for this pattern of curriculum development are varied but a few points take precedence:

1. The language difficulties of the hearing impaired are seen as so profound that curricula for normally hearing children are considered fundamentally inappropriate.
2. Science curricula routinely expect too rapid a mastery of content for most hearing-impaired students.
3. Individual science curricula do not meet the unique needs of the majority of hearing-impaired students. Judicious selection of topics and support materials from a number of curricula blended into a locally designed product is the most productive procedure.

4. Many science teachers in programs for the hearing impaired are teachers of the deaf first and teachers of science by assignment or interest rather than training. They lack extensive and intensive familiarity with contemporary curricula.

### Language Difficulties

Point 1 summarizes a basic concern of all teachers working with hearing-impaired students. The vast majority of such students are simply unable to read materials prepared to explain and support regular curricula due to syntactic, lexical, and semantic complexity. The acknowledged language difficulties mean, for many educators, that specialized curricula must be prepared.

Even those who favor adapted curricula are faced with the demon of language as is apparent in Sunal's (1984) warning that science teachers must resist the temptation to totally rewrite curricula selected for adaptation. Methods of dealing satisfactorily with the problem of language deficiency are few, and all call for considerable thought on the part of the person charged with teaching science. Sunal's (1984) ideas for adapted curricula were discussed earlier. In addition, a number of techniques for specialized curricula are suggested:

1. Avoid introducing formal terminology until students have been familiarized with activities using known vocabulary (Owsley, 1968).
2. Introduce science slowly from a concrete level, making use of experiences that might normally be taken for granted as part of a child's background knowledge (Leitman, 1968).
3. Prepare students for the language needs of a topic prior to introduction of the topic.
4. Choose supporting materials that best suit the language levels of the hearing-impaired group to be taught (Clarke School for the Deaf, 1975).

That teachers find the language needs of the hearing-impaired population to be particulary challenging is apparent in responses to the Lang and Propp (1982) survey mentioned earlier. Teachers across the United States stressed a need for language-controlled material and a K–12 curriculum designed to meet the needs of hearing-impaired students. "Having textbooks and workbooks written at a language level that hearing-impaired students can comprehend" was given the highest ranking (4.62 in a 5-point scale) in an evaluation of factors contributing to a successful science program.

### Pace of Curricula

Science curricula, in concert with other curricula, are designed in anticipation that an average student will master the material of the curriculum at a predictable rate. This rate is reflected in the number of topics to be introduced in a school-year period. It is the position of a number of educators that hearing-impaired students encounter significant difficulty proceeding at this rate. Therefore, curricula for the hearing impaired must be written specifically for them. These curricula will contain yearly amounts commensurate with the abstractive and language abilities of the hearing impaired. As Hayden and Woodward (1968) noted, expecting children to take in language and concepts before the appropriate time will result in "learning to equate verbalism with understanding and memorization with knowledge. Intellectual curiosity is stifled by the desire to please a teacher who is asking the wrong questions and setting the wrong goals." To ensure that students proceed in keeping with their cognitive and language abilities, curricula specifically taking into consideration the limitations imposed by hearing impairment are necessary.

### Dilution of Content

An unavoidable consequence of the aforementioned reasoning is a pruned-down science curriculum. Topics are included according to their perceived relevance to the needs of the hearing-impaired group being taught. The depth to which topics are explored is contingent on student needs and the materials available, to say nothing of the teacher's interest in the topic. As Leitman (1968) stated, "Because of the nature of the problem of teaching deaf children language and speech, forces are sometimes present in a classroom or school that unintentionally limit the range of educational experiences of the deaf child." This position was reinforced by the finding of Sunal and Burch (1982) that locally designed curricula had structural defects, most significantly in appropriate cognitive levels. To Leitman the most appropriate solution is the collating of activities and ideas that might be used within curriculum development and the concept of "the workshop classroom," in which students would have plentiful opportunity to explore social and physical reality. Leitman emphasized the hands-on approach as being particularly suited to those with limited language. To the curriculum planners of the Clarke School for the Deaf (1975), the method of choice was to lay-out a series of units in biology, chemistry, physics, and earth and space science, and then select various science text series to support the units. These are simply two examples of well-reasoned but quite different approaches. Whatever the merits of these and alternative selective approaches to meet the unique needs of hearing-impaired students, the fact remains that in curricular terms they are selective. Some pruning or avoidance of contemporary curricular design and content is the result.

### Insufficient Teacher Background

A final point given earlier dealt with the training of teachers in science. As has been emphasized, the teaching of language is the first concern of most educators of the hearing impaired. Other concerns, even the adequate preparation of teachers for "content" subjects, is secondary. This point may be readily substantiated by reference once more to the Lang and Propp (1982) survey. Of the 470 respondents to this survey of science teachers in programs for the hearing impaired, 31.4 percent indicated that they had no training in science and 41.7 percent indicated that they had less than a minor concentration in science. Only 15.2 percent listed science as their subject area for certification.

The situation, with regard to uniformity in teaching science, is graphically outlined by Sunal and Burch (1982) in their review of science programs for hearing-impaired students. They found that of 47 schools with hearing-impaired children aged 2 to 14 years, 45 percent used commercial public school curricula, 34 percent had local curricula, and 21 percent had no science curricula. In addition, only 17 percent had process-oriented goals. Some 66 percent did not use adapted methodological strategies for teaching hearing-impaired students, whereas 21 percent had no particular science instruction methodology.

## CONTEMPORARY CURRICULAR CONCERNS—SUMMARY

From the preceding discussion emerge a number of concerns related to the development of science curricula for hearing-impaired students. Some of these are not unique to the area of science. All pose significant challenges to those engaged in this particular aspect of education. The concerns can be summarized as follows:

1. Should curricula be adapted from those designed for normally hearing students or should they be written specifically for the hearing impaired?
2. To what degree should terminology and language be simplified?
3. Should curricula focus on concrete rather than abstract approaches?
4. To what degree should factors beyond hearing impairment (e.g., support materials) influence curriculum design?
5. Should science curricula for the hearing impaired reflect a process or content orientation?
6. How can adequate training in science be provided for teachers of the hearing impaired?

Discussion on each of these points with arguments for and against each has been presented briefly in earlier passages. It is obvious that the area of science in general and the preparation of appropriate curricula have not been of primary concern within the field of education of the hearing impaired. For a significant body of educators it would appear that it has not been even an area of secondary concern. This situation is changing, at a slow but perceptible rate. Among the reasons for change are the integration of an increasing number of hearing-impaired individuals, the continual evolution of teacher preparation, and the realization that hearing-impaired individuals must be knowledgeable about the world about them to a greater degree than was common in past years. As these dynamics and others affect education of the hearing impaired, the study of science will receive increased attention. As this attention is turned to curricular design the concerns and views mentioned earlier will serve, in part, as guidelines to the generation of improved curricula.

## TYPE SCIENCE RESOURCES IN REVIEW

*Controlled Language Science Series* P. Fleury (1979a, 1979b, 1979c, 1979d, 1979e, 1982a, 1982b, 1982c, 1982d, 1982e, 1982f, 1982g, 1982h, 1982i)

*Science* Clarke School for the Deaf (1975)

*Science for Deaf Children* A. Leitman (1968)

*Science Curriculum*, St. Mary's School for the Deaf M. Amo, M. Burk, M. Karol, J. Kohl, N. Moore, and A. Petrillo (1985)

*Science for the Hearing Impaired* D.W. Sunal and C.S. Sunal (1981a, 1981b)

## *CONTROLLED LANGUAGE SCIENCE SERIES*

### P. Fleury

*Publisher*:

Dormac, Inc.
P.O. Box 752
Beaverton, Oregon 97005

Dominie Press Limited
345 Nugget Avenue, Unit 15
Agincourt, Ontario MIS 4J4

*Skills taught*: Introduction to the scientific study of insects (praying mantis, the house fly, and the honey bee) and reptiles (turtle, alligator, snake, and lizard)

*Age/grade range*: Students must be at a second grade reading level. Upper elementary, intermediate interest level

*Group size*: Class group

**THEORY:** No theoretical orientation is given for the selection of topics. The series is not intended as a complete curriculum but simply as an introduction to the study of insects and reptiles. Although no particular theoretical orientation is discussed, examination of the materials indicates more concern with content than with process.

Fleury has adopted a particular approach to the language required for the study of science. Language is controlled through the control of vocabulary, the rate of introduction of vocabulary, and the number and type of linguistic structures used. Vocabulary was selected from the Dolch 220 word list and the linguistic structures from those acquired by 3-year-old children. Structures are processed in transformational grammar style.

**DESCRIPTION:** The series consists of seven science readers, *The Praying Mantis, The House Fly, The Honey Bee, The Turtle, The Alligator, The Snake,* and *The Lizard*), a student workbook and teacher's guide for insect study, and a teacher's guide and individual workbooks for reptile study. The workbooks are devoted entirely to expression of content knowledge. Teacher's guides contain overview of teaching units, transformational analyses of all structures used in the three insect-study readers, references and sources for support materials, and an answer key for student workbooks. Each reader contains a series of sections composed of introductory vocabulary pages followed by a few pages of content reading. There are numerous colorful, pleasing illustrations with accompanying text. Frequently the illustrations do little to support or illuminate the text.

Each teaching unit for insects is organized under specific concept, materials needed, materials needed for supplement, and an unvarying instructional procedure of eight steps. Teaching units for reptiles are organized under specific concepts and an unvarying instructional procedure of eleven stages. Each teaching unit relates to one reader section composed of introductory vocabulary pages and following content page(s). Instructions are straightforward. Supplemental activities are suggested for each unit and support materials noted in the guides.

**EVALUATION:** The *Controlled Language Science Series* is much too limited in scope to be considered a curriculum, even within the restricted scope of a curriculum for the introduction of the insect and reptile study. The author does not claim that it fulfills the function of a curriculum. No discussion of its role within the study of science is given. Few would argue with the need for control of the language of instructional materials for any population. In the instance of this series, however, the teaching of science appears almost subordinate to the need to control language.

The units presented are covered with sufficient attention for introductory study. The pedagogical approach is predominantly a concrete-oriented rather than process-oriented approach. This may be partially the result of the decision to control vocabulary and language structure.

A quite straightforward lesson format is presented. Lessons are of an acceptable length, and the facts presented relate well to one another and proceed in logical fashion. The readers are bright and interesting, and the student workbook is well-organized. The teacher's guide has paid insufficient attention to the placing of these units of study in a general approach to science instruction for hearing-impaired students.

The *Controlled Language Science Series* has limited utility, but is a valuable experiment in the control of instructional language. As such it is worthy of extension.

## *SCIENCE*

### The Clarke School for the Deaf

*Publisher*:
The Clarke School for the Deaf
Northampton, Massachusetts 01060

*Skills taught*: Biology, chemistry, physics, and earth and space science
*Age/grade range*: Grades 2-8; Clarke Middle and Upper Schools

*Group size*: Class groups

**THEORY:** No fundamental theoretical orientation is provided in this curriculum and the committee charged with the design chose to outline a number of units of study in the fields of biology, chemistry, physics, and earth and space science. The design of units outlined in some detail suggests a content orientation coupled with explanatory activities. A variety of texts are suggested as resources. The theoretical positions adopted by the authors of these texts would appear to be the ones influencing individual units of study.

**DESCRIPTION:** The Clarke School *Science* program covers levels (or grades) 2 to 8, which constitute Clarke's middle and upper schools. The content of units in biology, chemistry, physics, and earth and space science for levels 2 through 5 is considered appropriate for students of all ability levels given teacher adaptation as necessary. Units 6 through 8 are designed for two tracks of students: Track A students would have higher reading ability than track B students. The program at each level is considered to be one year's work.

Units for each discipline are outlined at each level. In the main the outlines consist of short statements of content and purpose. Some introductory statements contain a "Teacher Suggestions" section noting instructional recommendations. Student texts with appropriate pages noted, teacher references, library books, filmstrips, and films are detailed in a Resources section. Unit outlines for track A and track B are the same.

At each level, one unit is outlined in some detail, and exact concepts to be taught and suggested activities are given. In addition, new vocabulary words are underlined. Introductory teacher suggestions and resource sections are provided, as they are for all units. Detailed outlines for track A and track B are the same.

An overview of the entire program noting number of units at each discipline level, appropriate texts, and the unit outline page number appears early in the curriculum. The entire program consists of a number of units for each level and discipline, as presented in Table 5-1.

Units are based on a variety of recommended texts. Texts may or may not be consistent for all units of study within a level. Exact pages of study are noted.

**Table 5-1.** Number of Units in Biology, Chemistry, Physics, and Earth and Space by Level in Clarke School Science Curriculum

| Level | Units | | | |
|---|---|---|---|---|
| | Biology | Chemistry | Physics | Earth and Space |
| 2 | 3 | 2 | 4 | 2 |
| 3 | 4 | 1 | 2 | 3 |
| 4 | 2 | 1 | 4 | 4 |
| 5 | 3 | 1 | 2 | 4 |
| 6A | 4 | 3 | 4 | 1 |
| 6B | 4 | 4 | 3 | |
| 7A | 3 | 2 | 2 | 3 |
| 7B | 1 | 3 | | 6 |
| 8A | 4 | 3 | 2 | 1 |
| 8B | 3 | 2 | 4 | 1 |

The Clarke School's *Science* curriculum contains a number of useful additional sections: One is a series of 18 brief suggestions for the science teacher using the curriculum. These suggestions range from the specific (the need to assign homework) to the general (an outline of the experimental report model). Additionally, space is devoted to teacher references and sources of media materials.

**EVALUATION:** Clarke School has produced a detailed, wide-ranging science curriculum. It is a locally devised curriculum but is based on selected units of commercial curricula. It avoids a number of pitfalls of other locally devised courses of study, because of its heavy dependence on science content as presented in mainstream education. Comparatively, it is more complete and better reasoned than many other curricula. Unfortunately, however, no discussion of theoretical orientation is provided. When a school depends on such a wide variety of published texts, with differing theoretical and instructional approaches, it is necessary to rationalize their use to lessen possible internal conflicts when teachers switch from resource to resource.

Particular strengths of the Clarke curriculum are the following: (1) two tracks for different reading abilities; (2) an overview of the entire program; (3) the detailed selected study units; (4) a considerable array of support materials; and (5) instructional suggestions provided throughout the curriculum. A particular area of concern is the apparent emphasis on content as compared to process. A well-trained teacher might be able to provide sufficient emphasis on process but, as noted earlier, many science teachers are not as well-prepared as might be wished.

One final note: The Clarke School *Lower School Five Year Curriculum Guide* contains information on science for the years preceding Level 2.

## *SCIENCE FOR DEAF CHILDREN*

**A. Leitman**

*Publisher*:
Alexander Graham Bell Association for the Deaf
3417 Volta Place, NW
Washington, DC 20007

*Skills taught*: Science activities and units of science study in an activity-based program.

*Age/grade range: Preschool (ages 3 to 6 years) to advanced level (12 to 17 years)*

*Group size*: Class group within an individualized approach

**THEORY:** Leitman (1968) developed teaching ideas on the basis of a hands-on, activity-centered approach to science. He noted that such an approach is in keeping with trends in science curricula development current in the United States in the 1960s. In his view his material, and that of the Science Curriculum Improvement Study (SCIS), the science program of the American Association for the Advancement of Science (AAAS), the Elementary School Science Project (ESSP), and the Elementary Science Study, possess common emphases on both direct activity by students and problem solving. He stated categorically that the need for direct experience is even greater for hearing-impaired students than for others.

The linch pin of the activity approach for Leitman is "the workshop classroom." He stressed the requirement for a classroom structure that allows for effective interaction of room, materials, and teacher. Materials will be available at a certain time, in appropriate quantity, and in appropriate places only because teachers have predecided the time, amount, and place of their need in response to the needs of the students. Combined with the workshop classroom concept is that of the individualized program. Any program must focus on the individual in a flexible fashion, although lessons are presented to groups.

Intertwined with the above is the position that the development of language takes precedence over all other educational activities. Leitman supports the natural approach to language instruction, indicating that this approach supports his activity-centered, child need-centered science schema. There exists in his formulation a place of early concrete experiences that will lead eventually to vocabulary acquisition, language enrichment, and abstract thought.

**DESCRIPTION:** Leitman cautions that his ideas do not form a curriculum plan but are the type of positions, activities, and units that are to be considered in curriculum planning. He further cautions that his ideas rise from experience in an oral environment. Finally, he notes that his materials and ideas may not be suitable for children with more than a minimum of central nervous system damage.

The bulk of Leitman's publication deals with program sequences and teaching ideas for four age ranges, from preschool through 16 or 17 years. The objectives and general content of each area follow.

For the preschool years (ages 3 to 6), the major objective is "To provide activities and materials that can be accessible to [students] non-verbally, yet, at the same time, stimulate and excite the children so that they will need more and more language to express their interests."

Activities and materials focus on the natural interests of preschoolers and their perceived developmental rate. Initial activities relate to the physical self, body and senses, self-perception, perception and relationships to others, and the integrated use of these pieces of information. Subtopics include the following:

1. *Children Study Themselves*: Activities to develop a sense of appearance, name, and relative size.
2. *Large Muscle Movements*: Activities to develop body control.
3. *The Senses*: Activities to develop the use of the five senses with increasing precision.
4. *Integrated Use of the Senses*: Activities to provide a base for the understanding of future science concepts (water play, clay play, woodwork, pets and plants, storytelling, and dramatic play, trips, activities with older children, painting).

The major objectives for the primary years (ages 6 to 9 ) are:

1. Ability to use observation for gaining information
2. Problem-solving ability
3. Broadening of interests
4. Primary skills in collecting and using various kinds of data.

Activities and materials continue to focus on the development of observational skills and discovery or understanding through an activity-centered approach. Major activity units include the following:

1. Animals
2. Plants
3. Ice cubes (heat, melting, insulation)
4. Light and shadows

## *SCIENCE FOR THE HEARING IMPAIRED*

**D.W. Sunal and C.S. Sunal**

*Publisher*:

Department of Curriculum and Instruction
College of Human Resources and Education
West Virginia University
Morgantown, West Virginia 26506

*Skills taught*: Variation, space and motion, interaction and energy, populations and interactions, exploring matter, patterns, exploring energy, environments, forces, motion, matter and energy, adaptations, models of matter, models, energy and ecosystems, population needs, looking at life, life systems and biological systems

*Age/grade range*: 9 years to 13 years approximately

*Group size*: Class group

**THEORY:** Sunal and Sunal (1981a, 1981b) consider that a process-oriented curricular approach is most appropriate for all students, normally hearing or hearing impaired. In their analysis locally developed special science curricula for hearing-impaired students do not focus sufficiently on skills and science processes, discovery and unknown results, and active participation in meaningful activities. Additionally, commercially prepared curricula for normally hearing students assumed language competency levels not routinely found among hearing-impaired students, were insufficiently visually oriented, and required supplementation of activities. However, commercially prepared curricula answered the need for a process-oriented approach and certain commercial curricula appeared amenable to adaptation for hearing-impaired students. Therefore, an adaptive approach to science education for the hearing impaired was selected.

Within the adaptive process-oriented approach, Sunal and Sunal wished to preserve the conceptual themes put forth by the National Science Teachers Association (NSTA).

1. There are structural patterns in all matter.
2. There is order in space and time.
3. Change and interaction are universal.
4. Living objects change and interact.

Woven through these major themes is the problem-solving approach of a process-oriented curriculum.

**DESCRIPTION:** The commercial curricula found to best combine the above approach, with promise of adaptability for the educational needs of the hearing impaired, were *Science* (Berger, Berheimer, Lewis, & Neuberger, 1979) and *Spaceship Earth* (McLaren, 1981), both published by Houghton Mifflin. *Science* was reorganized in four levels (3 to 6) for the hearing impaired with each level having one unit focussed on the NSTA major conceptual themes as follows:

1. There are structural patterns in all matter.
   Level 3 Unit 1: Variation
   Level 4 Unit 2: Exploring matter
   Level 5 Unit 2: Forces
   Level 6 Unit 3: Models of matter
2. There is order in space and time.
   Level 3 Unit 2: Space and motion
   Level 4 Unit 3: Patterns
   Level 5 Unit 3: Motion
   Level 6 Unit 2: Models
3. Change and interaction are universal.
   Level 3 Unit 3: Interaction and energy
   Level 4 Unit 4: Exploring energy
   Level 5 Unit 4: Matter and energy
   Level 6 Unit 4: Energy and ecosystems
4. Living objects change and interact.
   Level 3 Unit 4: Population interactions
   Level 4 Unit 1: Environments
   Level 5 Unit 1: Adaptations
   Level 6 Unit 1: Population needs

*Spaceship Earth* was reorganized into three units: (1) Looking at Life; (2) Life Systems; and (3) Biological Systems.

Reorganization included alteration in the order of some lessons to promote initial concrete experiences, omission of those lessons considered too abstract, and the addition of activities to increase concrete experiences in lessons retained. Effort was made to maintain the integrity of the original texts and to accomplish their basic objectives.

A specific lesson sequence was created to achieve the dual objectives of reaching original text objectives and meeting the learning needs of hearing-impaired students. This sequence is:

1. Introduction–a concrete, active experience designed to gather information, to call on previous experience, and to promote discovery.

2. Development–presentation of new skills and concepts on an activity base.

3. Application-use of the new concept on additional examples to promote internalization and generalization through practice effect.

4. Evaluation-generalization of concepts and skills to new problem situations.

Throughout all levels certain skills are emphasized to assist in reaching objectives. These are coupled as observing-describing, investigating-manipulating, organizing-quantifying, and generalizing-applying.

*Science* and *Spaceship Earth* texts are used with lessons except where specifically noted. The teacher is expected, as necessary, to rewrite the text, paraphrase content, or read the text to the students inserting appropriate modifications and explanations. Certain words and phrases are noted for each lesson as requiring emphasis by the teacher and internalization by the students. A videotape of these *key words and phrases* is available. To further assist the students' learning the authors suggest that important lesson objects be labelled (identification cards) and that sentences and questions are written on cards (language cards). Audiovisual materials to accompany the *Science* series and *Spaceship Earth* are noted where appropriate.

All of the previously mentioned lessons are planned in considerable detail in teachers' guides for each level. Each lesson is outlined under (1) development; (2) purpose; (3) advance preparation; (4) teaching suggestions; and (5) desired learning outcome. In addition lessons are clustered under subtopics for each unit of each NSTA conceptual theme. In the case of Level 3, Unit 1: Variation, the sub-topics are (1) variation in objects, with a cluster of four lessons; (2) variation in matter, with a cluster of two lessons; and (3) variation in interaction, with a cluster of two lessons. A lesson-cluster outline provides text reference pages, teaching strategies, lesson titles, teaching time required, and notes on materials required or recommended.

**EVALUATION:** Sunal and Sunal have written a useful science curriculum. Their decision to adapt existing commercially available texts ensures maintenance of instruction parallel to that of normally hearing students. It also allows them to emphasize a process-oriented approach as opposed to the content-oriented approach common to many locally created curricula.

The detailed teachers' guides are a boon to many teachers. Every need is anticipated. Planning is all but done and all the teacher has to do is organize the materials and follow the outline. While useful such detailed guides also contain drawbacks. Major among these is the removal of planning responsibility from the teacher. It should be quite possible for a teacher to work through each lesson without obtaining an understanding of how lessons relate to one another, or of the process orientation of the whole. This point may be especially telling when it comes to the application and evaluation steps of the lesson.

The adaptations suggested by Sunal and Sunal will not be new to most teachers of the hearing impaired. The focus on language and the need to explain the text crosses all subjects. One possible result of this focus could well be a preoccupation with vocabulary and language to the detriment of the content of the lesson.

All in all, however, *Science for the Hearing Impaired* is an excellent effort. It lays out important guidelines for others to follow in adapting existing curricula for this population.

## REFERENCES

American Association for the Advancement of Science. (1963). *Science—A process approach*. Washington, DC: Author.

Battaglia, M., Scouten, E., & Hamil, F. (1982). A teaching strategy for the science laboratory. *Volta Review, 84,* 34-38.

Berger, C.F., Berheimer, G., Lewis, L.E., Jr., & Neuberger, H. (1979). *Science*. Boston: Houghton Mifflin.

Clarke School for the Deaf. (1975). *Science*. Northampton, MA: Author.

DeWalt, P.A. (1968). Adaptations of the scientific method for the deaf child. In H.G. Kopp (Ed.), *Curriculum: Cognition and content* (Monograph) Washington, DC: Alexander Graham Bell Association, pp. 26-30.

Fitzgerald, M.A. (1968). Trends in science education. In H.G. Kopp (Ed.), *Curriculum: Cognition and content* (Monograph) Washington, DC: Alexander Graham Bell Association, pp. 17-21.

Fleury, P. (1979a). *Controlled language science series: Student workbook*. Beaverton, OR: Dormac.

Fleury, P. (1979b). *Controlled language science series: Teacher's guide*. Beaverton, OR: Dormac.

Fleury, P. (1979c). *The honey bee*. Beaverton, OR: Dormac.

Fleury, P. (1979d). *The house fly*. Beaverton, OR: Dormac.

Fleury, P. (1979e). *The praying mantis*. Beaverton, OR: Dormac.

Fleury, P. (1982a). *The alligator*. Beaverton, OR: Dormac.

Fleury, P. (1982b). *The alligator: Student workbook*. Beaverton, OR: Dormac.

Fleury, P. (1982c). *The lizard*. Beaverton, OR: Dormac.

Fleury, P. (1982d). *The lizard: Student workbook*. Beaverton, OR: Dormac.

Fleury, P. (1982e). *Reptile: Teacher's guide*. Beaverton, OR: Dormac.

Fleury, P. (1982f). *The snake*. Beaverton, OR: Dormac.

Fleury, P. (1982g). *The snake: Student workbook*. Beaverton, OR: Dormac.

Fleury, P. (1982h). *The turtle*. Beaverton, OR: Dormac.

Fleury, P. (1982i). *The turtle: Student workbook*. Beaverton, OR: Dormac.

Grant, W.D., Knight, D.L., & Rosenstein, J. (1973). *Final report on a project to determine the feasibility of BSCS's Me Now for hearing-impaired children*. Washington, DC: Model Secondary School for the Deaf.

Grant, W.D., Rosenstein, J., & Knight, D.L. (1975). A project to determine the feasibility of BSCS's Me Now for hearing-impaired students. *American Annals of the Deaf, 120,* 63-69.

Hayden, J.S., & Woodward, H.M.E. (1968). Rationale for a science program. *Volta Review, 70,* 159-165.

Hedges, H.G. (1968). Natural science for all students. In H.G. Kopp (Ed.), *Curriculum: Cognition and content* (Monograph) Washington, DC: Alexander Graham Bell Association, pp. 11-16.

Lang, H.G., & Propp, G. (1982). Science education for hearing-impaired students: State-of-the-art. *American Annals of the Deaf, 127,* 860-869.

Leitman, A. (1968). *Science for deaf children*. Washington, DC: Alexander Graham Bell Association.

McLaren, J.E., Stasik, I.H., & Levering, D.F. (1981). *Spaceship earth*. Boston: Houghton Mifflin.

Owsley, P.J. (1968). Development of the cognitive abilities and language of deaf children through science. In H.G. Kopp (Ed.), *Curriculum: Cognition and content* (Monograph) Washington, DC: Alexander Graham Bell Association, pp. 21-25.

St. Mary's School for the Deaf. (1985). *Science curriculum*. Buffalo, NY: Author.

Scouten, E.L. (1979). The laboratory report: An instructional module for technical English. *American Annals of the Deaf, 124,* 377-380.

Sunal, D.W. (1984). Without reinventing the wheel. *Perspectives, 2,* 16-18, 28.

Sunal, D.W., & Burch, D. (1982). School science programs for the hearing impaired. *American Annals of the Deaf, 127,* 411-417.

Sunal, D.W., & Sunal, C. (1981a). *Science for the hearing impaired: Introduction to the program*. Morgantown, WV: West Virginia University.

Sunal, D.W., & Sunal, C. (1981b). *Science for the hearing impaired: Teacher's guides for level three to seven*. Morgantown, WV: West Virginia University.

Sunal, C., & Sunal, D.W. (1981c). *Adapting science for hearing-impaired early adolescents* (final report). Morgantown, WV: West Virginia University.

# CHAPTER 6

# *Speech Curricula*

Education for hearing-impaired children and adolescents has an extensive, and frequently controversial history that dates back several centuries (Bender, 1960; Moores, 1978; Scouten, 1984). Many of the early issues and controversies were directed at teaching the severely and profoundly hearing-impaired students to communicate orally, and those same debates have continued decade after decade. Although there have been many educational concerns for hearing-impaired students, the mode of instruction and the teaching of speech have been among the most obvious issues for educators, parents, and related professional groups. The purpose of this chapter, however, is not to review the pros and cons of arguments on modes of communication. The basic position taken here is that the vast majority of professionals, parents, and hearing-impaired individuals agree that ability to communicate through speech is a desirable goal, and that a planned curricular approach toward that goal is likewise necessary. Mulholland (1981) clearly stated the rationale for speech instruction:

> The most obvious deviancy in the child with deafness from early life is the lack of speech, oral or spoken language, through which the child normally structures reality, organizes his experiences to understand and to control his environment, labels his experiences, and increases his discriminating and differentiating ability, thus attaining higher levels of conceptualization. (p. 27)

## PROBLEMS OF SPEECH CURRICULA

The particular problems which do arise in the area of speech and exert general influence on the practice of the art are:

1. Effectiveness of instruction
2. Adequacy of teacher preparation in speech
3. Heterogenous nature of the hearing-impaired population

These influences are interrelated rather than clearly dichotomized. Nevertheless, they will be discussed separately here to highlight salient points contributing to their effect on speech instruction.

Even when it comes to choosing a preferred approach to speech instruction, no particular difficulty arises. Over the past many years two general systems for teaching speech have developed. One is the analytic or elemental. The other is the natural or whole word approach. The analytic approach was reflected in the methods of programs such as that at the Clarke School and epitomized in Yale's *Formation and Development of Elementary English Sounds* (1946). In this system attention is focussed on the exact articulation of individual sounds. These are combined into words as mastery is attained. Haycock's *The Teaching of Speech* (1936) taught the natural approach in which concern with accent, rhythm, and phrasing was equally as important as the mastery of individual vowels and consonants. Today most programs adopt an eclectic method combining aspects of both general systems. Depending on the philosophical and practical beliefs of those responsible for speech curricula and implementation of speech instruction, either the analytic or the natural method receives greater emphasis.

### Effectiveness of Instruction Problem

The reality of speech instruction in the past is that it has not been successful in producing acceptable levels of intelligibility in the majority of hearing-impaired individuals with severe to profound losses. Whereas a number of speech and hearing clinics, classes, and schools have reported significant success, this success has not been generalized. Markides' (1970) finding that only 30 percent of words spoken by residential deaf students were intelligible to experienced listeners is typical of findings in intelligibility studies. It is this lack of generalized effectiveness that has become the central argument for the substitution of alternate communication systems for speech or for their use simultaneously with speech. The fact that these alternate systems are not markedly advantageous in the academic and vocational sense has not been a matter of central concern.

Bishop (1979) presented an interesting point relating to effectiveness of speech instruction for adolescents. He advised viewing speech training in the dual perspective of both the likelihood of developing intelligible speech and what other possible aspects of education would be sacrificed to provide time for speech instruction. According to Bishop, motivation on the student's part is the controlling factor in whether or not to offer speech instruction. He coupled this argument with previous achievement in speech implying that previous success leads to motivation for continued effort. In Bishop's words:

> The critical variable now is motivation. At this stage of development it is not unusual to find students who are either "turned on" or "turned off" regarding speech. Their attitude has been shaped by many factors: parental involvement, teacher attitudes and techniques, peer and adult pressures, and the number of successful or defeating experiences.

Generalized effectiveness and the concept of choice bear on curriculum development in speech. If, indeed, speech instruction is not effective, why continue with the effort to improve and implement curricula? That the present situation is not as positive as might be desired was underlined by Ling (1981).

> If our current methods of developing oral communication were truly effective, our efforts with totally deaf and profoundly hearing-impaired children would be as successful as with those with hard-of-hearing youngsters. In general, they are not.

Those familiar with Ling's impressive contribution to speech curricula would be astounded if this view of the situation in speech instruction were interpreted as implying cessation of effort. Ling, and many other professionals, would argue for continued work on curricula, meaningful integration of speech curricula with the student's needs and life, and improved teacher education in speech instruction as ways to increase effect. These points will be addressed later in the chapter.

Bishop's point would raise eyebrows in many quarters as well. In effect he suggests redefining speech curricula as appropriate for specific audiences and not as an across-the-board offering. Whereas he focusses on the adolescent-to-adult stage, others would argue that it is possible to separate potentially "good" and "poor" speakers at earlier ages. Such a line of argument suggests reduced need to develop speech curricula, most particulary for those with severe and profound losses and additional handicaps.

In summary, the lack of effectiveness may have two results. Some professionals appear to argue that the effort is one of futility and should be abandoned except for those showing promise of acceptable speech intelligibility and those motivated to study speech. Others point out variables that interfere with acquisition of intelligibility in the majority of hearing-impaired individuals and urge continued curricular efforts.

### Teacher Education Problem

Historically, teachers of hearing-impaired students have been charged with being everything to all hearing-impaired students. As a consequence of this philosophy, teachers were expected to understand and be able to implement speech instruction curricula as part of their daily activities, and to be able to implement such curricula appropriately. Mulholland (1981) highlighted this position in her discussion of philosophical bases of oral education mentioned earlier. Her statement that "The staff must recognize and believe that each teacher is responsible for instruction in speech, language, and listening" is unequivocal. Every teacher is a teacher of speech. That this view is held generally in the field was documented in a study of personnel preparation by Subtelny, Webster, and Murphy (1980). Of responding professionals in programs in education of the deaf, 96 percent indicated they had taken courses in teaching speech to the deaf and 87 percent had undertaken clinical practica in teaching speech to the hearing impaired. In a study of state certification standards (Moulton, Roth, & Winney, 1983), 26 of 28 states detailing standards indicated that preparation in speech was a specific requirement.

In the comparatively recent past, a second group of professionals has become involved in speech instruction for hearing-impaired students on a routine basis. The field of speech pathology and audiology views hearing-impaired children as a target population for their services. Increasingly, programs for the education of hearing impaired are placing speech and language pathologists on staff to complement the activities of teachers. Increasingly, as well, professionals in speech and language programs are undertaking specific preparation for work with the hearing impaired. In the Subtelny et al. study (1980), 50 percent of respondents from speech and language pathology indicated that they had included courses in teaching speech to the deaf in their studies while 71 percent had participated in clinical practica in speech with hearing-impaired individuals.

Despite the apparent and widespread view that both teachers and speech and language pathologists are responsible for speech instruction and the related development of speech curricula, and are participating in courses in speech for the hearing impaired, the quality of their work is considered less than satisfactory on the average. Ling and Ling (1978) made no bones about their view of the goals of speech instruction and the ability of instructors to achieve them.

> The goal of teaching speech production skills is to provide the child with the means to express himself fluently and effectively through spoken language in a variety of social situations. Speech teaching is worthless unless it is directed to this goal. Failure to reach this goal is common because speech training is, in general, appallingly inadequate.

Hogan (1980) pointed a finger at professional preparation programs in hearing impairment as explanatory, in part at least, for inadequate instructor skill levels. She suggested that "It would appear that students graduating from teacher education programs having limited contact in speech-related experiences with deaf children are poorly prepared to engage in the difficult task of teaching speech to deaf children." Boothroyd (1980) reinforced Hogan's criticism in noting that preparation programs in the area of speech fail to swiftly and effectively incorporate new and existing knowledge in their offerings.

A final point bearing on teacher effectiveness is how adequate for the task teachers perceive themselves to be or are perceived to be. Dale (1971) noted that speech was the area where teachers feel most inadequate. Ling (1976) echoed this statement in his curricular text on speech instruction. Subtelny et al. (1980) reported that 13 percent of both professionals in hearing impairment and speech and language preparation programs felt some deficiency in speech. At the same time, those in hearing-impairment programs reported that 25 percent of students at the master's level had less than good knowledge of speech training of the hearing impaired. Those instructors at the master's level in speech and language programs consider that 71 percent of students possess less than good knowledge.

In summary, speech instruction is believed to be the responsibility of both teachers and the speech and language pathologists working with hearing-impaired individuals. However, it is the widespread consideration of knowledgeable professionals that preparation in speech is less than satisfactory. Additionally it is the opinion of many teachers and pathologists that they are less than strongly capable of carrying out the task of speech instruction. Such a situation suggests both hesitation and insufficient ability to design and implement speech curricula with the necessary fervor.

### Heterogenous Population Problem

Professionals and lay people routinely refer to the deaf or the hearing-impaired population as if it were a grouping of like individuals. Speech curricula are commonly designed on this same principle. Nevertheless, there is little truth to the concept of homogeneity in the hearing-impaired population. Even a superficial consideration of the issue reveals that population differs on a number of significant variables. Central among these are: (1) Degree of hearing impairment; (2) Educational placement; and (3) Multihandicapping conditions.

The relationship of speech intelligibility and a number of variables was investigated by Jensema, Karchmer, and Trybus (1978). Their findings documented conclusively that speech intelligibility was more strongly related to degree of loss than to any other variable: the greater the hearing loss, the less the speech intelligibility. Obviously, the possibility of preparing specific curricula or parts thereof for differing loss groups must be considered.

Educational placements for hearing-impaired students range from residential placement in a school for the deaf, day attendance in a residential school for the deaf, attendance in a day school, and attendance in a full-time day class, to participation in an integration program. Enrollment in any one of these programs is directly related to degree of hearing loss (Jensema, Karchmer, & Trybus, 1978) on the average. Residential schools are populated primarily by students with profound losses (65 percent), and the losses decrease in the earlier noted programs, finishing with only 18.5 percent who have profound losses in integrated programs. Degree of speech intelligibility changes by programs, though the controlling factor is degree of hearing loss rather than type of program. Again, the possible need for different curricula for different programs must be considered. Obviously this consideration and that of hearing-loss-based curricula cannot be separated.

The final major contributor to the heterogeneity of this population is presence or absence of additional handicapping conditions. Shane (1985) noted that the "Presence of the more extreme or severe form of speech apraxia or dysarthria (referred to as anarthria) quite often results in the clinical decision to introduce an augmentative communication system." Stremel-Campbell (1982) concluded that for mentally retarded deaf children, the goal of speech as an ultimate communication ability "may be unrealistic for many children who do not have potential or do not have the oral mechanism for speech." The numbers involved here are not to be disregarded. Vernon (1982) reported the following incidences of additional handicaps in a hearing-impaired population: cerebral palsy and hemiplegia, 15.8 percent; mental retardation, 12.2 percent; aphasoid disorders, 21.9 percent; visual defects, 29.8 percent; orthopedic defects, 4.8 percent. The presence of these, and other handicaps to such extent in this population, cannot be ignored in preparation of any curricula. Speech instruction is no exception to this rule.

It was noted earlier that speech curricula have been designed as if a homogenous hearing-impaired population existed. The foregoing discussion outlines three areas that indicate such a view is overly simplistic. The import of the discussion here is that such factors should be considered both in the design and delivery of speech curricula. Degree of loss, educational placement, and the presence of additional handicaps are too relevant to the development of speech communication in the hearing-impaired individual to be ignored.

## Summary

It is incontestable that the area of communication method is the most controversial topic in education of the hearing impaired. It is also incontestable, that, as far as curriculum design or delivery is concerned, the arguments churning around communication method are irrelevant. Speech instruction curricula do exist, they require implementation, and they will benefit from continued improvement.

That which is significant is the question of what major factors presently influence the design and delivery of speech curricula. These factors have been identified as:

1. Effectiveness of instruction
2. Adequacy of teacher preparation in speech
3. Heterogeneity of the hearing-impaired population

These factors overlay any consideration of speech curricula. They define the primary influences affecting need to continue effort on speech curricula and the milieu in which this need will be judged. They are the factors against which the future state-of-the-art will be decided as it extends from the present.

## PRESENT STATE OF THE ART

Instruction in speech has altered significantly since the 1960s. Traditional methods emphasized a phoneme-by-phoneme procedure, an appreciation of the movement of the articulators, a reliance on syllable drills, and the use of taction and visible feedback within a generally multisensory framework. Of particular import to teachers of speech to deaf children in the first half of the 20th century were two publications. The first was Haycock's (1933) treatise in which the principles and practices of *natural* speech were presented in an organized lucid fashion. Even today, *The Teaching of Speech* serves as a reference book for many professionals. The second publication was Yale's (1946) *Formation and Development of Elementary English Sounds,* in which the Northampton or Yale charts, that underlie the element method in speech instruction, were presented. From earlier beginnings such as these a number of contemporary approaches have emerged. Calvert and Silverman (1975) presented a useful categorization of the primary general systems.

### Auditory Global Method

The auditory global method is known by a number of titles: chief among these are the aural-oral, the auditory, the acoustic, the acoupedic, and the unisensory. Within this approach, there is jointly a rejection of multisensory techniques and an adherence to the practice of stimulation of residual hearing as the only productive path to acceptable speech. Closely connected to the concept of auditory stimulation are comprehensive intervention on an ecological level and the pursuit of connected speech (Calvert & Silverman, 1975). Various advocates of the auditory global method have espoused it as the one fruitful method yet devised, and as a radical departure from other, lesser methodologies (Pollack, 1964, 1970; Stewart, Pollack, & Downs, 1964). Griffiths (1967), for example, stirred considerable controversy with her suggestion that sufficiently early intervention with the auditory global method would reverse hearing impairment.

Calvert and Silverman (1975), as noted earlier, have described the method in detail. It is not intended that their fine work simply be replicated here. However, their description of the method can serve as a guideline for curriculum developers who select the auditory global approach as the basis for speech instruction. Their discussions of the need for comprehensive intervention and the need for comprehensive speech will be found to be of most value in curriculum development. In these two areas the central points are:

Comprehensive intervention, including (1) Stimulation in home, school, and community, in the total environment; (2) Positive response to speech attempts by all in the environment; and (3) Reinforcement of speech by constant, appropriate modeling.

Connected speech, which includes (1) Normal amounts of connected speech input; (2) Maintenance of natural rhythm, expansions of student's utterances, and consistent modeling by those in the total environment; and (3) Specific direction of connected speech to the student using the auditory mode as the primary signal system.

These points, while serving as general guide-points for the curriculum developer, are not independent of appropriate amplification and other such ways of ensuring reception of the best possible auditory signal. These allied aspects may not be featured in a speech instruction curriculum, but they must not be taken for granted, forgotten, or reduced in importance in any way. Calvert and Silverman presented these aspects as crucial to the auditory global method.

## Multisensory Syllable Unit Method

Many aspects of the auditory global method may be found in the multisensory syllable unit method. It differs, however, in a number of ways. As defined by Calvert and Silverman (1975) and Silverman, Lane, and Calvert (1978) these are:

1. Multisensory stimulation for speech. Seeing the similarities and differences among speech sounds and feeling their tactile characteristics is considered supportive of auditory feedback.
2. Focus on development of speech sounds. Speech sounds are taught directly and in a laid-out sequence.
3. The syllable is the basic unit of instruction. Specific use is made of syllables as the smallest speech unit carrying voice quality inflection, and stress. It is also sufficient for work on coarticulation of phonemes without overstressing motor memory.

In terms of curricular development, the major aspects of the auditory global approach are accepted, but the limitations of one sensory avenue and connected speech alone are rejected. Daily, spontaneous speech and elicited connected speech are supplemented by an expansion of the modalities employed, a daily speech period focussed on speech development, correction of spontaneous speech attempts, repetitive practice, and the use of an orthographic system as a teaching tool.

### Association Phoneme Unit Method

Calvert and Silverman (1975) viewed their division of speech instructional strategies as being a division of methods based, to some degree, on the ability of individual hearing-impaired students to benefit through a particular instructional approach. Certain children would learn effectively through the auditory global approach and it was recommended particularly as the approach of choice for younger students. Others would benefit from more carefully structured teaching systems. Among this latter group many would succeed under the multisensory syllable unit method, but still others would require an even more prescribed approach. The association phoneme unit method, derived from the work of Mildred McGuiness with first deaf, and then aphasic, children, is suggested as effective with some who fail to progress under other methods.

This highly specific method has the following characteristics:

1. Speech production associated with other language modalities. Individual phonemes are taught directly and precisely with emphasis on the development of motor memory. Correct production is immediately reinforced and associated with other forms of the phoneme through reading the graphic form, speechreading the sound, and writing, repeating, and listening to the sound.
2. The phoneme is the basic unit of instruction. Individual breath and voice phonemes are practiced to articulatory mastery. Once a number of phonemes are mastered they are blended in syllable form and drilled. Mastery of syllables leads to extension to words but does not replace individual phoneme practice.
3. Small increments of progress. A progression from phoneme to syllable to word is followed. As new phonemes are mastered in the prescribed sequence new syllables are learned and then new words. As words are mastered, simple sentences are introduced.

### Summary

Other professionals have suggested other terms and groupings for general approaches to speech instruction. However, those suggested by Calvert and Silverman (1975) are sufficiently inclusive to serve as guides for curriculum developers and speech instructors. They also reinforce a point made earlier: the hearing-impaired population is markedly heterogenous. A method suitable for one child, or for many, may not be suitable for others. This finding underlines the fact that speech curricula must be sufficiently flexible to meet many needs. Unfortunately, it is more often the case that a curriculum based on one approach is designed and it is left to the students to be flexible. Given the reality that most programs may not have the resources to develop a variety of curricula for students with varying needs, that it may not be possible to prepare teachers in discretely different methods, and the philosophy of some professionals that almost all students can benefit sufficiently under one curricular approach, it might well be decided to go with one basic system. Such a decision may not be reasonably argued against, but those taking it should be aware that others may see a need for a continuum of curricula to meet a continuum of needs.

## STATE OF KNOWLEDGE

Significant progress has been made in the recent past in the development of curricula, the improvement of auditory aids, the utilization of residual hearing, and the involvement of allied professionals in speech instruction with the hearing-impaired population. Nonetheless, respected professionals such as Moores (1982) have felt no qualms in advancing such statements as "Although most program directors view their approaches to the teaching of speech as eclectic, a better descriptor might be haphazard," and "A period of generations apparently has brought no improvements in techniques of teaching speech to the deaf." Countering this somewhat pessimistic view is that of other professionals in speech instruction who, with Ling (1976), would aver that "speech communication is a worthwhile goal and that high standards of speech production can be achieved through informed, systematic, and sustained effort," despite very real stumbling blocks to the attainment of that goal.

These stumbling blocks are of concern to those professionals charged with developing curricula which, properly implemented, will result in acceptable standards of speech production. A number of these, use of alternative communication systems, lack of proven effect, inadequacy of teacher preparation, and the heterogenity of the target population, have been reviewed. Others have been nominated as well.

1. Lack of knowledge about the processes of speech acquisition in the face of hearing impairment (Moores, 1982).
2. Lack of substantial relationship to and assistance from other general areas of study (Vorce, 1971).

3. The nonempirical nature of much of the research in speech (Calvert, 1986).

4. Insufficient use of available research information and clinical knowledge in speech assessment and development (Pronovost, 1979).

5. "Inadequate understanding, in qualitative and quantitative terms, of the speech of deaf children" (Moores, 1982).

6. Lack of follow-up studies to determine lasting effects of speech instruction (Silverman, Lane, & Calvert, 1978).

7. Paucity of theoretical models for instruction in speech for the deaf (DiCarlo, 1964; Moores, 1982).

8. Over-reliance on the teacher as the jack-of-all-trades in education of the hearing impaired, including being a sophisticated teacher of speech (Ross, 1976).

With such sizable obstacles in the path to acceptable speech production, it is surprising that so much progress has been made. At the end of this chapter specific curricula are reviewed. These have been found quite effective in many programs. Their authors have gathered up the various pieces of knowledge in speech instruction and produced workable curricula. It should not be argued that these have yielded across-the-board success, but many teachers, speech pathologists, and parents have found them effective. Before proceeding to these reviews, it will be valuable to examine general considerations in the design of any speech curricula.

## DESIGN OF SPEECH CURRICULA

Vorce (1971) pointed out that one characteristic that sets the designing of speech curricula apart from planning in other areas is a lack of "experimentation in speech content and methodology" and of models on which to base a curriculum. Vorce's point has been echoed by Calvert (1986), Erber (1980), Ling (1976), Moores (1982), and Silverman, Lane, and Calvert (1978) among others. It is accurate to say that models of speech acquisition among hearing-impaired individuals are few, and that the area of speech acquisition and development in general is relatively unresearched. Despite these shortcomings, a number of guidelines for the design of curricula are available. There has been an accretion of experience that may be shaped into principles and practice. These vary from the quite broad to the specific.

## The Environment

It is considered necessary to set broad conditions as a framework for the speech curriculum. There must be an environment conducive to the acquisition and development of speech for speech attempts and speech instruction to thrive. Magner (1971) stressed that "The child's parents, teachers, and peers must share in establishing an environment wherein the child might gain a desire and receive adequate practice in the utilization of speech as his chief means of communication." Vorce (1971) considered it essential that school and home together establish an environment in which the desire to talk is consistently stimulated and in which speech is the expected form of communication. Silverman, Lane, and Calvert (1978) noted the necessity of an environment "in which speech is experienced as a vitally significant and successful means of communication" be created.

Calvert (1986) listed five conditions for programs serious about speech instruction. These were:

**A POSITIVE INSTRUCTIONAL ATTITUDE TOWARD SPEECH.** If speech instruction is to succeed, those offering it must be convinced that it will succeed. This means that not only must teachers and parents be convinced, but that all others associated with the student must share this positive conviction. If such a condition exists, the child will respond positively as well.

**OPPORTUNITIES TO USE SPEECH WITHOUT MANUAL COMMUNICATION.** Central to this point is the expectation that every child will encounter individuals who do not use manual systems. The child must be aware of this and recognize and accept that speech will be the expected mode of communication in such situations. Calvert suggests that some individuals in the immediate environment with whom the child communicates should specifically not understand manual communication.

**ALL TEACHERS CONTRIBUTE TO TEACHING SPEECH.** Many professionals have believed and continue to believe that a "true" teacher of the hearing impaired is a teacher of speech. From our earlier discussion it is apparent that not all teachers believe themselves adequately prepared to teach speech. However, Calvert does not suggest that all *teach* speech. The suggestion is that all *contribute* and that this contribution might take various forms. The idea that all maintain a positive attitude and involve themselves in speech as appropriate for their abilities and training is put forward. Searls (1981) has offered comments on how the hearing-impaired teacher, too, can contribute to speech instruction in a realistic fashion. No teacher is to be left out.

**SOME STAFF MEMBER RESPONSIBLE FOR EACH CHILD'S SPEECH.** The concept here is that speech instruction, knowledge by all interested parties of speech progress, and continued effort will be facilitated if one person coordinates the individual program and is responsible for it being carried through. In this way no child will be left out and no program allowed to drift for lack of direction.

**MONITORED USE OF ACOUSTIC INFORMATION.** If speech instruction is to be given the maximum opportunity for success, the child must have maximum opportunity to use every available auditory clue. Regular attention to the routine provision of an auditory environment, to the availability of appropriate aids, and to the maintenance of those aids is required.

The aforementioned conditions are necessary aspects of providing an appropriate environment, particularly in programs where manual systems are also employed.

## Delineation of Objectives

In Chapter 1 it was noted that the choice of objectives governed much of curriculum design. Earlier in this chapter the point that the hearing-impaired population is a heterogenous one was made also. These two contentions come together in the design of speech curricula in a complex, yet simple, fashion. It is absolutely necessary, as Vorce (1971) stated, to declare general and specific objectives in speech curricula. Without such objectives a curriculum would lack guideposts for direction. Yet variables of hearing level, primary communication system, educational placement, teacher or pathologist expertise, and multihandicapping conditions suggest that different objectives might be necessary for different groups. This would introduce a formidable complexity into speech curriculum development. Simplicity, on the other hand, appears to be the choice of those stating objectives. The variables reviewed above are ignored and objectives are stated as if there were a homogenous hearing-impaired population. This may be the most sensible approach given the variety of possibly relevant determiners and the difficulty of producing a single well-designed curriculum, not to mention an array of differentiated curricula in one area.

Siebert (1980), Buckler (1980), and Cusack (1980) have provided a useful series of articles in which objectives from preschool through secondary school are presented. Together the articles suggest that there are common objectives across age levels, but that objectives do change both in type and emphasis. Siebert (1980) advanced the position that objectives derive from underlying principles that connect speech instruction at all levels. The principles of speech development of the St. Joseph Institute for the Deaf may be paraphrased as:

1. Speech is the right of all hearing-impaired children, regardless of individual differences.
2. Every teacher is a teacher of speech and responsible for the speech program of children in an assigned class.

3. Children have unique needs that must be considered in any program of speech instruction.
4. Individual strengths and weaknesses must be determined for appropriate application of the speech curriculum.
5. Speech development must proceed in an orderly manner, as it does in the nonhearing-impaired child.
6. Evaluation must be routine to determine areas of need, emerging skill, and established skill.
7. Auditory ability must be maximized and supplemented by visual and tactile systems as appropriate.
8. Careful attention must be paid to motor skills that control intelligible speech.
9. Speech must be taught directly with sufficient practice to result in mastery provided.
10. A relaxed yet demanding speech environment will best support speech development.

Without guiding principles, whether one agrees with these specifics or not, it will be difficult to develop a logically ordered and clear curriculum. Objectives must share common and acknowledged roots, if a rationalized curriculum is to result from any planning attempt.

Once guiding principles for a program are set out, more specific, though yet general, objectives may be stated. There is a process of working from the philosophical level of setting principles, to that of stating general and then more and more specific objectives (see Fig. 6-1). It is this process of increasing specificity that provides the teacher and pathologist with both the framework from which to work and the detailed objectives around which to plan individual lessons.

An example of this process may be found in tracing the sequence from general principle to specific lessons. Siebert (1980) stated the principle that speech is a learned skill and requires direction and practice. She also presented the general objective "To develop good breath control," and correct and precise breathing patterns are compulsory for intelligible speech. These patterns do not occur naturally and must be taught and practiced over a period of years according to some speech professionals. Instruction and practice are initiated early in speech work and continued as long as necessary. Ling (1976) operationalized the general objective of obtaining appropriate breath control into three parts:

1. The maintenance of a steady breath flow for continuous vocalization

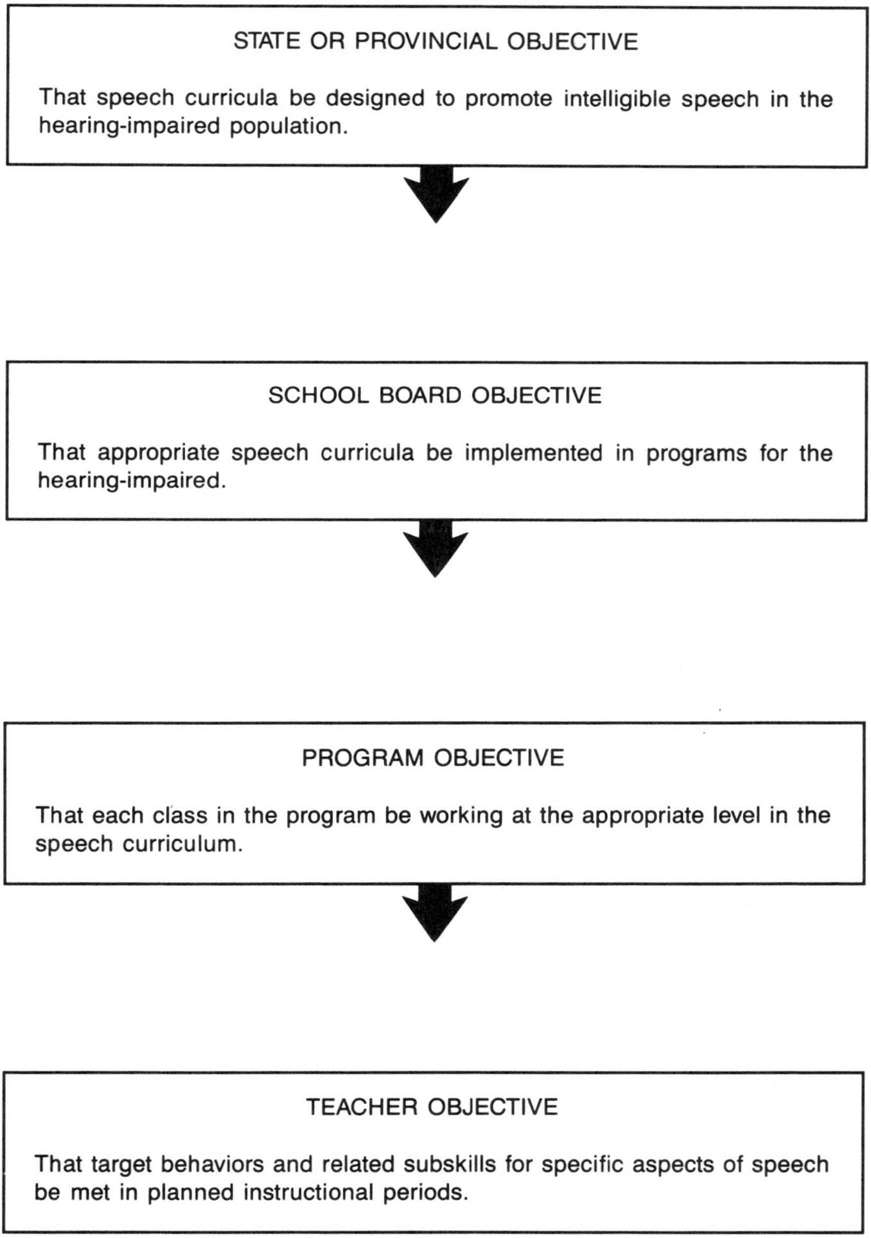

STATE OR PROVINCIAL OBJECTIVE

That speech curricula be designed to promote intelligible speech in the hearing-impaired population.

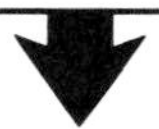

SCHOOL BOARD OBJECTIVE

That appropriate speech curricula be implemented in programs for the hearing-impaired.

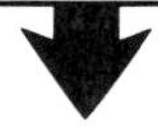

PROGRAM OBJECTIVE

That each class in the program be working at the appropriate level in the speech curriculum.

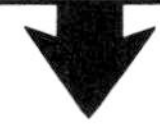

TEACHER OBJECTIVE

That target behaviors and related subskills for specific aspects of speech be met in planned instructional periods.

**Figure 6-1.** The process of object setting from general to specific for speech instruction.

2. The production of a pulsed breath stream in coordination with laryngeal and articulatory valving for sounds and syllables in running speech
3. The organization, through feedforward control, of intake and expenditure of breath in relation to the linguistic structure of the utterance

Ling then cited more detailed objectives and exercises suggested by Hudgins (1937). This process of moving from level-to-level in setting objectives is mandatory in the establishment of any worthwhile curriculum.

A particular difficulty interfaces with the easy accomplishment of this task, and it relates to the earlier-mentioned analytic and synthetic approaches to speech instruction. The practice of setting objective after objective in an accretional approach to the final assembly of some speech skill is attractive and practiced by a good many teachers. However, one can be overly analytical pursuing the mastery of splinter skills without due regard to synthesizing skills for adequate social communication. This must be discouraged.

Additionally, many areas requiring the statement and definition of objectives are not to be found for normal populations of speakers. This situation results in a conundrum for those who espouse adherence to developmental patterns of speech planned through contemporary psycholinguistic study for normally hearing individuals. What patterns does one follow when models are not to be found in other populations?

The statement of objectives presents a significant challenge to instructors in this area. In many ways the science is yet in its infancy with a great variety of areas yet to be clarified.

## Speech Development Models

One area that has attracted relatively little attention over the years is the elaboration and testing of a model of speech development in hearing-impaired individuals (Ling, 1976; Moores, 1982). Traditional practice has been to lay out a developmental schema for the sequential acquisition of phonemes in either isolation or combination, and to build to words and sentences in an analytic fashion while also encouraging spontaneous speech attempts. Though this practice may be considered to produce rather simplistic models that fail to utilize much presently available research information, such early models continue in use in many programs. The most popular sources for models of this type in the first half of the 20th century were Haycock (1933) and Yale (1946). Haycock suggested a sequence of sound development according to his appreciation of: (1) The nature of the sounds themselves and the organic activities involved in their production; and (2) The mental and sensory equipment of the child. Yale (1946) laid out a sequence of acquisition based on expediency of a "judicious order of teaching." Both arbitrary sequence models were accompanied by attention to aspects such as accent, rhythm, phrasing, and breathing.

Vorce (1974) presented a speech development model originally laid out by Van Riper (1963). This model followed generalized steps in normal speech development, moving from early reflex sounds and babbling to the specific stimulation and development of articulation, voice, rhythm, and language. From preschool-level informal work incorporating various sounds in guided utterances, the Vorce curriculum proceeded later to structured work with conscious practice on, and refinement of, vowels and consonants in substantially normal acquisitional order. Accompanying the early informal work and eventual structured work, is effort on voice quality, phrasing, and rhythm.

Ling (1976) offered a speech teaching model incorporating "the serial and parallel orders in which speech patterns are developed as well as economic and precise evaluation procedures which allow us to determine what phonetic and phonological patterns have been learned." The Ling model lays out seven acquisition stages at both the phonetic and phonologic levels. The first stage focusses on vocalization on demand, and stage two on development of suprasegmental patterns forming a general vocalization category. Stage three involves the teaching of all diphthongs and vowels and may be considered a category in itself. The final four stages involve teaching aspects of consonant production. Ling specified a number of target behaviors for each of the seven stages with each target behavior supported by a series of subskills. All of these contributed to the elaboration of a speech-teaching model considered by Ling to satisfy the philosophical and instructional beliefs of proponents of both natural or the synthetic approach. Following its publication in 1976, this model, and with it Ling's approach to the teaching of speech, became widely acclaimed and accepted. Ling's *Speech and the Hearing-Impaired Child* presently serves as the basic speech curriculum document in the majority of schools with a serious commitment to a speech program.

This short review of various models for the teaching of speech is not presented as anything other than a brief description of models that underlie curricula in various programs to various extent. It is presented to emphasize the fact that curriculum developers must have a model for the development of speech in mind. Curricular objectives and curricular activities rise directly from the model in use. The model forms the skeleton upon which the curriculum developer builds the body of the curriculum. If the model is simplistic, the curriculum may also be simplistic with all the implications for teaching and success implied by simplicity. Conversely if the model is elaborate, that, too, has implications for the curriculum. The importance of the selection of a model and the importance of a clear understanding of the philosophical and instructional implications rising from it cannot be overemphasized.

## SUMMARY

Speech instruction is an area of controversy in the education of hearing-impaired individuals and will continue to be so into the foreseeable future. Contributing to this controversy are the lack of overall success in obtaining intelligible speech and the availability of rather more easily mastered alternative communication methods. Other dynamics, such as the quality of teacher and pathologist preparation in speech and the variegated nature of the hearing-impaired population, also add to the controversy and to the general difficulty of ensuring continued effort in the speech instruction area.

These things, however significant, should not deter attempts to improve and to implement speech curricula. Speech is accepted as a desirable objective by the great majority of professionals working with hearing-impaired individuals. If it is to be an attainable objective, even for one hearing-impaired individual, logically planned, effective curricula must be available. In this respect, it is advisable to consider the types of curricular approaches and emphases in present use. It is not necessary to reinvent the wheel completely nor is it efficient, but it is necessary to consider evaluation of existing curricula, the principles that underlie them, models of speech development, and other major and minor areas related to speech instruction. At the same time, it is valuable to be aware of, and work on, less directly related areas, if speech instruction is to be as effective as possible.

## TYPE SPEECH RESOURCES IN REVIEW

*Speech* (Curriculum) The Clarke School for the Deaf (1971)

*Speech and Deafness* (Text and Curriculum) D.R. Calvert and S.R. Silverman (1975)

*Speech and the Hearing-Impaired Child* (Text and Curriculum) D. Ling (1976)

*Teaching Speech to Deaf Children* (Curriculum) E. Vorce (1974)

## *SPEECH*

### The Clarke School for the Deaf

*Publisher*:
The Clarke School for the Deaf
Northampton, Massachusetts 01060

*Skills taught*: Voice quality, articulation, speech rhythm

*Age/grade range*: Lower school, middle school, upper school; four years to seventeen years

*Group size*: Individual and group

**THEORY:** No statement of theory is made in the Clarke School speech curriculum beyond an indication "that profoundly deaf children can acquire the use of intelligible speech and that they have the right to learn the necessary oral skills in a manner as nearly like that of children with normal hearing as possible." Examination of the curricula reveals the belief that an environment conducive to oral communication can and must be established. In addition, a purely natural approach to speech instruction is considered most appropriate for the first few years of school. The analytic approach is introduced in time on an individually determined basis and then serves as the primary tool for speech development and correction. The natural method, though lessened in direct instructional importance, is continued as well.

**DESCRIPTION:** The Clarke School curriculum is pragmatic. It spends little time on philosophy and considerable time on the specifics of speech instruction.

The first section of the book is devoted to what might be termed the framework for the speech program. This framework includes:

1. A statement on how speech is coordinated throughout the school
2. The scheduling of speech (daily classes and lab work)
3. Systems for diagnosis and assessment
4. General aims for all levels and general approaches at each level
5. Detail of the Northampton vowel and consonant charts that provide the developmental model for the speech program.
6. Detail of the role and use of a dictionary system including a diacritical system.

These major aspects of the system, their purpose, and an indication of how they are used are described succinctly. Discussion of how these contribute to the development of an oral environment, to a natural approach, or to an analytic approach is minimal.

Delineations of problems, causes, and remediation techniques for each of voice, articulation, and speech rhythm form the midsection of the curriculum. Each of these three sections begins with a statement of the quite general objectives. Next problems, causes, and remedial techniques for type problems (omission of syllables, lack of accent, etc.) are detailed. Under the topic of voice, the problems addressed are:

Strength: (1) lacking voice; (2) lacking control of volume; (3) weakness; (4) harshness; and (5) breathiness.

Resonance: (1) hypernasality; and (2) hyponasality.

Placement: (1) high pitch; (2) low pitch; (3) gutteral voice; and (4) erratic changes.

Inflection: (1) lacking variation; and (2) erraticness.

Articulation problems are noted as:

General: (1) development or production of specific sounds; (2) knowledge of, and application of, Northampton charts; (3) grouping sounds in words and phrases; and (4) inappropriate movements.

Vowels: (1) duration; and (2) distinguishing between similarly formed vowels.

Consonants: (1) distinguishing between types of consonants; (2) consonant substitution; (3) arresting consonants; and (4) compound consonants and malarticulation.

Syllabification: (1) omission; and (2) addition.

Accent: (1) lack of accent; and (2) misplaced accent.

The problems of speech rhythm are: (1) lack of rhythm; (2) unnatural rhythm; and (3) rate of utterance.

The final chapter of the curriculum is given to the development in detail of a series of instructional practice exercises under:

1. Speech breathing
2. Voice
3. Articulation
4. Speech rhythm

The articulation section is supplemented by the presentation in an appendix of the classification, formation, and development of the Northampton Chart vowels and consonants.

**EVALUATION:** The Clarke School curriculum is a bare bones, no-nonsense curriculum. It is specific in detailing the bases of speech instruction at Clarke in the early 1970s, particularly the heavy reliance on the Northampton Charts and analytical methods of instruction. Though natural methods and the need for an oral environment are mentioned, the curriculum does not deal with their development to any real degree. A major strength of the curriculum is the careful specification of common errors of voice, articulation, and speech rhythm, possible causes of each, and suggested remedial techniques. The teacher or pathologist seeking a "how to" resource will find the Clarke curriculum attractive.

The curriculum may be criticized on a number of fronts. Those with an instructional philosophy favoring natural methods will find the analytical emphasis a problem. Those wishing a clear explication of a speech development model and a set order of teaching for vowels and consonants will not find them here. In addition, the heavy reliance on a visual coding system, such as the Northampton Charts, will make many uncomfortable. There is evidence that visual coding may interfere with the planning of oral utterances and speculation that over-reliance on a visual coding system will reduce attention to suprasegmental aspects of speech (Ling, 1976). Finally, some readers will find insufficient attention paid to assessment and diagnosis.

## *SPEECH AND DEAFNESS*

**D.R. Calvert and S.R. Silverman**

*Publisher*:
Alexander Graham Bell Association,
3417 Volta Place N.W.,
Washington, DC 20007

*Skills taught*: Aspects of speech, speech development, and the teaching of speech

*Age/grade range*: Preschool through secondary school

*Group size*: Individual or group

**THEORY:** Calvert and Silverman (1975) endorse the auditory global theory and method described earlier as the method of choice for all beginning hearing-impaired learners and for those who, at older ages, continue to benefit from this approach. They note that some individuals may reveal specific needs that suggest eventual use of the multisensory syllable unit method or the association phoneme unit method.

Underlying this acceptance of one preferred method with possible alternatives, is a view of the child as a person with varying needs, abilities, and potentialities. To the greatest degree possible, the teacher and parents must create an oral environment taking these characteristics into account, while pursuing natural language and speech acquisition.

**DESCRIPTION:** *Speech and deafness* is more than an attempt to present a speech instruction curriculum. Although it does present sections on methodology, phoneme development, and articulation, it also deals with topics providing the teacher education background necessary for the study and practice of speech instruction. It is a discussive text rather than a prescriptive one.

Speech and the production of speech provide the content of Chapter 1. Articulation, voice, and rhythm are nominated as the primary factors influencing intelligibility and are reviewed in some detail. Under articulation phonemes, orthographic systems (largely the Northampton Chart system), place of production (functions of physical parts of articulatory mechanism), manner of production (stops, fricatives, affricatives, and resonants), perceptual features of articulation, and coarticulation are discussed. The section on voice includes production and perceptual features of voice. Production of rhythm, rhythm features, and perceptual features of speech rhythm fall under the rhythm section in the concluding section of the chapter.

Significant influences on speech (the student, the environment, and the school program) are reviewed in Chapter 2. Selected characteristics and attributes of the student are presented as requiring consideration. Among these are physical growth and maturation, sensory abilities, and learning abilities. Environmental factors are noted as language-generating experiences, oral environment, and carry-over from classroom to total environment. Lastly an oral environment in the school and systematic instruction as basic to a speech instruction program are discussed.

Ling contributed Chapter 3 on amplification for speech. The utility of the hearing aid as a tool for the development of speech is noted and a review of technical aspects of hearing aids offered. A short section on auditory cues, such as intensity in voicing and feature recognition, follows. This, in turn, is followed by an examination of acoustic cues, hearing aids, and hearing levels. An imposing amount of technical information is presented in a few packed pages.

Chapter 4 deals with the production of individual phonemes. Each phoneme is reviewed under five areas:

1. Production
2. Internal feedback information
3. Sensory instructional possibilities
4. Suggestions for development
5. Common errors and suggestions for improvement

Methods of developing speech provide the focus of Chapter 5. The auditory global method, the multisensory syllable unit method, and the association phoneme method are reviewed in terms of fundamental characteristics, which method to choose, and when. The authors present four guides for the choice of method:

1. The method should be appropriate for very young children whenever they are identified.
2. The method should provide maximum opportunity for each child to develop his or her hearing ability, regardless of early estimates of the nature and degree of hearing loss.
3. The method should provide an opportunity to identify other disabilities that might affect speech development.
4. The method should provide sufficient experience for assessing progress in speech development (Calvert & Silverman, 1975).

The final chapter treats the continuance of speech instruction past initial development to speech improvement. The need to signal the occurrence of speech errors, to specify identifying characteristics of an error, and to correct the error is stressed. The balance of the chapter is devoted to methods of correction (errors of articulation, voice, and rhythm), the maintenance of speech, and some final comments on diagnosis.

The *scales of early communication skills for hearing-impaired children* are presented in a short appendix. The text concludes with an annotated bibliography of resources and suggested readings.

**EVALUATION:** Speech and deafness provides a valuable examination of a variety of topics related to speech instruction as well as presenting curricular material directly related to that topic. To some degree the text is so wide-ranging that the curricular materials appear to be secondary to such issues as the need to use amplification appropriately and to understand the characteristics of alternate instructional methods.

The decisions to include considerable allied material, to include in chapter form details on phoneme production better relegated to an appendix, and to not include a discussion of one particular model of speech development lent a somewhat unfocussed air to the book. On the other hand the emphasis on a natural approach, the use of all available sensory avenues, and the realization that no one instructional approach is appropriate for all are strong points.

This text would serve as a valuable resource for curriculum development and as a support reference for practitioners.

## *SPEECH AND THE HEARING-IMPAIRED CHILD: Theory and Practice*

**D. Ling**

*Publisher*:
Alexander Graham Bell Association
3417 Volta Place N.W.
Washington, DC 20007

*Skills taught*: Theory, practice, and evaluation of speech instruction

*Age/grade range*: Preschool through secondary school

*Group size*: Group and individual

**THEORY:** Ling supports the position that hearing-impaired children with a range of hearing losses can learn to speak intelligibly if appropriate methods of instruction are employed by appropriately trained professionals and speech is expected by teachers, parents, and others. It is assumed that language acquisition will proceed in a normal development pattern and that the phonetic and phonologic levels of speech will be acquired through stimulation and direct teaching in parallel order.

A model for speech acquisition is put forth. Through it speech is viewed as a developmental process consisting of seven sequential stages. These are:

| Phonetic Level | Phonologic Level |
|---|---|
| Vocalizes on demand | Vocalization for communication |
| Development of suprasegmental patterns | Meaningful use of suprasegmental patterns |
| Development of vowels and diphthongs with voice control | Use of different vowels to approximate words |
| Development of consonants by manner | Clear use of some words with good voice patterns |
| Development of consonants by manner and place | Continued addition of words said clearly and with good voice patterns |
| Development of consonants by manner, place, and voicing | Continued addition of words said clearly with good voice patterns |
| Development of initial and final blends | Generalized intelligible speech with natural voice patterns |

Each stage is developed and reinforced through a series of target behaviors reached by attention to requisite subskills.

Ling suggests that his model is independent of any particular approach to speech instruction and will fit equally well into a natural or analytic system.

**DESCRIPTION:** The text may be divided roughly into two sections: The first deals with a review of existing knowledge in speech production and provides a base for a developmental model and the second presents the model and details teaching needs and procedures.

Ling does a masterful job of compiling and presenting both research knowledge and knowledge gained through extensive experience in the first chapters of his text. They are examined in critical fashion. As a result of this wide-ranging review Ling suggests that sufficient knowledge is available for considerable success in speech instruction, even though some areas remain inadequately researched. The general low levels of progress in speech are attributed to insufficient application of existing knowledge and poor teaching. Topics covered in this early section are:

1. Studies of speech production
2. Sense modalities in speech reception
3. Multisensory speech reception
4. Feedback and feedforward mechanisms in speech production
5. Sense modalities in speech production
6. Levels of speech acquisition and automaticity
7. Teaching order
8. Evaluation of speech

Ling's speech model is described in Chapter 10, the first chapter of several that are focussed on the actual teaching of speech. In this chapter the relationship of target behaviors and subskills to a stage within the model is addressed. Subsequent chapters deal directly with major aspects of speech development, proceeding from stage one to stage seven of the model. The majority of these chapters present target behaviors, subskills, and teaching strategies. There is sufficient discussion of such points as the mechanisms of breathing and voicing, the acoustic properties and sensory correlates of consonants, and the treatment of deviant patterns in development to render this section more than a simple iteration of teaching needs and ideas. Indeed, throughout the text, care is taken to explain clearly, without patronizing the reader, and to expand as required for clarification and coherence.

**EVALUATION:** *Speech for the Hearing-Impaired* child is by far the leading curricular resource in speech. The development of a speech model for hearing-impaired children is clear and logical, if not always based firmly on sufficient research knowledge. The delineation of target behaviors, subskills, and teaching strategies will gladden the heart of any teacher of speech. Although it is possible to criticize aspects of this text (DiCarlo, 1976; Springer, MacDougall, & Mattingly, 1977; Moores, 1982), the criticisms offered will not detract from the value of the publication in the eyes of most frontline professionals.

## *TEACHING SPEECH TO DEAF CHILDREN*

**E. Vorce**

*Publisher*:
Alexander Graham Bell Association,
3417 Volta Place N.W.,
Washington, DC 20007

*Skills taught*: Voice quality, rhythm and phrasing, articulation of vowels and consonants

*Age/grade range*: Preschool through secondary school

*Group size*: Individual and group

**THEORY:** Speech is the spoken component of language that precedes and controls speech. Although the hearing-impaired individual requires a longer period of time to develop speech, the manner and order of acquisition are basically similar to that of the normally hearing child. The auditory, visual, tactual, and kinesthetic channels contribute to speech acquisition in a multisensory system, with auditory amplification of prime importance, as it is mandatory for consistent and acceptable self monitoring.

Speech develops according to the following sequence:

1. Reflex sounds
2. Babbling
3. Socialized vocal play
4. First words
5. Phrases and sentences; jargon
6. Articulation; voice; rhythm; language

At each of these levels teacher and parent intervention and stimulation is required to facilitate acquisition of pleasant voice quality, rhythm and phrasing, and eventual correct articulation and pronunciation.

**DESCRIPTION:** *Teaching Speech to Deaf Children* is divided into three definable sections: theory, process, and overall plan; speech plans for school divisions; and teaching ideas and evaluation.

Chapter 2, on theory, process, and overall plan, is devoted to a discussion of how an environment conducive to the development of speech is established. The need to regard speech as the vocal component of language is emphasized. Work on phonological skills is bereft of meaning unless that work is directed toward the development of functional language. The goal of speech work is realized only "when the child is able to *use* his ability to produce the phonemic and prosodic features of speech to *communicate his ideas and feelings to others*" (Vorce, 1974).

This goal is reached through considerations of, and action on, a number of features in the environment. Among these are:

1. Psychological aspects: The teacher and parents must affirm that the child is valued beyond the ability to acquire speech.
2. School variables: The school must accept and fulfill its responsibilities with regard to human and material resource.
3. Teacher skill: Teachers must be skilled and must hold consistent realistically high expectations in speech.
4. Philosophy and teaching model: The school must develop a philosophy focussed on speech and language acquisition. To enact this philosophy a comprehensive teaching model for development and correction of speech is suggested. Vorce supplies ideas for setting a daily schedule, routine checking of hearing aids, and the planning of speech work.

Chapter 3 presents an organizational plan for speech work. Van Riper's (1963) developmental model (noted under theory) is briefly described. Short discussions of aspects of work on voice, rhythm and phrasing, articulation, and pronunciation are provided. The balance of the chapter provides general listings of a hierarchy of skills (vocalization, intonation, producing the correct number of syllables, and accurate phonemic and phonetic content), teacher behavior, teaching strategies, levels for phoneme development (imitation, localization, localization for manner, localization for place, analogy for manner, analogy for place, and manipulation), and levels for correction (awareness of communication process, vocalization for attention or communication, understanding of the communicative process, specialized vocal play, application of speech skills, specific speech work, and direct application). Through these discussions and listings, the major features contributing to an organizational plan are nominated, though it would be perhaps too interpretive to state that a cohesively ordered plan is described.

Vorce uses the school divisions of the Lexington School as the framework for her discussion of speech plans for school divisions, a specified developmental plan for the teaching of speech. Separate and relatively detailed outlines for the speech work of preschool, lower school, intermediate school, and secondary school are provided. For all areas, comments specific to the teaching of voice, phrasing and rhythm, articulation of vowels and consonants, and pronunciation are noted. In addition, aspects specific to any one school division are presented.

The final two chapters of the Vorce curriculum focus on aspects related to speech instruction in supportive fashion. First among these is a series of activities and resources that might contribute to speech instruction. Among these are teaching ideas for using records and tapes, language masters and auto flash cards, commercial visual materials for articulation practice, displays and instruments useful for speech monitoring, and speech material.

Speech evaluation is the topic of the second-to-the-last chapter of the curriculum. The need for consistent evaluation and the maintenance of complete records is emphasized. Varieties of school-wide reports and the content of departmental or school division reports are noted in detail. No discussion of how to evaluate speech or which instruments might be most useful are given, though the need for careful selection of methods and tools is stressed.

**EVALUATION:** Vorce produced a valuable curriculum that continues to serve as a resource to many programs and can serve well as one of a number of guides to the writing of future curricula. The emphasis on use of a natural method of speech instruction and the linking of speech and functional language are positive points. Also positive is the emphasis on utilization of residual hearing and the concept of establishing a conducive auditory and speech environment. Teaching suggestions for school divisions, particularly those relating to phonological-level work, are clear and logical.

*Teaching Speech to Deaf Children* suffers at times due to a lack of sufficient closure in some main areas. Listings of points and ideas, though valuable in themselves, are not firmly wrapped up and interrelated. Also, philosophical points are not precisely linked to teaching ideas. This is not a major problem but it contributes a choppiness to the text, and is particularly characteristic of those chapters dealing with process and organizational plans.

The section on evaluation is somewhat disappointing. After quite valuable, teacher-oriented suggestions throughout the latter half of the text, the discussion of evaluation appears as administratively oriented and general. This is not to suggest that what is said is not of value. It is. The comments on the place of speech intelligibility assessment in evaluation are quite helpful. However, the teacher or pathologist who looks for specific recommendations for techniques or tools will look in vain.

This resource remains one of the primary contributions to the field.

## REFERENCES


Bender, R. (1960). *The conquest of deafness.* Cleveland, OH: Press of Case Western Reserve University.

Bishop, M.E. (1979). Mainstreaming: A goal or a process? In M.E. Bishop (Ed.), *Mainstreaming*. Washington, DC: Alexander Graham Bell Association, pp. 33-47.

Boothroyd, A.L. (1983). Pre-conference recommendations. In. J.D. Subtelny (Ed.), *Speech assessment and speech improvement for the hearing impaired.* Washington, DC: Alexander Graham Bell Association, pp. 395-397.

Buckler, J. (1980). Speech training for the hearing impaired: Principles, objectives, and strategies for the intermediate level. In J.D. Subtelny (Ed.), *Speech assessment and speech improvement for the hearing impaired.* Washington, DC: Alexander Graham Bell Association, pp. 111-117.

Calvert, D.R. (1986). Speech in perspective. In D.M. Luderman, *Deafness in perspective.* San Diego, CA: College-Hill Press, pp. 166-191.

Calvert, D.R., & Silverman, S.R. (1975). *Speech and deafness.* Washington, DC: Alexander Graham Bell Association.

Clarke School for the Deaf. (1971). *Speech.* Northampton, MA: Author.

Cusack, M. (1980). Speech training for the hearing impaired: Principles, objectives, and strategies for the secondary level. In J.D. Subtelny (Ed.), *Speech assessment and speech improvement for the hearing impaired.* Washington, DC: Alexander Graham Bell Association, pp. 118-126.

Dale, D.M.C. (1971). Social aspects of speech. In L. Connor (Ed.), *Speech for the deaf child: Knowledge and use.* Washington, DC: Alexander Graham Bell Association, pp. 183-204.

DiCarlo, L.M. (1964). *The deaf.* Englewood Cliffs, NJ: Prentice-Hall.

DiCarlo, L.M. (1976). *Speech and the hearing-impaired child: Theory and practice* (Review). *Volta Review, 78,* 228-230.

Erber, N.P. (1980). Speech correction through the use of acoustic models. In J.D. Subtelny (Ed.), *Speech assessment and speech improvement for the hearing impaired.* Washington, DC: Alexander Graham Bell Association, pp. 222-241.

Griffiths, C. (1967). *Conquering childhood deafness.* New York, NY: Exposition Press.

Haycock, G.S. (1933). *The teaching of speech.* Washington, DC: Volta Bureau.

Hogan, J.H. (1980). Pre-conference recommendations. In J.D. Subtelny (Ed.), *Speech assessment and speech impovement for the hearing impaired.* Washington, DC: Alexander Graham Bell Association, pp. 390-395.

Hudgins, C.V. (1937). Voice production and breath control in the speech of the deaf. *American Annals of the Deaf, 82,* 338-363.

Jensema, C., Karchmer, M., & Trybus, R. (1978). *The rated speech intelligibility of hearing-impaired children.* Washington, DC: Office of Demographic Studies, Gallaudet College.

Ling, D. (1976). *Speech and the hearing-impaired child: Theory and practice.* Washington, DC: Alexander Graham Bell Association.

Ling, D. (1981). A survey of methods in English speaking countries for the development of receptive and expressive oral skills. In A.M. Mulholland (Ed.), *Oral education today and tomorrow.* Washington, DC: Alexander Graham Bell Association, pp. 81-94.

Ling, D., & Ling, A.H. (1978). *Aural habilitation.* Washington, DC: Alexander Graham Bell Association.

McGinnis, M.A. (1963). *Aphasic children.* Washington, DC: Alexander Graham Bell Association, pp. 25-45.

Magner, M.E. (1971). Techniques of teaching. In L.E. O'Connor (Ed.), *Speech for the deaf child.* Washington, DC: Alexander Graham Bell Association, pp. 245-264.

Markides, A. (1970). The speech of deaf and partially-hearing children with special reference to factors affecting intelligibility. *British Journal of Disorders of Communication, 5,* 126-140.

Moores, D. (1978). *Educating the deaf.* Boston: Houghton Mifflin.

Moores, D. (1982). *Educating the deaf* (2nd ed.). Boston: Houghton Mifflin.

Mulholland, A.M. (1981). The philosophical bases of oral education. In A.M. Mulholland (Ed.), *Oral education today and tomorrow.* Washington, DC: Alexander Graham Bell Association.

Pollack, D. (1964). Acoupedics: A unisensory approach to auditory training. *Volta Review, 66,* 400-409.

Pollack, D. (1970). *Educational audiology for the limited hearing infant.* Springfield, IL: C.C. Thomas.

Pronovost, W. (1979). Speech assessment and speech improvement for the hearing impaired. *Volta Review, 81,* 511-514.

Ross, M. (1976). Verbal communication: The state of the art. *Volta Review, 78,* 324-328.

Scouten, E.L. (1984). *Turning points in the education of deaf people.* Danville, IL: Interstate.

Searls, S.C. (1981). Classroom management of speech instruction by a hearing-impaired teacher. *Directions, 2,* 49.

Shane, H.C. (1985). Selection of augmentative communication systems. In E. Cherow (Ed.), *Hearing-impaired children and youth with developmental disabilities.* Washington, DC: Gallaudet College Press, pp. 270-292.

Siebert, R. (1980). Speech training for the hearing impaired: Principles, objectives, and strategies for preschool and elementary levels. In J.D. Subtelny (Ed.), *Speech assessment and speech improvement for the hearing impaired.* Washington, DC: Alexander Graham Bell Association, pp. 102-110.

Silverman, S.R., Lane, H.S., & Calvert, D.R. (1978). Early and elementary education. In H. Davis & S.R. Silverman (Eds.), *Hearing and deafness.* New York, NY: Holt, Rinehart, & Winston, pp. 433-482.

Springer, S., MacDougall, J.C., & Mattingly, S. (1977). Speech and the hearing-impaired child: Theory and practice (Review). *American Annals of the Deaf, 122,* 305-306.

Stewart, J., Pollack, D., & Downs, M. (1964). A unisensory approach for the limited hearing child. *American Speech and Hearing Association, 6,* 151-154.

Stremel-Campbell, K. (1982). The development of language in the mentally retarded hearing-impaired child: Instructional methods. In D. Tweedie & E.H. Shroyer (Eds.), *The multihandicapped hearing impaired.* Washington, DC: Galludet College Press, pp. 211-248.

Subtelny, J.D., Webster, P.E., & Murphy, L.C. (1980). Personnel preparation for teaching speech to the hearing impaired: Current status and recommendations. In J.D. Subtelny (Ed.), *Speech assessment and speech improvement for the hearing* impaired. Washington, DC: Alexander Graham Bell Association, pp. 366-388.

Van Riper, C. (1963). *Speech correction: Principles and methods* (4th ed.). Englewood Cliffs, NJ: Prentice-Hall.

Vernon, M. (1982). Multihandicapped deaf children: Types and causes. In D. Tweedie & E.H. Shroyer (Eds.), *The multihandicapped hearing impaired*. Washington, DC: Gallaudet College Press, pp. 11-28.

Vorce, E. (1971). Speech curriculum. In L. Connor (Ed.), *Speech for the deaf child: Knowledge and use*. Washington, DC: Alexander Graham Bell Association, pp. 221-244.

Vorce, E. (1974). *Teaching speech to deaf children*. Washington, DC: Alexander Graham Bell Association.

Yale, C.A. (1946). *Formation and development of elementary English sounds.* Northampton, MA: The Clarke School for the Deaf.

# CHAPTER 7

# *Aural Habilitation Curricula*

It is commonly assumed that a hearing-impaired individual cannot hear but must use visual, tactile, and kinesthetic information in order to learn. In reality, hearing impairment is not an "all-or-nothing" phenomenon. It can range from a mild deficit that causes little handicap to total loss of the sensory function, which is extremely rare. Most hearing-impaired persons have some residual hearing and many, depending on how much and how successfully that hearing can be amplified and processed by the individual, may be able to learn through the auditory sense. It is the task of teachers and therapists who work with hearing-impaired students to design effective aural habilitation curricula to maximize the use of residual hearing. Degree of residual hearing is determined in the following manner.

During audiological testing, the audiologist presents pure tones through ear phones to the child to determine how loud a sound must be at each frequency in order for the child to detect it. Each ear is tested individually and plotted on a graph called an audiogram. The right ear is represented by O-O-O and the left by X-X-X. Hearing aids are fitted and the test redone. The aided response, that with the hearing aids on, is plotted using the symbols A-A-A. The hearing aid with the most beneficial characteristics is then recommended. Sometimes a child can be amplified into the normal range of hearing; but more often, a gap is still apparent between the loudness needed by the hearing-impaired child to detect sound and that needed by a person with normal hearing. This gap between the aided responses and normal hearing limits is called the sensitivity gap. The aided responses help to indicate how well or poorly a hearing aid is helping the child detect sound. It is not a measure of how well the child uses his amplified hearing to discriminate, identify, or comprehend speech but may indicate his potential to do so. A teacher or therapist can use the aided response information to set auditory goals (Fig. 7-1).

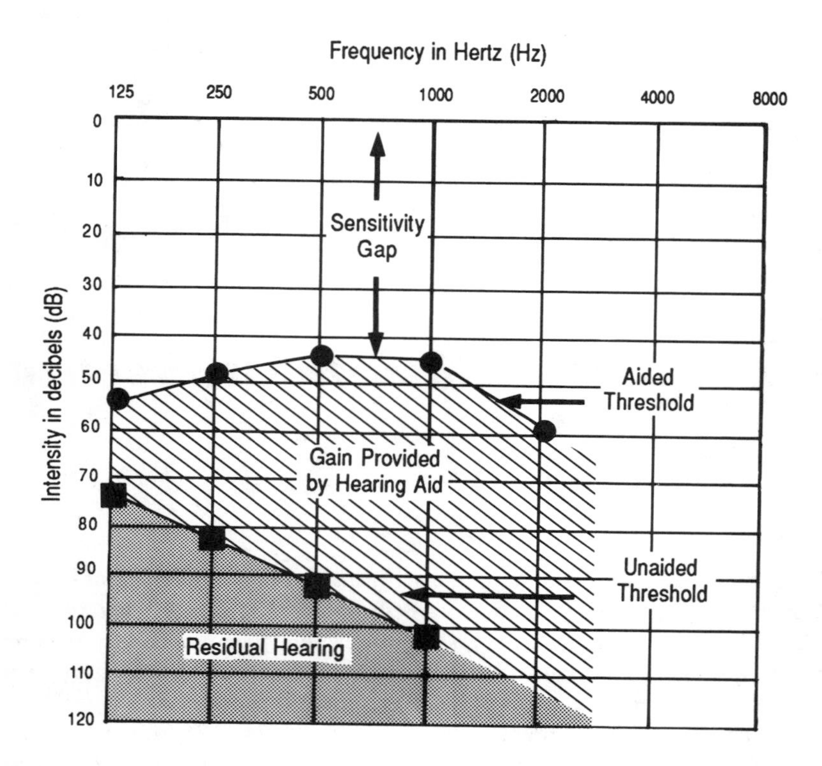


**Figure 7-1.** An audiogram showing the unaided and aided hearing thresholds of an individual. The difference between the two is a measure of gain provided by the hearing aid. The fact that a hearing aid cannot fully compensate for the loss is indicated by the sensitivity gap. From Ling, D., and Ling, A.H. (1978). *Aural habilitation.* Washington, D.C.: Alexander Graham Bell Association. © 1978 by the Alexander Graham Bell Association. Reprinted by permission.

Aural habilitation is the process of reproducing for a deaf child, as nearly as possible, the conditions by which a hearing child learns to hear and talk (Whetnall & Fry, 1971). A hearing baby listens to language and responds with smiles, gestures, and babbling sounds for many months before beginning to use speech for communication. A hearing-impaired child, once amplification is in use, needs to hear speech at levels in excess of background noise, and in meaningful situations, for many months before expressive language can be expected. As with the hearing child, he or she needs time to listen and play with new sounds, to gather meaning from sounds and develop a need for both verbal and nonverbal communication. Ling and Ling (1978) considered aural habilitation to be the foundation for verbal learning. Audition is the natural sense for speech reception and its role can be given primary emphasis even with the hearing-impaired child. This primary emphasis may be achieved through the process known as aural habilitation.

Aural habilitation requires fitting the child with the most appropriate hearing aids, having good audiological management, supporting and educating the parents, and supplying the child with auditory experiences of spoken language that are meaningful and appropriate to the child's age and interests. Lenneberg (1967), Harris (1973), Pollack (1970), Vaughan (1981), Erber (1982), and Paterson (1982) all discussed the importance of using audition as it is the fastest, most economical means of acquiring spoken language. Most hearing-impaired children have intact central nervous systems and therefore the brain capacity for processing spoken language (Lenneberg, 1967; Ling & Ling, 1978; Paterson, 1982). Most have residual hearing and obtain benefit in language development from amplification (Boothroyd, 1976; D. Ling, 1976; Ross & Giolas, 1978). Consequently, since cognition and language are essential to learning (Piaget, 1955), it is wise to make as much use as possible of residual hearing. Ling & Ling (1978) stated that:

> The central nervous system of a hearing-impaired child, unless severe brain damage is also involved, is tuned by nature to process spoken language patterns. The problem faced in aural habilitation is, essentially, how best to supply the child's central nervous system with verbal patterns that are sufficiently clear and sufficiently frequent to activate this processing capability and to develop it.

The concept of using residual hearing is relatively new. Goldstein, (1939), was one of the earliest to try to teach children using an acoustic method. He used ear trumpets to amplify sound directly into a child's ear. He was convinced that the child would hear if only the sound was loud enough. He had some success but mostly used environmental sounds rather than seeking comprehension of speech.

In the 1940s people became interested in a multisensory approach (combining lipreading, auditory, and vibrotactile information). The development of hard-wired amplification (children under headphones connected to a teacher's microphone) provided even very deaf children with the opportunity to augment their lipreading skills with amplified acoustic information. This system was used during lesson-time only and amplification was still not an all-day, integral part of the child's auditory system. Most of the day the child remained in a signal to noise environment that was not adequate for hearing language. The multisensory approach continued to be promoted as the curricular approach of choice (Ewing & Ewing, 1961; van Uden, 1977; Whetnall & Fry, 1971). Success was experienced by many children with moderate and severe hearing impairments when visual information tended to fill-in what was missing auditorily. Less satisfactory results were obtained by the profoundly deaf. To achieve maximum benefit in all areas of the child's life, teachers began to involve parents more as natural teachers of their hearing-impaired children.

This was an important development as it placed the child in a more optimal listening and learning environment all day and not just when the teacher of the deaf was present.

In the 1960s and 1970s, the expanding electronics industry led to miniaturization of hearing aids and to higher powered aids. Children began to use binaural fittings more routinely. This allowed the two ears to complement each other by using whatever ear had the better threshold at each frequency. There is a binaural summation effect of wearing two hearing aids that allows a sound presented at a given intensity to be heard as louder than the same sound presented to one ear. Children require less output from two aids in order to reach a comfortable listening level. It also appears that optimal development of both hemispheres of the brain can be better realized when information enters through both ears.

A further beneficial development at this time was the design of several types of wireless systems for classroom use—magnetic induction loops, radio frequency transmissions and infrared radiation. These devices improved the acoustic environment considerably, allowed greater mobility, and, therefore, more natural interaction between teacher and child.

Because the multisensory method was not uniformly successful and because of better amplification, instruction shifted to a unisensory or acoupedic approach. More babies were diagnosed and aided, so that very early training could begin. Pollack (1970), Grammatico (1975), and Beebe, Pearson, and Koch (1984) were among the first who advocated a new curricular approach emphasizing unisensory methods. Individual instruction rather than group work was encouraged. Full mainstreaming into regular classrooms became a major goal. Hearing aids were worn during all waking hours and mothers became the primary teachers under the guidance of a teacher therapist. It remains controversial whether or not all hearing-impaired children can learn by this method (Erber, 1982). However, it does seem plausible that children with hearing across all frequencies could be expected to do better using an acoupedic method than ones with a left-corner audiogram (Ling, 1978). Many feel all children, regardless of the amount of residual hearing, should begin with an auditory learning program in order to develop language in the most natural way possible. Our language is acoustic in nature and the more one can learn through listening, the more complete one's language can be.

More sophisticated hearing aids, superior earmolds, the use of mold and tubing adaptations, hearing aid filters, and upcoming digital aids, are constantly changing our expectations of what a hearing-impaired child can hear and use to increase his or her awareness of speech and language. The development of cochlear implants (House, 1976) is giving the totally deaf person a new opportunity to detect and discriminate timing and intensity cues. Although this is very limited information, it can be enough to alert deaf individuals and allow them to feel more secure in their environment. Pickett and McFarland (1985) discussed the success of single-channel versus multichannel cochlear implants. Multichannel implants of various kinds are under intense evaluation with groups of postlingually deaf adults. All implants give useful timing and intensity cues, but the question remains whether or not a multichannel system would give more speech information than a single-channel system. In all experiments, results varied widely. There were some star subjects who did very well. Pickett and McFarland (1985) suggested that success may depend on the listener's use of word predictability and knowledge of sentence structure, and to the listener's individual auditory nerve response to the electrical stimulation.

Some children have now been fitted with single channel House implants and have learned to discriminate auditorily between one- and two-syllable words. Children have not yet received multichannel implants. Experimentation will continue on postlingually deaf adult subjects who can be tested accurately before multichannel implant and who have language skills to draw on.

Implants are invasive and have possible potential for damaging the auditory system (Schein, 1984). Pickett and McFarland (1985) suggested that high-gain hearing aids often function like vibrators for the profoundly deaf. Perhaps even higher gain aids should be developed and fitted on deaf children before implants are permanently inserted. More development and experimentation needs to be done before we can clearly evaluate the impact cochlear implants may have for the profoundly deaf individual in the future.

Technological changes in equipment have a continuing positive impact on our expectations for hearing-impaired children and it is essential that teachers regard this as part of their continuing education. For all of these technological and pedagogical reasons, aural habilitation has become a major focus of contemporary curricular attempts.

## AN AURAL HABILITATION PROGRAM

An aural habilitation program includes providing an environment for hearing-impaired children in which they can use auditory information to develop verbal communication skills. Once the environment is optimal, a premeditated language and speech program, based on what is known about normal language development, is presented. This can be done in a structured or natural way depending upon the learning style of the child. Teachers with a firm understanding of normal language and speech development must be flexible in their style to meet the individual needs of the child.

Audiological management, including the use and care of appropriate hearing aids, is the first and major part of any aural habilitation program. If the aids are not in use, not appropriate for the individual, or are broken, one cannot expect the habilitation to succeed. The audiogram must be studied carefully and the aided responses of each child compared to the acoustics of speech. It must be assured as much as possible that the child can detect and discriminate what is asked of him. Many teachers have been unrealistic in the past by failing to acknowledge that each child has limits to his auditory potential. Conversely, many teachers have failed to recognize the auditory potential of their pupils and offered visual information when auditory would have succeeded (Table 7-1). However, an audiogram can be misleading and requires checking. A technique such as the Ling 5 sound test (Ling, 1978) will identify which frequencies the child can detect. Curricula must provide examples of, or references for, such techniques to assist teachers and therapists in understanding the auditory abilities of their students.

One must also provide a good acoustic environment (quiet, little reverberation, and a teacher who is close to the child), a wide range of normal auditory experiences, and finally, auditory training, to formally teach skills that should be acoustically available to the child, but for one reason or another are not learned in a natural way. Ling (1978), emphasized that the greater the hearing loss the more important auditory training becomes.

Auditory training consists of a hierarchy of speech detection, discrimination, identification, and comprehension of language, skills that are described later in detail. It can also include memory and localization skills.

Aural habilitation is an all-and everyday activity. Although it is easy to prepare the requirements of a good aural habilitation program, it is difficult to assure its appropriate implementation. Everyone involved with the child must become knowledgable and participate in developing auditory learning skills. Attention must be paid to the following basic components of an aural habilitation curriculum:

1. Early diagnosis of the hearing loss and early training
2. Consistent use of appropriate amplification
3. Good acoustic environment
4. Natural auditory experience
5. Auditory training
6. Knowledgeable and flexible teachers and parents

## Early Diagnosis

Many researchers have stressed the importance of early diagnosis of the hearing loss as relating to successful language acquisition (Fry, 1978; Fry & Whetnall, 1954; Lenneberg, 1967; Moores, 1981; Rhoades, 1982). Both hearing and hearing-impaired infants begin crying, cooing, and babbling during the first six months of life. Hearing infants get pleasurable feedback from their efforts and proceed to imitation and parroting sounds. Hearing-impaired infants do not receive this feedback without amplification, and so discontinue their

**Table 7-1.** Aided Response Auditory Expectations: An Interpretation of the Acoustics of Speech when Superimposed on a Child's Aided Audiogram.

| If the Aided Responses are within the speech banana to this Frequency. | The child should have the Potential to: |
|---|---|
| 500 Hz | Detect the fundamental frequency; discriminate duration, loudness, and pitch; discriminate voiced/voiceless contrasts |
| 1000 Hz | Detect all vowels; discriminate consonant manner contrasts |
| 3000 Hz | Discriminate all vowels |
| 4000 Hz | Discriminate consonant place of articulation contrasts |

babbling. Stoel-Gammon and Otomo (1986) reported that hearing-impaired babies with early amplification demonstrated babbling that was near normal and language acquisition proceeded. Hasenstab (1983) suggested that language acquisition is enmeshed with cognitive, social and emotional development and can enhance or restrict all components of growth. Koegel and Felsenfeld (1977) suggested that lack of early and systematic auditory stimulation caused neurological deterioration. This implies that the earlier amplification is in place and stimulation begun, the better the outcome might be. Erber (1982) demonstrated that the main objective of aural habilitation is to help hearing-impaired children learn to communicate through speech, and the best speech results come from the use of early and consistent acoustic methods.

In reality, many hearing-impaired children are not diagnosed early, or even within the critical first 3 years of life, and so early training is often not an option. Many curricula assume early diagnosis (Beebe et al., 1984; Pollack, 1970; Sitnick, Rushmer, Arpan, Melum, Sowers, & Kennedy, 1985) and offer nothing for the older child. Paterson (1982) agreed that early aural habilitation is best, but demonstrated that many late diagnosed children have more residual hearing, are more mature and attentive, have wider interests and knowledge of the world, and perhaps more highly developed cognition with which to integrate auditory training.

All experienced teachers have taught children whose diagnosis came late and yet successful language learning still took place. Vernon and Koh (1972) studied both children who had graduated from the John Tracy preschool program and a matched group who had no early intervention; they found no differences in speech, speechreading, reading, or academic skills. Auditory skills were not assessed. Stein, Benner, Hoversten, McGinnis, and Thies (1980), offered appropriate activities for older children at each level of difficulty but did not mandate the use of audition throughout the day. They provided no indication objective of aural habilitation curricula. The danger is that a teacher will foster daily listening activities and record progress only to find the student unable to apply his listening skills in real-life situations. Although some late diagnosed children are successful, we know that the earlier the hearing loss diagnosis is made and accepted, the less critical language learning time is lost. This makes it easier to develop a habilitation program that follows the child's natural cognitive and social development.

## Appropriate Consistent Amplification

The second requirement for an aural habilitation program is that the child wear appropriate amplification consistently. The audiologist tests and fits the child, but teachers and parents need to be knowledgeable in order to assess and monitor the day-to-day functioning of the aids. Grammatico (1975) suggested that hearing aids should be evaluated and chosen by a team consisting of an audiologist (clinical input), a teacher (functional school input), and a parent (functional home input). Lenneberg (1967) pointed out that language acquisition cannot begin until a child is exposed to it. In other words, time of amplification is the beginning of a child's listening age. Time for receptive language to develop must not be rushed. A premature expectation for expressive language may hinder development of the child's inner language (Bunch, 1975).

The need for appropriate, consistent amplification is highlighted in the many curricula for preschool children that discuss how hearing aids work and how to do a quick listening check. A hearing aid listening check consists of the following steps:

1. Check the body of the aid for loose screws, connections, dirt or broken parts. Clean the earmold of accumulated wax and dirt.
2. Test the battery on a battery tester. It is best to do this at bedtime rather than first thing in the morning to avoid a false recovery reading.
3. Insert a working battery into the aid.
4. Attach a listening tube to the aid.
5. Set the switch to *M* (microphone on) and turn the volume to what is recommended for the child. Say the following sounds into the microphone; *oo, ah, ee, sh, s.*
6. Continue speaking while moving the volume control up and down. Listen for intermittency and distortion.
7. Shake the aid gently and listen for any unusual noise or breaks.
8. If the aid is not functioning correctly take it to the audiologist for an electroacoustic analysis.

Clarke School for the Deaf (1971), discussed the problems and solutions of getting the equipment used consistently. Parents need to have a positive attitude towards their children's hearing aids, be firm but matter-of-fact about their consistent use, and explain to the curious what they are. If the child rejects the aids, they may be too powerful or not powerful enough, the earmold may not fit comfortably, or the child may need quiet, short wearing periods until he adjusts.

Unfortunately, wearing aids consistently is only the first hurdle. Gaeth and Lounsburg (1966), studied elementary school children's hearing aids electroacoustically, but found most of their data was meaningless because such a high percentage of the aids were defective. In a two year study, Zink (1972), found 27 percent of new hearing aids and 58 percent of newly repaired aids were not functioning to specifications. Musket (1981), in her comprehensive review, concluded that on any given day, up to 50 percent of children's hearing aids were malfunctioning. Both Rhoades (1982) and Pollack (1984) found that children are more often than not using ineffective amplification. Unfortunately, one often sees auditory lessons begun without any check of either the child's personal hearing aids or wireless auditory system. Intervention at this point is essential if aural habilitation is to succeed. It means that parents and teachers must have knowledge and equipment available to ensure that the amplification is in working order every day. Even something as simple as wax clogging the earmold can substantially cut back on the reception of the important high frequency information.

Teachers and parents are usually pleased to see higher powered hearing aids coming on the market because they produce better aided responses. However, one wonders if power aids could result in more hearing loss for the child. According to Whetnall and Fry (1971) there is no indication that this is true. Rintelmann and Bess (1977) when reviewing the research on this topic, however, reported contradictory results. Some studies reported threshold shifts from high-powered amplification and others did not. It appeared that children with moderate-to-severe losses presented a greater risk to increased threshold shift than those with profound losses. It appeared impossible to state a universal maximum safe acoustic output for all hearing aids and many audiologists judge this on the tolerance of individual children. Some hearing impairments are progressive in nature and it is difficult to control for this fact in research studies. To be conservative most hearing aid Saturated Sound Pressure Levels (SSPL) should not exceed 130 decibels (dB). Binaural fittings are usually considered superior and allow for a slightly lower gain to obtain the same results (Ling & Ling, 1978; Urbantschitsch, 1982; Whetnall & Fry, 1971).

Hartbauer (1975) pointed out that infants need auditory feedback cues to develop inner language, and even imperfect (distorted) information is better than none. As speech is a clear acoustic signal, good amplification all day seems to be essential in order for the hearing-impaired child to match what he hears to what he produces (Fry, 1978).

## Good Acoustics

Ross (1978) felt that poor classroom acoustics for mainstreamed hearing-impaired children may be a major factor responsible for their poor performance.

The signal-to-noise ratio needs to be better than +12 dB even with very low reverberation (Finitzo-Hieber & Tilman, 1978). Classrooms usually fail to meet this criterion even though children are being mainstreamed more and more. Plomb (1986) suggested we are placing children in environments where their hearing aids are not effective and a wireless auditory trainer is essential. Ross (1978) offered ways to overcome noise by having more teacher input into the child's room placement, closing windows and doors, checking the kinds of ventilation and heating systems installed, and encouraging the use of carpet, acoustic tile, and soft drapes. Børrild (1978), reminds us that lipreading is important in the mainstream classroom and, if available, helps compensate for some of the acoustic problems. Very few of the available auditory curricula address the problem of noise interference or suggest training in noise. Some children can benefit from training in noise but others cannot tolerate it. Such simple techniques as making tapes of white noise and competing speech messages to use with material that has been mastered in quiet may be of benefit. Given the reality of the signal-to-noise ratio of most mainstream classrooms, training in noise may be an area of concern for curriculum writers.

## Natural Auditory Experience

Two components are considered essential if an environment of natural auditory experiences is to be developed for the hearing-impaired child. These are a structured adult and an unstructured child (Northcott, 1978). The adult ensures that the hearing aid is working and that the acoustic environment is satisfactory, and then uses meaningful situations to draw the child's attention to sound. Listening doesn't just happen when the hearing aid goes on, it has to be nurtured and the child's interests exploited. Auditory experience develops speech perception through meaningful situations (Paterson, 1982). Normal children's games and activities (Gordon 1970, 1972), give many hours of fun, repetition, and learning to the child. Redundancy is a natural part of language (Fry, 1978; Sanders, 1971), and the repetitive nature of a baby's routine lends itself especially well to exploiting this redundancy (Ling & Ling, 1978). Following the child's interests to develop, auditory memory and auditory speech responses are encouraged. A natural conversational style of turn-taking, waiting, prompting, and encouraging interactive communication is considered the most appropriate approach (Manolson, 1985, Northcott, 1978, Sitnick et al., 1985).

Even the child with the left-corner audiogram benefits greatly from good auditory experience. He or she can develop the use of the suprasegmental aspects of speech—duration, loudness, and pitch—that are extremely important and meaningful for developing more intelligible speech and comprehending language strings. The suprasegmentals are only available through audition and not through vision or touch. A child who develops a deaf voice often does not have sufficient low-frequency gain on his hearing aids and not enough auditory experience. Maassen (1986) found that the intelligibility of deaf speech could be improved by adding pauses to coordinate the timing patterns with the syntactic phrasing of each utterance. This suggests that even children who do not articulate correctly and only have usable hearing to 500 Hz, can improve their speech communication by monitoring the suprasegmentals through audition. van Uden (1977), considered training normal rhythms, breathing patterns, and music to be essential for deaf children and best done through natural play activities. while auditory experience sounds easy and natural, it requires knowledge, programing, and evaluation skills on the part of the adult. It is relatively easy to integrate natural activities if the child is very young and the parents are naturally interactive. It is far more difficult if the child is older and the style of the parents is not interactive, or if everyone has grown discouraged over the years.

### Auditory Training

While auditory experience may be described as natural, auditory training is appropriately described as structured. It should be viewed as a supplement to auditory experience and as an integral part of language and speech training (Ling & Ling, 1978). Auditory training alone, a series of listening exercises that may or may not be related to the child's interests or study areas, is often the only component of aural habilitation offered regularly or spasmodically to hearing-impaired children. Many curricula have as their major component lists of activities for auditory training (Stein et al., 1980; Whitehurst, 1978). Some are strong on using the child's normal play routines for auditory training (John Tracy Clinic 1972; Northcott, 1978; Sitnik et al., 1985), but still rely on a sensitive teacher to choose what suits each child best.

Grammatico and Miller (1974) recognized the folly of using separate curricula for hearing-impaired and normally hearing students and developed a preschool program based on the regular school curriculum. If a child is mainstreamed, then a teacher should sensibly use the regular classroom curriculum for building auditory skills through training. It is often a very helpful and successful technique to have a teacher or parent preteach classroom material in a quiet one-on-one environment and allow the hearing-impaired child auditory experience with the vocabulary before receiving it in the regular classroom.

Auditory training is made up of four distinct and perhaps hierarchical skills of listening: (1) detection; (2) discrimination; (3) identification; and (4) comprehension. Detection of sound requires a simple yes or no response. One either hears something or hears nothing.

Discrimination between sounds requires a person to hear two sounds and tell whether they are the same or different. Identification of sound may require repeating what was said or answering a question (active response), or pointing to a picture, word, or sentence representing what was heard (passive response). The most difficult, but the most important level, is comprehension of sound. This can be as simple as following a command or as difficult as understanding a lecture with no contextual or visual clues. Ling (1978) emphasized that comprehension should be meaningful to the child and parallel to cognitive growth.

It is unclear whether one should begin training with detection tasks and move-up to comprehension of language, or begin with complex language strings and remediate as needed. Probably one needs to move up and down the hierarchy to fit the needs of individual children (Fig. 7-2). Normally we deal with strings of language, not individual words or phonemes and coarticulation effects are clues that hearing-impaired people can learn to perceive. Although sentence comprehension may be easier in some respects, it does assume the person has a good language base (Erber, 1982).

Auditory training tasks should be based on what the child can hear and what he needs to hear—suprasegmentals, phonemes, words, phrases, sentences, and stories. Evaluation of a child's auditory skills should be made before programing is done. Time must not be wasted on identification tasks if a child can comprehend the material at a higher level of language.

Suprasegmentals must be taught auditorily. Some children pick them up during natural experiences, others need specific training. They are very important and carry considerable language information. Use of regular school vocabulary (e.g., pencil, glue, scissors) and usual classroom commands (e.g., line-up, turn off the lights, sit down) can be utilized to build-up listening exercises that are useful and meaningful.

During training it is important that the child use an active rather than passive response to develop auditory memory, auditory sequencing, and self-monitoring skills (Bess & McConnell, 1981, Hirsh, 1970, Northcott, 1978, Paterson, 1982). This active response (imitation) is considered to develop auditory-articulatory encoding processes in the brain. Caution in this interpretation is necessary as the benefits for comprehending spoken language may be doubtful and should not be assumed (Ling, 1978). Auditory training should use meaningful stimuli, follow the normal stages of language acquisition (Paterson,

| **Auditory training response tasks** | **Hearing activity** |
| --- | --- |
| Comprehension | Cog/linguistic Store |
| Identification | Working memory |
| Discimination | Iconic/Echolic memory |
| Detection | Use of senses |

Figure 7-2. Auditory training tasks are described as requiring detection of sound, discrimination between sounds, identification of sound and comprehension of sounds. It is unclear whether a bottom up or top down sequence is the preferred order or if movement up and down is necessary. Based on tables developed by Dr. D. Ling, London, Ontario: Faculty of Applied Health Sciences, University of Western Ontario. Reprinted by permission.

1982), and offer the hearing-impaired child plenty of opportunities to listen, match with known language, and make reasonable guesses (Fry, 1978). A useful resource in this area is a videotape produced by Edwards and Estabrooks (1985). Examples of auditory training exercises at the levels of detection, identification, and comprehension for children of all ages and abilities are demonstrated.

Many auditory training programs begin with detection and discrimination exercises involving environmental sounds (Clarke School for the Deaf, 1971; Stein et al., 1980; Whitehurst, 1978). Although it is useful for safety reasons that a city child be able to identify a subway train, or a country child a cow bell, there is no evidence that suggests this ability promotes improvement in speech discrimination (Bess & McConnell, 1981; Ling & Ling, 1978; Paterson, 1982) A.H. Ling (1976) pointed out that environmental and speech sounds are processed in different hemispheres of the brain and that perceptual and memory strategies used for one are inappropriate for the other.

Auditory training is usually done using audition alone. Ling (1978) suggested that visual input certainly supplements auditory information but may not be wise to use in early childhood if a child is to make the best use of his residual hearing. Although Rollins (1972) advocated a multisensory approach, many others believe this results in a sensory overload, causing slowness, and may, in reality, be more difficult than a unisensory approach (Ling, 1978; Ling, Ling, & Pflaster, 1977; Pollack, 1970). However, realism is necessary. When there is not enough auditory information for a particular child, then other modalities should be added. Leung (1986) found that tap dancing was fun for children and offered kinesthetic and sensory inputs to emphasize the rhythms of speech and developed a child's memory for sequencing. Ross (1978) pointed out that while we focus on audition, bisensory intelligibility scores are typically better than single modality scores. He suggested that we must make visual information available, particularly in the mainstreamed classroom. Erber (1982) presented three approaches to auditory training: (1) natural conversational; (2) moderately structured; and (3) specific task practice. The natural conversational approach allows the child to build self confidence in a relaxed, natural environment in which there is little pressure. Many opportunities occur in which the child is encouraged to make guesses within the context of a specific subject. The moderately structured approach is based on the experience chart story format (e.g., a planned activity, a discussion, and writing words and sentences to describe the activity). These words or sentences should differ acoustically so that identification through audition can be made. Specific task practice consists of stimulus-response activities covering detection, discrimination, identification, and comprehension of sound.

Telephone use requires auditory-only skill and is ignored in most curricula. Erber (1982, 1985) has developed a comprehensive auditory program for telephone training that should be part of a school-age child's program. Use of the telephone is universal in our society and hearing-impaired children are anxious to use it to the best of their ability.

Auditory training supplements auditory experience, allowing skills that are not learned in a natural way to be presented in a more structured environment. The results of auditory training can be readily measured, which makes this component of aural habilitation popular with both writers of curricula and teachers. The component of figure-ground interference is often not addressed, nor are methods to ensure transference of the new skills to everyday experiences.

### Parents and Teachers

Parents and teachers play fundamentally important roles in an aural habilitation program. A combination of positive attitude and vigorous action from them is considered essential to the appropriate implementation of a curriculum. Rollins (1972) commented that attitude to residual hearing may be compared to perceiving a cup as being half empty or half full. The positive view is to be preferred to the negative view. Rhoades (1982) suggested that if we look at the aided responses and expect a deaf child to respond as hard-of-hearing we immediately have higher expectations for that child. Research bears out the notion that what one expects is what one gets (Jones, 1977). Sitnick and associates (1985) insisted that the attitude of the adults helping the hearing-impaired child develop listening skills is one of the most important factors in that child's success. Northcott (1978) warned that "It is unfortunately true that if our expectations are too low the child may not progress as rapidly as his potential would allow."

There is no doubt that curricula must convey a consistently positive attitude to those who will use them.

Some of the most successful auditory curricula use parents as the primary teachers and professionals as guides and evaluators (Beebe et al., 1984; John Tracy Clinic, 1972; Pollack, 1970; Sitnick et al., 1985). A.H. Ling (1977) developed a check-list for parents to help monitor their child's auditory, speech, and language development. The audition schedule includes the use of the hearing aid, the child's response to sound at a preverbal level, and auditory discrimination of speech patterns at the verbal level. Professionals need to prepare parents for their task as teachers (Ling, Ling, & Pflaster, 1977) through such checklists, and, also, in other ways. Whetnall and Fry (1971) emphasized this point when they stated that efforts at developing auditory skills were futile without the parents' participation. In response to this belief a number of guidelines for parental participation have emerged in this area. They have recognized that parents spend the most time with their child and have the best opportunity to offer natural auditory experiences (Rhoades, 1982; Sitnick et al, 1985).

However, many parents are not able to give the time and effort auditory programs require. They may be overburdened with other responsibilities, they may not speak English, or they may want professionals to take over the training of their child. There are many reasons why parents may not be able to assume the teacher role. Unfortunately, many aural habilitation programs rely on parent commitment and fail to offer a substitute for it. Thus, when parent participation is not obtained, it is impossible to implement the curriculum as it was designed.

Teachers and therapists must remember that most parents care about their children, know them in a very intimate way, and are ultimately responsible for them. Therefore:

1. Parents must never be isolated from their child's program.
2. Parents must be involved with the professional team.
3. Parents must be listened to.
4. Parents must be given all possible knowledge about their child's development.

### Programs: Group Versus Individual

Many auditory programs emphasize the need for early diagnosis and early training (Beebe et al., 1984; Grammatico, 1975; Pollack, 1970; Sitnick et al., 1985) so that advantage can be taken of the critical years for language learning. All of these programs involve the parents and instruct them in hearing impairment, hearing aids, language and speech acquisition, and auditory training. All use a one-to-one teaching model rather than a group lesson. Pollack (1970) stated that a one-to-one approach is the most effective way to assure a quiet, intensive, individually geared program.

Not all agree, however, that the individual approach is always to be preferred. Erber (1982) illustrated that group lessons are less expensive, less tiring, more natural, and teach such social interaction skills as turn-taking, waiting, and helping others more effectively than do individual programs. Alpiner, Amon, Gibson, and Sheehy (1977) tell parents to talk, talk, talk to their children. Alternatively, Bess and McConnell (1981) suggest we shouldn't be bathing the child in sound, but rather, engage in quiet, meaningful play. Again, the implication for curriculum is that we should be using material of interest or importance to the child, planning it carefully and presenting it in as natural a way as possible.

### Success Factors

A variety of factors, believed to contribute significantly to the success of aural habilitation programing, have been identified. Ling (1978) suggested that the best results obtained by aural habilitation programs occur when the child is identified early, there is good audiological management, the teacher is well-trained in assessing and programing, and educational provision is supportive of auditory programs. Northcott (1978) indicated a successful auditory learner must have supportive parents, residual hearing, and the ability to integrate what is heard. Ross (1978) felt that the lack of appropriate and working amplification and poor room acoustics may be major factors affecting a hearing-impaired child's auditory skills and school performance. Pollack (1970) and Ling and Ling (1978) agreed that aided responses on the audiogram, intelligence, parental skill, and involvement all help predict a child's success or failure. Ling and Ling (1978) also considered teacher skill, suitability of materials used, and consistency and frequency of the program to be contributing factors. Important success factors may be summarized as follows:

1. Early identification of the hearing loss
2. Good audiological management
3. Well trained teachers
4. Supportive parents
5. Aided responses on the audiogram
6. Intelligence of the child
7. Consistency and frequency of the program

## Summary

It is obvious from the preceding discussion that a variety of factors influence a child's ability to learn through an impaired auditory sense. However, we do not know which factors are most critical: A considerable amount of careful and controlled research is required before we draw any useful conclusions. We do, however, recognize the link between auditory perception, auditory comprehension, and language learning. We can agree that we want hearing-impaired children to develop their residual hearing to the best of their abilities. We can also agree that technological changes in hearing aids have meant better auditory reception for many. It is the task of teacher therapists to assure on a daily basis that the equipment is functioning appropriately and that our expectations are based on what we know the child can hear. This can be done through a listening check of the aids and then using such procedures as the five-sound test (Ling, 1978), or the Glendonald Auditory Screening Procedure (GASP) (Erber, 1982). Both these tests present consonant–vowel syllables to the child across the frequency range for detection purposes. Variation from typical response helps the teacher to quickly determine whether or not the aids are functioning normally. It cannot be over-emphasized that aural habilitation can only be successful if you know what the child hears and program accordingly.

Many hours have been wasted by teachers who are anxious to get on with a lesson and fail to realize that the child's amplification equipment is broken.

An auditory program should contain activities relating to the child's experience and interests and fall within his cognitive ability. They must be well-planned and presented within listening range and with redundancy. Auditory skills should be tied to speech skills so that memory, sequencing, and self-monitoring can develop (Ling, 1976, Paterson, 1982, Cole & Mischook, 1985). Figure-ground environments should be included in training as soon as a child has mastered material in quiet. Selective attention is very difficult to obtain and needs training. Assessment of skills in the areas of speech reception and production, and language must be carried out regularly so that programs can be adjusted. It is not clear whether auditory training should begin with detection tasks (Clarke School for the Deaf, 1971; Sitnick et al., 1985; Stein et al., 1980; Whitehurst, 1978) and move up to discrimination, identification, and comprehension tasks, or begin with comprehension (Erber, 1982; Grammatico, 1975), and remediate to lower tasks as needed. Curriculum designers must make an informed choice on conflicting positions such as these.

Perhaps no one teaching approach will ever be right for every child. Perhaps we should not seek such a program, but rather be eclectic, sensitive, and flexible to meet the needs of each individual child. The need to employ these characteristics in designing aural habilitation curricula appears evident in this particularly demanding and important area.

## TYPE AURAL HABILITATION RESOURCES IN REVIEW

*Auditory Skills Curriculum* D. Stein, G. Benner, G. Hoversten, M. McGinnis, and T. Thies (1980)

*Auditory Training* Clarke School for the Deaf (1971)

*Auditory Training* N.P. Erber (1982)

*Curriculum Guide: Hearing-Impaired Children and Their Parents* W. Northcott (1977)

*Listening Skills Curriculum* S.C. Baldwin, J.B. Nielsen, R.M. Ochs, and S.L. Porter (1975)

*Parent-Infant Communication* V. Sitnick, N. Rushmer, R. Arpan, A. Melum, J. Sowers, and N. Kennedy (1985)

*The Ski-Hi Model* T.C. Clark, and S. Watkins (1985)

## *AUDITORY SKILLS CURRICULUM*

### D. Stein, G. Benner, G. Hoversten, M. McGinnis, and T. Thies

*Publisher*:
Foreworks
Box 9747
North Hollywood, CA 91609

*Skills taught*: A comprehensive package of auditory skill activities arranged in order of difficulty and including figure-ground training. Appropriate activities at each level are offered for older as well as younger children.

*Age/grade range*: Infant to high school.

*Group Size*: Individual and small group.

**THEORY:** The *Auditory Skills Curriculum* is designed to make hearing-impaired children's auditory skills sharper and to help them develop their own strategies for the perception of auditory patterns. Training activities are based on language used in the pupils' everyday academic and social surroundings. They assume the use of consistent and appropriate amplification.

The authors have based their program on the theories of the redundancy of language, the motor theory of speech production, the importance of language chunks, or strings, and the matching of usable hearing to the acoustics of speech. Early training is based on contrasting suprasegmental information. Stimuli are presented within meaningful linguistic contexts to preserve the intonational features, the natural boundaries, and the coarticulation effects.

**DESCRIPTION:** There are four major areas in the curriculum to be developed concurrently. They are discrimination, memory sequencing, auditory feedback, and figure-ground.

The discrimination section includes attention to sound, discrimination of nonverbal sounds, discrimination of the suprasegmental aspects of speech, linguistic messages with contextual clues, and discriminating words on the bases of segmental features.

Memory sequencing includes recalling and sequencing critical elements in a message, demonstrating auditory cognitive skills within a structured set, and showing auditory cognitive skills within a conversation.

Auditory feedback includes preverbal behaviors, imitating vocal productions, and modifying vocal productions.

Figure-ground presents material at varying distances in quiet, in normal classroom noise, and with verbal distraction.

A child's base level is assessed by using the intermediate performance objectives or by using the companion assessment tool, the *Test of Auditory Comprehension* (TAC) (1976). The TAC is normed on hearing-impaired children (4-to-17 years, with moderate-to-profound losses) and contains ten subtests presented on tape. These are linked to the curriculum objectives.

The curriculum activities are presented in sets (closed, limited, and open). Factors affecting the difficulty of the set include the number of choices and the presence or absence of situational and contextual clues. The activities are designed for preschool, primary-, intermediate-, or secondary-level pupils at all levels of difficulty.

**EVALUATION:** The curriculum is well-founded on a theoretical base, is easy to use, and is one of the few that presents material that is suitable for older students. After skills have been mastered in quiet, the teacher is encouraged to repeat the activity with distance added between the listener and speaker and the point of noise interference. The activities are based on normal everyday happenings and can be matched to the cognitive development of individual pupils. The authors suggest beginning some activities, using new language concepts, in a multisensory mode and gradually withdrawing visual and tactile cues instead of beginning with audition alone and adding other modes if needed. This is only common sense, as one should not be training listening skills using unknown language.

This is not a curriculum to use sequentially from beginning to end. It relies on knowledgable and creative teachers to pick and choose activities as needed to train specific skills. However, because the activities have been carefully matched to normal developmental interests it should be easy to link natural auditory experience to these activities and, therefore, achieve more successful transference of the skill to everyday understanding and use.

## *AUDITORY TRAINING CURRICULUM SERIES*

### Clarke School for the Deaf

*Publisher*:
The Clarke School for the Deaf
Round Hill Road
Northampton, MA 01060

*Skills taught*: Information is given about audiograms, equipment, auditory training exercises, developing an auditory environment, and parent information.

*Age/grade range*: 5 to 12 years

*Group size*: Individual and small class

**THEORY:** *Auditory Training* is defined as the structuring of an individual's environment to facilitate the development and use of sound perception. Structuring refers to many aspects of the environment including wearing hearing aids, participating in auditory training exercises, focusing attention on meaningful environmental sounds, modifying a teacher's behavior, and advising parents on hearing impairment.

**DESCRIPTION:** Chapter 1 presents a history of persons advocating the exploitation of residual hearing in deaf children and the various methodologies employed. In Chapter 2 audiological testing, audiograms, and educational implications of hearing loss are discussed. Chapter 3 is a discussion of hearing aids and early classroom systems and includes a short discussion of what creates problems in the environment for a hearing-impaired listener. Some of this information needs updating. Chapter 4 is a discussion of hearing and how to develop it in the deaf. The parameters of detection, discrimination, recognition, and comprehension are perceived as sequential. It is suggested that a general approach to training is necessary and more successful than is greater emphasis on special exercises. However, young children are given a variety of special exercises beginning with closed sets of environmental sounds, names, colors, numbers, and days with gradual movement to open sets. This approach recommended for the first 4 years of school when one would then enter a more general approach or an all-day, learning-to-listen program. No extended explanation or theoretical base is given for this procedure. Chapter 5 contains a collection of auditory training exercises that are explained under the headings of sound detection, discrimination, recognition and comprehension. The activities are general in nature and lend themselves well to adaptation to the child's environment. They are presented in a unisensory mode first, then with lipreading, then with print. It is stressed that exercises are only a part of providing an all-day listening environment. The child needs to listen in order to participate. Chapter 6, "Hearing and Hearing Aids," has not been revised and so has very little usable information. All equipment discussed is outdated and even the discussion of a child's potential from his audiogram is misleading because it does not take new technology into consideration.

**EVALUATION:** Although this is not really a curriculum, it does lay out a sequential list of auditory training activities that are easy to use with young children. The need to have a consistent auditory expectation within the child's environment is appropriately emphasized. As with many older curricula, it does presume that learning about environmental sounds somehow leads into understanding speech sounds.

The parental attitude section and suggestions for family communication are strong. There is a useful auditory evaluation form at the end but it should be extended and a criteria level on 2-choice answer sections of 8/10 be required. It does not test comprehension of a story nor how a child copes with added distance or noise.

It is disappointing that the Clarke School for the Deaf has not revised this book since 1971, as whole sections on hearing aids and testing procedures remain as they were while the field has moved on. Attitudes of parents and suggestions for the family, however, are succinct and helpful.

## *AUDITORY TRAINING*

**N.P. Erber**

*Publisher*:
Alexander Graham Bell Association
3417 Volta Place, N.W.
Washington, D.C. 20007

*Skills taught*: A look at auditory training and ways to make service delivery meaningful to the child and teacher. It includes assessment techniques, telephone training, and three styles of auditory training.

*Age/grade range*: Preschool through high school.

*Group size*: Individual and class groups

**THEORY:** Erber's intent is to provide sufficient background information and auditory instruction strategies to enable a parent, teacher, rehabilitationist, or audiologist to develop their skills as auditory instructors. He offers practical suggestions on how to make a program successful in a nontechnical presentation. The ideas are based on laboratory experiences at the Central Institute for the Deaf, in St. Louis, Missouri, and classroom experiences at the Glendonald School for Deaf Children located in Kew, Victoria, Australia.

**DESCRIPTION:** Chapter 1 gives a historical overview of auditory training and amplification. In Chapter 2, speech perception and speech production are viewed as closely related in a stimulus-response relationship. Visual and auditory perception are discussed. Chapter 3 outlines goals, concepts, and methods for auditory training and a sequence for auditory evaluation:

1. audiometric examination
2. selection of hearing aids
3. speech discrimination testing
4. diagnosis of perceptual strengths and weaknesses (auditory, visual, and tactile).

The sequence of auditory tasks (detection, discrimination, identification, and comprehension) and speech stimuli (speech elements, syllables, words, phrases, sentences, and connected discourse) are discussed. A teacher may begin anywhere on the matrix and judge whether the levels of stimulus and response are too easy or too difficult and modify as needed. Chapter 4, "Screening Auditory Abilities" describes in detail the Glendonald Auditory Screening Procedures Test (GASP). It tests a child's auditory ability to detect phonemes, identify words, and comprehend sentences. It can be administered quickly and can be used to initiate auditory training. In Chapter 5, examples are given of three general styles of auditory training: a conversational approach, a moderately structured approach, and practice on specific tasks. The author suggests using all three approaches and lists many activities one might use. Chapter 6 discusses the merits and disadvantages of group versus individual instruction. The use of vibrotactile aids and the auditory versus auditory visual methods are reviewed. Chapter 7 gives ideas about how to use various recording machines for auditory training activities. Chapter 8 covers the use of the telephone; Chapter 9, speech development; and Chapter 10, important communication factors. A comprehensive list of teacher responsibilities and adaptive techniques are included.

**EVALUATION:** Although this book does not presume to be a full curriculum, it does offer the teacher some clear and easy to use assessment tools, and a framework for developing auditory skills. It is clearly written, and light on jargon and method bias. It does not stress early diagnosis, auditory expectation, or natural auditory experience factors. Its discussion of assessment is useful and gives pertinent, functional information quickly. The chapter on telephone training is easy to use and has practical suggestions for children with wide auditory abilities. This information is difficult to find elsewhere and one could program directly from it.

This work does rely on teacher skill and creativity, but assuming one has that, it is a useful reference for building auditory learning programs.

## *CURRICULUM GUIDE: HEARING-IMPAIRED CHILDREN (0–3 YEARS) AND THEIR PARENTS*

**W.H. Northcott (Editor)**

*Publisher*:
Alexander Graham Bell Association
3417 Volta Place, N.W.
Washington, D.C. 20007

*Skills taught*: Parent-teaching program for hearing-impaired infants to develop early auditory skills and language.

*Age/grade range: 0 to 3 years*

*Group size*: Individual

**THEORY:** This curriculum is based on the educational philosophy and practices of the Minneapolis Public School Family-Oriented Infant/Preschool Special Education Program. It suggests that parents are a child's natural teachers, but that parents of handicapped children need counselling and guidance in order to teach their children effectively. The home and community are a child's natural environment for learning. The family becomes responsible for providing listening and learning opportunities within the child's natural environment and range of activities. The curriculum identifies cognitive, social, and linguistic development in normally hearing children and follows this continuum. The emphasis is on language rather than speech and on listening skills rather than speechreading, but, most of all, on using a natural rather than a formal approach. It is practical and functional and uses an interdisciplinary team of professionals and parents. It assumes positive acceptance of binaural amplification when prescribed, and an auditory oral method of instruction.

**DESCRIPTION:** This curriculum makes substantial use of techniques suggested by Pollack (1970) and relies on assessment evaluations from an interdisciplinary team. The goals are auditory and verbal communication skills, and a regular education placement. It stresses early diagnosis so that listening can become part of the child's whole personality. The child is taught to detect, discriminate, identify, comprehend, localize, and imitate sounds. Emphasis is placed on the auditory environment with attention to distance and noise factors. Gross sounds, environmental noises, music, and speech are developed concurrently. Active responses from the child are encouraged to develop an auditory feedback system, auditory memory, auditory sequencing, and self-monitoring abilities. Objectives and check lists are provided for parent, teacher, and child.

**EVALUATION:** This program is limited in scope to infancy and relies on early identification of the hearing loss. It follows normal language, social, and cognitive developmental norms. It offers excellent lesson ideas that are fun for the child and meaningful for the adult. There is very little information about audiological management or advocacy for the hearing-impaired child. It assumes success of every child and does not discuss alternative approaches.

One might wrongly assume that success with this program leads automatically to continued success in the regular school system.

## *LISTENING SKILLS CURRICULUM*

**S.C. Baldwin, J.B. Nielsen, R.M. Ochs, and S.L. Porter**

*Publisher*:
Utah School for the Deaf
846 Twentieth Street
Ogden, UT 84401

*Skills taught*: Auditory training activities with some information about hearing aids and telephone use.

*Age/grade range: Preschool and school age*

*Group Size*: Individual and small group

**THEORY:** This program was developed to take into account new linguistic research and advances in hearing aid technology. The authors question the sequence and hierarchy of teaching auditory skills and conclude that several skills must be taught simultaneously. They are aware of the link between listening and speaking and the importance of developing a feedback system through active responses. Early training is considered best but it is suggested that all children, regardless of age, benefit from auditory training. Listening is considered an all-day activity and the parents are viewed as the most appropriate teachers for young children.

**DESCRIPTION:** The parameters of auditory skills are listed as perception, feedback, discrimination, and comprehension. The sequence of teaching is difficult to determine and several objectives are identified at one time. Lesson plans and activities are laid-out for teachers and parents. Brief discussions are included on hearing aids and trouble shooting, telephone and tape recorder skills, and behavior-reinforcement techniques.

**EVALUATION:** Although the authors suggest this program is appropriate for older children (a lesson plan for secondary students is included), most activities are for preschool and primary students.

The curriculum is well-founded on theory but the flow-chart of auditory phases makes use of linguistic jargon that a lay-person would experience difficulty following. The evaluation forms are very general and subjective in nature. The authors emphasize that all children (oral or total communication [T.C.]) benefit from developing listening skills and that one needs to apply these skills throughout the day. Each teacher is left to develop his or her own techniques for generalizing auditory skills.

## *PARENT-INFANT COMMUNICATION*

**V. Sitnick, N. Rushmer, R. Arpan, A. Melum, J. Sowers, and N. Kennedy**

*Publisher*:
Infant Hearing Resource
Good Samaritan Hospital
1015 N.W. 22nd Ave.
Portland, OR 97210

*Skills taught*: Information for parents about hearing loss, hearing aids, development of language and listening skills, behavior management, how to observe and record, and how to teach through play. A program of activities for developing auditory and communication skills in hearing-impaired infants.

*Age/grade range*: 0 to 4 years

*Group size*: Individual

**THEORY:** *Parent–Infant Communication* is based on developmental scales of acquiring communication skills in normal children and draws ideas from many curricula for the hearing impaired (Clarke School for the Deaf, 1971; John Tracy Clinic, 1972; Northcott, 1978; Pollack, 1970).

**DESCRIPTION:** Auditory activities are listed in a developmental sequence but parents are advised to follow the child's lead. All activities are easy to carry out in a home setting.

The manual for parents consists of information handouts describing the importance and care of hearing aids, information about hearing impairment, how to develop normal communication skills in the child, the difference between receptive and expressive language, and how to modify the child's behavior. Parents are also taught how to advocate for their child in the school system and how to record their child's progress.

The program is geared to early identification of hearing loss and consistent use of amplification.

The parameters of auditory skills include detection, discrimination, identification, and comprehension. The activities are based on natural life situations and play set ups. The goal is voice and speech comprehension.

**EVALUATION:** *The Parent–Infant Communication* manuals have made an excellent attempt to organize auditory learning activities for very young children in the context of home and play. This natural way for parents and children to interact is lacking in many programs.

The manuals are clearly written and the parent handouts are particularly good. In particular, assessment and record-keeping sheets are useful. Parents are encouraged to learn about a technical subject without being overwhelmed with jargon. Alternative methods of communication are discussed and auditory success is not assumed for all children.

## *THE SKI-HI MODEL*

**T.C. Clark and S. Watkins**

*Publisher*:
Project Ski-Hi Outreach
Utah State University
Logan, Utah 84322

*Skills taught*: A preschool home program that includes parent guidance, a hearing aid program, total communication, language, auditory training, and speech training.

*Age/grade range*: 0 to 36 months

*Group size*: Individual

**THEORY:** The *Ski-Hi Model* is based on the belief that every hearing-impaired child should be given the opportunity to use his or her residual hearing to full potential. It bases its program on the critical period for learning language research and the fact that auditory experience is linked to language learning. In order to offer an appropriate program, the following goals must be met:

1. Language learning must begin as close to birth as possible.
2. Audiological management must be appropriate.
3. A natural language development continuum is best.
4. Parents in the home make the best teachers.
5. The teacher of the deaf acts as a model.
6. Residual hearing must be trained regardless of educational methodology.
7. Language lessons should be natural rather than structured.
8. Psychological support should be offered to the parents.

**DESCRIPTION:** This is a program for hearing-impaired infants through amplification and home intervention. The model has three main components: administrative (child identification and program management), direct service to family (hearing aids, assessment, and auditory skill training), and supportive services (audiological, hearing aid, educational materials, psychological support, and child development information).

Parent and child objectives are identified for each of the 20 lessons. Materials and activities are clearly listed for easy reference. The 20 lessons are divided into 4 phases of listening skills. They are:

1. Attending to sound and vocalizing
2. Recognizing and locating sound and vocalizing with inflection
3. Training with fluctuating distance and loudness and producing vowels and consonants
4. Vocal discrimination and comprehension of words and phrases, and speech showing discrimination between vowels and using a variety of consonants

**EVALUATION:** This program assumes early identification and full-time use of appropriate amplification. The auditory part of this curriculum ties-in well with natural language and speech goals. It incorporates verbal responses in auditory activities and fosters the use of audition throughout the day. It does not have a communication method bias and emphasizes that developing listening skills is important for all hearing-impaired children.

## REFERENCES

Alpiner, J.G., Amon, C.F., Gibson, J.C., & Sheehy, P. (1977). *Talk to Me*. Baltimore, Md.: The Williams and Wilkins Co.

Baldwin, S.D., Nielsen, J. B., Ochs, R. M., & Porter, S. L. (1975). *Listening skills curriculum*. Ogden, Utah: Utah School for the Deaf.

Beebe, H.H., Pearson, H.R., & Koch, M.E. (1984). The Helen Beebe Speech and Hearing Center. In D. Ling (Ed.) *Early intervention for hearing-impaired children: Oral options*. (pp. 15-63) San Diego, Calif.: College Hill Press.

Bess, F.H., & McConnell, F.E. (1981). *Audiology, education, and the hearing-impaired child*. St. Louis, Missouri: Mosby.

Boothroyd, A. (1976). *The role of hearing in education of the deaf*. Northampton, Mass.: Clarke School for the Deaf.

Børrild, K. (1978) Classroom acoustics In M. Ross and T. Giolas (Eds.). *Auditory Management of Hearing-Impaired Children*. (pp.145-179.).

Bunch, G.O. (1975) *Evaluation of natural and formal language approaches for hearing-impaired children*. Unpublished doctoral disertaion, University of British Columbia.

Clark, T.C., & Watkins, S. (1985). *The Ski-Hi model* (4th Ed.). Project Ski-Hi outreach. Logan, Utah: Utah State University.

Clarke School for the Deaf. (1971). *Auditory training*. Northampton, MA: Arthur Boothroyd.

Cole, E.B. & Mischook, M. (1985). Survey and annotated bibliography of curricula used by oral preschool programs. *Volta Review 87,* 139-153.

Edwards, C., & Estabrooks W. (1985) *Sure I can Hear* (Video). Toronto, Ontario: VOICE for Hearing-Impaired Children

Erber, N.P. (1982). *Auditory training*. Washington, D. C.: Alexander Graham Bell Association for the Deaf, Inc.

Erber, N. P. (1985). *Telephone communication and hearing impairment*. San Diego, California: College Hill Press.

Ewing, I.R., & Ewing, A. W. G. (1961). *New opportunities for deaf children*. London: University of London Press Ltd.

Finitzo-Hieber, T., & Tilman, T.W. (1978). Room acoustics effects on monosyllabic word discrimination ability for normal and hearing-impaired children. *Journal of Speech and Hearing Research 21,* 440-458.

Fry, D.B. (1978). The role and primacy of the auditory channel in speech and language. In M. Ross and R. Giolas (Eds.) *Auditory management of hearinq impaired children* (pp.15-41). Baltimore Md.: University Park Press.

Fry, D.B., & Whetnall, E. (1954). The auditory approach in the training of deaf children. *Lancet, 1*: 583-587.

Gaeth, J. H., & Lounsburg, E. (1966). Hearing aids and children in elementary schools. *Journal of Speech and Hearing Disorders. 31,* 283-289.

Goldstein, M. (1939). *The acoustic method*. St. Louis: Laryngoscope Press.

Gordon, I.J. (1970). *Baby learning through baby play*. New York: St. Martins Press.

Gordon, I.J. (1972). *Child learning through child play*. New York: St. Martins Press.

Grammatico, L.F. (1975). The Development of Listening Skills. *Volta Review, 77,* 303-308.

Grammatico, L.F., & Miller, S.D. (1974). Curriculum for the preschool deaf child. *Volta Review, 76,* 280-289.

Harris, G. (1973). *Auditory training for verbal communication.* Paper presented at the first National Convention of Canadian Teachers of the Deaf. Belleville, Ontario.

Hartbauer, R.E. (1975). *Aural habilitation.* Springfield, Illinois: Charles C. Thomas.

Hasenstab, S. M. (1983). Child language studies: Impact on habilitation of hearing-impaired infants and preschool children. *Volta Review, 85,* 88-100.

Hirsh, I.J. (1970). Auditory training In H. Davis and S. Silverman, (Eds), *Hearing and deafness.* (pp. 346-359), New York: Holt, Rinehart and Winston.

House, W.F. (1976). Cochlear implants. *Annals of Otology, Rhinolology and Laryngology, 85,* 1-93.

John Tracy Clinic (1972). *John Tracy Clinic correspondence course for parents of pre-school deaf children* (Revised). Los Angeles: Author.

Jones, R.A. (1977). *Self-fulfilling prophecies: social, psychological effects of expectancies.* New York: Wiley.

Koegel, R.L., & Felsenfeld, S. (1977). Sensory Deprivation. In S. Gerber (Ed.), *Audiometry In Infancy.* (pp 247-262), New York: Grune and Statton.

Lenneberg, E.H. (1967). *Biological foundations of language.* New York: John Wiley and Sons.

Leung, K. (1986). *Facilitating speech, language and auditory training through tap dancing and creative movement.* Paper presented at the 64th Annual Convention Council for Exceptional Children, New Orleans, Louisiana.

Ling, A.H. (1976). The training of auditory memory in hearing-impaired children: Some problems of generalization. *Journal of American Audiological Soc. 1,* 150-157.

Ling, A.H. (1977). *Schedules of development in audition speech language communication for hearing-impaired infants and their parents.* Washington, D C: Alexander Graham Bell Assoc. for the Deaf, Inc.

Ling, D. (1976). *Speech and the hearing-impaired child.* Washington D C: Alexander Graham Bell Assoc. for the Deaf, Inc.

Ling, D. (1978). Auditory coding and recoding. In M. Ross and R. Giolas (Eds.) *Auditory management of hearing-impaired children* (pp. 181-216). Baltimore Md.: University Park Press.

Ling, D., & Ling A.H. (1978). *Aural habilitation.* Washington D C: The Alexander Graham Bell Assoc. for the Deaf, Inc.

Ling, D., Ling, A., & Pflaster, G. (1977). Individual educational programming for hearing-impaired children. *Volta Review, 79,* 204-230.

Maassen, B. (1986). Marking word boundaries to improve the intelligibility of the speech of the deaf. *Journal of Speech and Hearing Research 29,* 227-230.

Manolson, A. (1985). *It takes two to talk* (2nd Revision). Toronto, Canada: Hanen Early Language Resource Centre.

Moores, D.F. (1981). *Educating the deaf: Psychology, principles and practices* (2nd Ed.) Boston, MA: Houghton Mifflin Company.

Musket, C.H. (1981). Maintenance of personal hearing aids. In M. Ross, R. J. Roeser and M. Downs (Eds.), *Auditory disorders in school children.* New York: Thieme and Straton, pp 229-248.

Northcott, W.N. (1977). *Curriculum guide hearing-impaired children (0–3 years) and their parents.* Washington DC: Alexander Graham Bell Association for the Deaf.

Northcott, W.N. (1978). *I heard that: A developmental sequence of listening activities for the young child.* Washington, DC: Alexander Graham Bell Association for the Deaf.

Paterson, M.M. (1982). Integration of auditory training of speech and language for severely hearing-impaired children. In D. Sims, G. G. Walter and R. L. Whitehead (Eds.). *Deafness and communication*, (pp. 261-270). Baltimore/London: Williams and Wilkins.

Piaget, J. (1955). *The language and thought of the child*. New York: Meridian Books.

Pickett, J.M., & McFarland, W. (1985). Auditory Implants and Tactile Aids for the Profoundly Deaf. *Journal of Speech and Hearing Research Vol. 28,* 134-150.

Plomb, R. (1986). A signal-to-noise ratio model for the speech reception threshold of the hearing impaired. *Journal of Speech and Hearing Research Vol. 29,* 146-154.

Pollack, D. (1970). *Educational audiology for the limited hearing infant*. Springfield, Illinois: Charles C. Thomas.

Pollack, D. (1984). An acoupedic program. In D. Ling (Ed.) *Early intervention for hearing-impaired children: Oral options.* San Diego, Cal: College-Hill Press.

Rhoades, E. (1982). Early intervention and development of communication skills for deaf children using an auditory-verbal approach. In K. Butler and L. W. Nober (Eds.) *Topics in language disorders: Communication skills for deaf children.* Vol. 2, No. 3, Rockville, Md.: Aspen Publications, Inc.

Rintelmann, W., & Bess, F.H. (1977). High-level amplification and potential hearing loss In F. Bess (Ed.) *Childhood deafness causation, assessment and management* (pp.267-293) New York: Grune and Stratton.

Rollins, J.C. (1972). "I heard that!" Auditory training at home. *Volta Review, 74,* 25-28.

Ross, M. (1978). Classroom acoustics and speech intelligibility. In J. Katz (Ed.) *Handbook of Clinical Audiology,* (2nd Ed. pp. 469-478). Baltimore: Williams and Wilkins.

Ross, M., & Giolas, T.G. (Eds.) (1978). *Auditory management of hearing-impaired children.* Baltimore: University Park Press, 1978.

Sanders, D. A. (1971). *Aural rehabilitation.* Englewood Cliffs, New Jersey: Prentice-Hall.

Schein, J. D. (1984). Cochlear Implants and the Education of Deaf Children. *American Annals of the Deaf Vol. 129 No.3* 324-332.

Sitnick S.V., Rushmer, N. Arpan, R., Melum, A., Sowers, J., & Kennedy, N. (1985). *Parent-Infant Communication.* (3rd Ed.). Portland, Oregon Infant Hearing Resource, Good Samaritan Hospital and Medical Centre.

Stein, D., Benner, G., Hoversten, McGinnis, M., & Thies, T. (1980). *Auditory skills curriculum.* North Hollywood, California: Foreworks.

Stoel-Gammon, C., & Otomo, K. (1986). Babbling development of hearing-impaired and normally hearing subjects. *Journal of Speech and Hearing Disorders 51,* 33-41.

Trammell, J.L., Farrar, C., Francis, J., Owens, S.L., Schepard, D.E., Witlen, R.P., Faist, L.H. (1976). *Test of Auditory Comprehension* (TAC). North Hollywood, CA: Foreworks.

Urbantschitsch, V. (1982). *Auditory training for deaf mutism and acquired deafness* (S. R. Silverman, trans.). Washington, D C: Alexander Graham Bell Assoc. for the Deaf. (Original work published 1895)

van Uden, A. (1977). *A world of language for deaf children* Part 1: Basic principles (3rd Edition). Amsterdam: Swets and Zeitlinger.

Vaughan, P. (Ed.), (1981). *Learning to listen* (Revised Edition). Don Mills, Ontario: General Publishing Co., Ltd.

Vernon, M., & Koh, S. (1972). Effects of oral preschool compared to manual communication in deaf children. In E. Mindel and M. Vernon, (Eds.) *They grow in silence.* Silver Spring, Md.: National Assoc. of the Deaf.

Whetnall, E., & Fry, D.B. (1971). *The Deaf Child.* London: Whitefriars Press.

Whitehurst, M.W. (1978). *Auditory training for children*. Washington, D C: Alexander Graham Bell Assoc. for the Deaf, Inc.

Zink, G. D. (1972). Hearing aids children wear: A longitudinal study of performance. *Volta Review, 74,* 41-51.

# CHAPTER 8

# *The Arts and the Curriculum*

There are only two ways to educate:
with torture or the fine arts —Oscar Wilde

## THE ARTS IN THE EDUCATION OF THE HEARING IMPAIRED

The arts in education have had a long, if not a somewhat discouraging, history. Perhaps reflecting the views of society in general, they have traditionally been seen as extras, cultural niceties that enhance and enliven our daily existence. Artists continue to fight for funding and support in their creative endeavors; people who support courses in the arts in educational settings continue to fight for recognition and status.

This traditional view however, may be changing. In a recent survey of provincial curricula of the arts in general education in Canada (Booth & Reynolds, 1983) the authors open with these thoughts:

> The arts are central to the students' experience. They should be experienced by all students as part of their education. They should impact on and enrich all areas of the curriculum and provide a concrete link between the school and the artists in that community. . . . The arts help people understand themselves in historical, cultural and aesthetic terms . . . provide people with broader choices about their environment and influence the way they do their work and live their lives . . . (and) . . . are instrumental in teaching basic skills as well as in furthering individual intellectual development.

Similar sentiments were reflected by 150 professional artists, educators, and performers who gathered at the First International Conference on the Visual and Performing Arts in the Education of Deaf Students in Phoenix, Arizona in 1986. The conference was designed to assist schools in discovering new ways to infuse the arts into the general curriculum, to develop the arts for arts' sake, and to stimulate the development of the total curriculum and the total teacher. Presentations were exciting and enriching experiences for the participants. The list of topics included workshops in teacher–child interaction skills, storytelling, mime, creative language experiences, music, theatre, psychodrama, dance, shadow interpreting, and television production. The full impact of these activities is yet to be felt within the classrooms of hearing-impaired children.

This chapter will focus on the inclusion of art, drama and theatre, dance and movement therapy, and music and rhythm in the education of hearing-impaired children. Before looking more closely at curricular content, however, it is first necessary to discuss some issues that are influencing the inclusion of the arts in the educational curriculum for both hearing and hearing-impaired children. These issues include discussions that center around these questions:

1. How much emphasis should be given to the arts in the teaching and learning process and within the various educational philosophies to which children are exposed?
2. Who is best qualified to teach the arts within the educational framework and to what extent can or should classroom teachers become involved?
3. Are there in existence, teaching strategies that enhance or inhibit education in the visual and performing arts? If so, are there differences in teaching style that are unique to educators of the hearing impaired?
4. Are there ways in which hearing-impaired children can especially benefit because of their unique learning style?
5. What are the benefits and goals as reviewed in the literature for the arts in the education of hearing children in general, and for hearing-impaired children in particular?

## ISSUES IN THE ARTS

### The Place of the Arts in the Curriculum

The arts do not enjoy the status of the core subjects in programs for either the hearing or the hearing impaired. Their presence in the educational program differs greatly from school to school. Indeed, even in schools where they have a place, the position of the arts varies greatly from year to year as budgets are renewed, and as staff with differing attitudes and skills come and go. It is only in those schools that have adopted a philosophy that regards the arts as a fundamental part of the program we can count on much stability.

Johnston and Kral (1979) have proposed 4 categories into which all subjects, including the arts, might be placed. These categories are: (1) enrichment; (2) minor part of the curriculum; (3) equal part of the curriculum; and (4) core of the entire curriculum. They indicate the importance accorded to each subject.

**ENRICHMENT:** Many schools have adopted the attitude that the arts should be included, but only for the purpose of enriching the other and more importnat business of schooling. This attitude is reflected in the use of national songs and folk art to illustrate certain subject matter, particularly in social studies, and in the use of facts and events studied in other disciplines as subject matter for drawing and painting.

**MINOR PART OF CURRICULUM:** The more progressive curriculum developers see the arts as important, but minor parts of the curriculum. In this case, instruction in specific art disciplines will be provided but will receive less emphasis than academic components of the curriculum.

**EQUAL PART OF CURRICULUM:** When the arts are seen as equal in importance to academic subjects, they become an integral part of the total curriculum program in the context of interdisciplinary learning.

**CORE OF THE ENTIRE CURRICULUM:** When the arts become the core around which a comprehensive curriculum is built, they provide the basic teaching and learning tools from which other academic learning is derived.

The majority of schools tend to place arts at the least important end of the continuum. Smith (1979) points out that usually, educators make "a bow to the potential of the arts in education by wedging a few minutes of music and the visual arts into the school week by occasionally 'putting on a play.' Creative drama is seldom included in the educational experience and dance almost never." Within the field of hearing impairment, with only a few exceptions, the arts are definitely regarded only as enrichment.

This may happen, however, for a very good reason. School administrators, in making budget decisions, must be convinced that their choice of priorities will provide maximum benefit for the students. When they turn to the literature for help in analyzing the role of the arts in education, they find articles that describe exciting programs, but very little in the way of substantive research. Arts programs, due largely to the popular view that they best serve as enrichment activities only, and the lack of empirical evidence to the contrary, tend to retain their somewhat frivolous identities.

Not all educators however, hold this limited view. Some believe that the arts do possess considerable educational value and feature them highly in their programs; these schools are notable exceptions. St. Michielsgestel in Holland offers a program that is based on Van Uden's (1977) sound perceptive method and provides music and rhythmical activities as a basis for the development of oral language. Work at the Rhode Island School in New York uses the visual and performing arts to help bring understanding to all areas of learning (Geisser,

1985), and the Phoenix Day School for the Deaf in Arizona offers art, music, and the theatre arts as an integral part of their curriculum. These will be referred to later in the chapter under the headings music, art, and drama.

## The Teacher

Arts specialists are usally found within educational systems for hearing students. They are hired to take responsibility for the music, art, drama, or dance program within that system. The specialist's role requires an understanding of the total curriculum and an awareness of the relevance of the arts program to the individual student. In schools for the hearing impaired, however, more often a trained teacher of the deaf with interest, ability, or willingness in some arts area has been delegated or has appropriated a role in developing an arts program. Very seldom has their specialized training as a teacher of the hearing impaired included training for this role.

These teachers often have created innovative and exciting programs, as witnessed by articles published in various journals (Atkins & Donovan, 1984; Chamberlain-Rickard, 1982; Davies, 1984; James & James, 1980; Kelly, 1980; Latimer & Vollmar, 1982; Olson & Horland, 1972; Silver, 1983; Volpe, 1979). For the most part these educators have believed in the benefits of music, drama, and art and have seen the need for instructional strategies to enhance both the motivation and the knowledge of their students. They have then created programs to meet these needs. Developed with or without specialist teachers, they are planned to enhance the world of the child in both the home and school setting. Some are taught throughout the school year; others have a summer school focus.

Individual teachers, including many who have not published their work, have long recognized the value of the arts and have incorporated music, drama, and art into their teaching according to their own abilities. This kind of flexibility can be exciting, "reflecting the varied backgrounds, interests of the individuals teaching and, above all, their own enthusiasm for the arts as an integral part of the education of hearing-impaired children" (Stern 1975). The program, however, thus rests heavily on the special talents of particular individuals. If no such individual is on staff or leaves the school, any program in the arts is in jeopardy.

There is a strong plea from many of those within the arts community to recognize the special talents, in terms of both skill and knowledge, needed to develop comprehensive, effective arts programs. Those who work directly with the arts, and who believe strongly in the educational merits for deaf children, advocate the use of trained specialists in these areas and more arts options for teachers in training programs. It has been suggested (Harrington & Silver, 1968) that it isn't the lack of potential, but lack of opportunity to develop potential that accounts for some findings that show hearing-impaired children may be lacking in some abilities that correlate highly with artistic development.

Educators of the deaf are constantly striving to improve the quality of their own communication skills and to improve the educational environment for hearing-impaired children. In order to train teachers of the hearing impaired, education programs tend to focus on areas of greatest difficulty–those of language development, reading, and communication skill development. It may indeed be extremely beneficial, to broaden the traditional perspective, and to include if not specific instruction, then at the very least an exposure to the benefits of the arts in the educational experience. Courses in the arts as options, or offered as workshop experiences, might provide teachers with new creative ways of teaching. As with educational administrators however, university training programs lack substantial research to support changes within their program.

## The Arts: The Teaching Method

Teachers of the hearing impaired may, in fact, be limiting the creative potential of their students by the style of teaching used in classrooms. The well-known deaf actor Bernard Bragg (1972) described his own schooling:

> We are products of a system that we remember as being largely learning by imitation–imitating skills, however useful and important, that we could not always sense or evaluate for ourselves. Achievement was often measured by this ability to imitate skills that were not real to us.

Research in the field of deafness that has examined classroom patterns of communication has direct relevance for the teaching of the arts. Not surprisingly, these studies show that much classroom activity is teacher-directed and teacher-dominated, very possibly limiting the development of communicative patterns and creative expression (Craig & Collins, 1970; Crandall & Albertini, 1980; Wood, Griffiths, Howarth, & Howarth, 1982). The responsibility for initiating communicative acts has been taken away from the students in the teachers' efforts to maintain control within that environment. At the same time, freedom to be creative and stray from the accepted norm most often is very limited.

For the arts teacher, however, one of the most important goals is the enhanced development of individual expression and experimentation. The recurring theme of education in the arts is that emphasis, for realization of creative potential, must be on the process; the product is secondary. Opportunity for developing that potential depends largely on the atmosphere created within the teaching and learning environment; art programs for the hearing impaired are often stifling reported Harrington and Silver (1968):

> Directive teaching, whether 'modern' or 'old fashioned', subtle or flagrant, inhibits creativity. It motivates the child through approval and generally produces similar works. It also destroys the opportunity of knowing what a child is like . . . . Freedom is consistent with

> responsibility, and self expression is consistent with aesthetic merit. The art class can be guided without being controlled.

An appropriate curriculum, along with appropriate teaching and learning strategies, can indeed provide an atmosphere conducive to the full development of potential.

## Focus on Abilities

One of the most interesting aspects of the literature dealing with the arts in education is the way it reflects the changing perceptions of the characteristics and competencies of individuals with hearing impairment. Historically, educators have had very low expectations for hearing-impaired people. It was known that achievement in academic areas was minimal for the average student. In the sustained effort to raise academic levels, little thought was spared for such "frivolous" activities as dance, painting, and drama. When the arts did appear, they did so in a negative framework. Pintner (1941) first encouraged art in the curriculum "with the hope of finding that deaf children are less handicapped in this area than in others"! Even with this pious encouragement however, schools were slow to include courses in the arts. Art supervisors felt that the work of deaf children was so inferior that "it would be unfair to compare their paintings with the work of hearing children" (Silver, 1978). This view continued despite the considerable achievement of a few hearing-impaired individuals.

Research in the 1960s and early 70s also focused on the disabilities of hearing-impaired individuals. The literature reported that the deaf encountered difficulty in abstract thinking and conceptual ability, were unimaginative and excessively concrete (Myklebust, 1964); had poor posture (Lawson, 1967; Lindsay & O'Neal 1976); were lacking in agility, locomotor coordination, hand-eye coordination, and the knowledge of and use of space (Auxter, 1971); lacked breath control and rhythmical body control (Van Uden, 1977); had high rates of emotional problems and were lacking in confidence and social skills (Arnheim, 1973; Jones, 1981; Wisher, 1974). The difficulties of achieving competency in the English language also permeated the literature. Development of curricula in the arts that required many of these missing skills was impeded by this view of the deaf as deficient.

Present day research, of course, is finding that many of the aforementioned problems are no more frequent than in the hearing population, are very often associated with problems other than hearing impairment itself, or were the results of findings based on competency in the English language. Hearing loss can and does impact greatly in many areas of development but these areas of difficulty are no longer being made as excuses for implementing programs in the arts. Because recent literature emphasizing differences in learning styles and information processing, and many educators of the deaf emphasizing the need for dynamic interactive learning experiences in language and cognition (Furth, 1966; Kretschmer & Kretschmer, 1978; Truax, 1978), it appears that educators in the arts are well placed for building on the potential strengths of hearing-impaired students. As Uhlin & DeChiara (1984) state, "the deaf may have greater interest potentially in the visual arts than the hearing, because it gives them the opportunity to express and communicate ideas through their strongest modality, the visual."

The achievements and abilities of hearing-impaired children in every area of the arts cannot be denied. Given ample opportunities to develop their potential, and given teaching methods that encourage creative thinking and openness to emotional experiences, hearing-impaired children compare very favorably with hearing children. Artistic abilities of hearing-impaired children, including imagination, originality, and abstract thinking skills are on a par with hearing children their own age and level when nonverbal instruments of assessment are used (Anderson, 1978; Silver, 1966). In fact, the deaf do better than the hearing in some areas and show significant gains in cognitive and creative skills.

In life beyond the school system one need not search far in order to see world-class artists, writers, actors, and dancers who are hearing impaired. Canadian artist Forrest Nickerson is widely recognized for his achievements and for his enthusiastic efforts to encourage the inclusion of the arts in educational and cultural programs. The photography of Annie Leibovitz, the fine acting abilities of Bernard Bragg, Emmy award winner Julianna Fjeld and academy award winner Marlee Matlin, the superb mime performances of Ricky Smith—all of these attest to the outstanding perseverance of individuals brought up through educational systems that only minimally supported or encouraged their emerging talents.

## Goals and Benefits

The goals and the benefits of arts programs differ greatly. It is worthwhile noting in the studies cited in the references that not one indicated that the performance of hearing-impaired students declined or that they were "worse off" after participating in an arts program. In an in-depth review of the literature in drama and theatre, Leaf (1979a, 1979b) found the same positive emphasis, referring both to specific benefits and to an improved quality of life.

The studies can be classified into three major types: (1) those that outline arts programs and describe content; (2) those which describe a specific program implemented for hearing-impaired children and which list the benefits and achievements that resulted; and (3) those that describe specific research projects including procedures, analysis, and results. The latter category is by far, the most meager.

Leaf (1979a) reviewed 74 items in the literature on exceptionality in general, and summarized the stated goals and benefits derived from drama/theatre activity between 1957 and 1979. Her review included 11 items directly related to the hearing impaired, the most on any of the handicapping conditions. The literature reviewed for this chapter and supplemented by this writer dealt mainly with hearing impairment, and although art, dance, and music were also included, findings are consistent with Leaf's. The following listing, based on Leaf's intensive review, serves to illustrate the many and varied areas of potential gain for hearing-impaired individuals.

1. Goals and benefits that center around the word "self," including self-understanding, self-development, self-awareness, self-esteem, self-exploration, self-acceptance, self-appreciation, self-confidence, and self-expression.
2. Goals referring to improvement in the area of such skills as verbal language and speech, body skills, or increased use of the senses. This area was heavily emphasized with hearing-impaired individuals. Music and dance have been especially noted for their use in teaching rhythmic concepts, developing auditory skills, and increased body awareness. All four areas—music, dance, drama, and the visual arts can be seen as creative vehicles by which language development can be enhanced.

   Silver (1979) has stated "Educators of deaf children often look for new ways to stimulate imagination but they usually have in mind verbal stimuli and they usually overlook art. To the extent that art experience can enable deaf children to engage in imaginary play, and possibly sustain or prolong it, it can provide opportunities for abstract thinking as well as reinforce patterns set by language and set patterns for language to follow.
3. Goals referring to cognitive skills; i.e., thinking in orderly sequence; promoting clarity of thought; increasing attention span; promoting problem solving; teaching fundamentals of drama and speech; learning concepts.

   Tomlinson-Keasy & Kelly (1978) have brought to our attention studies of the perceptual abilities of deaf children. "If, as suggested here, deafness means that the information processing system of the child takes a decidedly different developmental turn, then it behooves us as educators of the deaf to construct and provide materials and experiences which mesh with that system . . . curriculum developments could also increase the focus of visual experiences, visual labels, and visual transformations of information in an effort to maximize the potential of visually constructed information processing system."
4. Goals and benefits referring specifically to creativity. Reference has been made to the tendency to teach hearing-impaired individuals didactically. The arts are perceived as a way of letting go of these more directive approaches and emphasizing the process, rather than the product.
5. Goals and benefits referring to working with others. For hearing-impaired children solving problems together, strengthening peer relationships, and social interactions were seen as very beneficial.

6. Goals and benefits referring to integration seemed especially meaningful when hearing-impaired children worked side-by-side with hearing children.
7. Goals and benefits referring to the participant as having a positive, safe, successful experience. Items were described as having fun, expressing ideas without fear of ridicule, trying out new feelings and alternate behaviors in a safe environment, having a sense of successful accomplishment and working to one's own standards and capacities.
8. Goals and benefits having a therapeutic value. On an informed basis, the arts were seen as allowing hearing-impaired individuals to channel emotions into constructive uses; and to allow the child to communicate more easily through nonverbal channels. Reference was also made to the use of psychodrama as a therapeutic technique and to the use of art forms as a tool for the diagnosis of possible emotional problems.
9. Goals and benefits referring to the arts as a means of exposing hearing-impaired individuals to literature and different art forms.
10. Goals and benefits as a means of teaching other curricular subjects (e.g., history, reading, and social studies).
11. Goals and benefits as a means of informing the public about hearing-impaired individuals and of changing public attitudes.
12. Goals and benefits as a leisure-time activity.
13. Goals and benefits pertaining to exploration of and increased awareness of the environment.
14. Goals and benefits related to the arts as a potential career: i.e., to produce deaf drama teachers; to show that the theatre is a source of career opportunities for the deaf.

These goals and benefits are indeed comprehensive and, at this point, it is worthwhile adding a note of caution. As stated previously, more substantive research is needed to support these claims. It is important to maintain an objectivity; or, as Timms (1985) succinctly notes, "the perspective held by those who are *not* True Believers in the Cause." For those who are looking at new and innovative ways to improve approaches to curricular concerns there is no doubt as to the exciting potential that lies within the framework of education in the arts. Under what conditions and in what ways this potential may be realized is still open to question.

It is also worthwhile noting the exciting and important influence of the arts in the culture of the hearing impaired. Deaf actors, painters, sculptors, and dancers are touring the world and giving outstanding performances. The Jazz Combo group from the Rochester Institute of Technology has performed in the States and in Denmark and is gaining an international reputation for their high-quality musical performances. The Access Theatre group, serving as a forum for the disabled and nondisabled together, has received awards for outstanding achievements in the United States and tours internationally. Their workshops on the use of the performing arts in educational settings for the hearing impaired are especially noteworthy. Hollywood has recognized the special talents of the deaf actor, Albert Ballin, who has coached many famous Hollywood stars in expressing emotion through movement (Clements & Clements, 1984).

It is of critical importance, as well, to recognize the impact of the development and recognition of American Sign Language itself. Not only has its acceptance as a language helped strengthen the cultural identity of the deaf community in North America, the development of American sign language is emerging as a "vibrant new art form, a visual poetry" (House, 1979). The beauty of movement is seen on stage in theatres across America, as well-known songs, and even opera, are being interpreted and appreciated by both deaf and hearing audiences. Shadow interpreting in dramatic productions is being developed to encourage a nonintrusive way of joining verbal and visual expressive language. In poetry, sign language is taking its place "in literary tradition as the creative means of expressing the feelings and experiences of deaf persons" (Rios, 1979).

Success in the arts, especially the performing arts gives the participant and the observer a sense of power and control, and with that an emerging new status (Panara, 1980).

> The deaf person who identifies with his deaf counterpart on stage or on television gets a psychological boost which serves to remove the "stigma" of deafness. He discovers a "new image" of himself—a person with self worth, with greater confidence, with a more positive attitude toward life and society.

The goals for the arts then, may be seen as educational, creative, recreational, or cultural. When the arts become infused into the traditional subject-matter areas, they become a means to an end. Instruction may also focus on the arts as an end in itself. Bernard Bragg, justly called "The Prince of Players of the Silent Stage" (Panara, 1980), summarizes most effectively the potential of the arts in education of the hearing impaired as a vehicle for which the deaf themselves become the prime players.

> Let us create for ourselves. Guide us in teaching ourselves. Open the doors for us to those fields where there are only differences, not success or failure. Give us work in which we learn by doing; by creating ourselves real images of the world and of each other. We will retain so much more because it is our own, and fun—is that such a dirty word? Let us hold on to our imaginations, our self-awareness, and pride in our own strengths and abilities. Give us something that is not imitative; something in which we work together but without competing; where we as individuals can excel and create—where our minds are constantly enlarging towards their full potential—and where we, as humans, cannot fail" (Bragg, 1972).

## Mainstreaming and The Arts

Hearing-impaired students are being educated in many different kinds of settings. The recent past has seen a decline in the number of students in the more traditional residential schools, and an increase in the numbers of students within the public school system. As a result two bodies of literature have emerged: research and articles that deal with the hearing-impaired child who is being taught with peers by a teacher of the deaf, and literature that deals with individual students in regular classes. The information in this chapter deals with both groups, but primarily with the former. It is of value to make some remarks specifically about the second.

The *curriculum*, for hearing-impaired students who are mainstreamed, tends to be consistent with that being offered to hearing children, and is therefore subject to the same strengths and weaknesses of any existing program. Texts dealing with the arts in education have broadened to include information for the arts teacher on how to adapt teaching methods to meet the needs of all handicapped children (Anderson, 1978; Birkenshaw, 1965, 1967, 1982; Clements & Clements, 1984; Evans, 1982; Hadary & Cohen, 1978; House, 1979; Juul, 1983; McCaslin, 1984; Nordoff & Robbins, 1971; Nocera, 1979; Robertson, 1979; Uhlin & Chiara, 1984). These books usually include some kind of background information regarding the special characteristics of special-needs children, and proceed to give examples of creative changes that can be made to the programs. For the hearing impaired, background includes information mainly on hearing loss, communication style, and behavioral characteristics. Adaptations usually deal with methods of communication and use of language.

In an interesting and exciting new twist, Hadary and Cohen (1978) have developed a curriculum that balances art with a science program. The purpose of their research, which began in 1972, was to "especially design, implement, test, evaluate and finally put into a mainstream situation a laboratory science and art program for blind, deaf and emotionally disturbed children that has intellectual development and fulfillment of human potential as its goal." It is a unique program based on an assumption that both disciplines (art and science) share common learning experiences, discovering, describing, and demonstrating. The book provides both background information on various handicaps and suggestions for working with the children in laboratory situations. In addition, detailed "lesson plans" provide a wealth of exciting and stimulating ideas for the regular classroom teacher.

Anderson (1978) focuses on art, and her book is filled with creative ideas. Appreciating the intrinsic value of the arts in and of themselves, "they enrich and enhance our lives because they *are*," she also included a comprehensive annotated bibliography. In the music area Birkenshaw (1982) is able to translate musical theory based on the work of composer and author Carl Orff, and provide practical experiences that help the teacher focus on developing language skills, short term memory, bodily coordination, and listening skills, among others. These creative works help teachers bridge the gap in regular classrooms, between the needs of disabled and nondisabled students.

In order to deal more specifically with the programs and curricular content that exist mainly for those children in the more traditional school setting, where classes of hearing-impaired children are learning together, the remainder of this chapter will be devoted to each of the four major areas of focus: drama and theatre; art; dance and movement; music and rhythm.

## DRAMA AND THEATRE

To be a good teacher of the hearing impaired, indeed, to communicate effectively, one needs to be an actor or actress to express visibly the emotional overlay that lies imbedded in the intonational speech patterns so difficult for many hearing-impaired individuals. For those of us who hear, our best teachers often are deaf people themselves, who are the experts at communicating with their bodies what their voices or words may be unable to do. Even those individuals who have a good amount of residual hearing, and whose speech is highly intelligible, are strongly aware of the role of body language in communication.

In order to discuss the role of drama and theatre in the curriculum, it is first necessary to emphasize the difference between the two and to define a third component, that of mime. Drama is "involved with the process of creation and can operate at all levels—from playing games like charades, to role playing, to improvisation. Its objective is not performance as such...but to explore whatever happens to the subject" (Tomlinson, 1982). Concerned with the players themselves, and the experiences they have while playing, there are no rights and wrongs, and "all experiences are valid" (Furth and Wachs, 1975, p. 237). On the other hand, theatre requires the performance of a rehearsed program and the presence of a usually nonparticipatory, passive audience (Furth and Wachs, 1975; Tomlinson, 1982). Another form of dramatic play, that of pantomime, has been described as "the silent form of drama which is developed by movement, gesture and facial expression" (Arnold, 1980). These three must be planned into the curricula for hearing-impaired students. It is not sufficient simply to expect them to occur.

There is no doubt that creative drama is used in almost every classroom in which hearing-impaired children are learning. "Acting out" takes on new meaning when it is used positively to express an emotion or communicate an idea. Apart from readings outside the field of deafness that deal with creative drama, the teacher is usually dependent on her or his own imagination supplemented with the noteworthy articles that describe existing programs in various classes for the hearing impaired (Cayton, 1981; Davies, 1984; Denis, 1966; Gaffney, 1952; Gerits, 1980; Gould, 1983; Seely & Camus, 1983).

For many years, writers in the field of cognition and language of the hearing impaired have supported the use of drama as a creative, interactive technique to enhance and develop pragmatic and semantic functions of language and to aid thinking skills (Furth, 1970; Kretschmer & Kretschmer, 1978; Perks, Shaw, & Stevens, 1981; Truax, 1978). Stemming from this theoretical base, an innovative research-oriented program has been developed by Timms (1985) at the Phoenix Day School for the Deaf in Arizona. The Ladders Curriculum, Language Arts Through Drama in the Developmental, Educational and Remediation Systems for deaf students originated as part of a study designed to develop, execute, and evaluate a creative drama and role-playing procedure designed to teach story structure to deaf students (Timms, 1985).

Many teachers of the hearing impaired will recognize immediately the difficulties inherent in developing the concepts involved in the structure of story form, i.e., exposition, character, motivation, conflict, and problem resolution. Through the practice of actively involving children in the creative process of pantomime and story enactment, and using the creative and spontaneous products of these children as a springboard to learning, Timms has been able to present a whole new world of challenge and excitement not only to the children but also to the teachers.

This author has experienced, first hand, the process that the students experience under Timms' guidance, and the potential inherent in this dramatic form would seem to be tremendous. If there is a weakness, it lies in the fact that teachers do not learn best in workshops. Therein lies its strength: we learn best by doing. Timms also uses the unfinished story technique and playback theatre as part of the process.

Theatre for the deaf has become much more visible in the educational field in recent years. This is due partly to Davies (1984) survey of the status of theatre in programs for the hearing impaired between 1965 and 1970. Theatre activities in classes and schools for the deaf did indeed exist, but on a rather small scale. Survey results suggested that deaf children must have the use of theatre both to learn and to create; that there is a need for both specialized teachers and specialized deaf teachers (Bragg, 1972); and that the distinction between formal and informal methods of teaching and exposure to drama as opposed to training in drama be recognized.

Because of their emphasis on providing theatre and drama classes and experiences for all handicapped individuals, the deaf theatre groups have been looked upon as leaders. The founding of the National Theatre of the Deaf in 1967, impacted greatly on the members of the American Theatre Association (ATA). In 1978 the ATA authorized a special Committee on Drama/Theatre and the Handicapped that included Bernard Bragg and others. In 1980, its convention was made "accessible for the first time to deaf, blind and motorically impaired members of the theatre community" (Shaw, Perks, & Stevens 1981).

Theatre performances by deaf people have gained national and international recognition and childrens' theatres for the deaf (Olson & Horland, 1972; Robertson, 1979) are gaining in popularity. The famous PBS series, *Rainbows End*, produced by Emmy award winner Betsy Ford, has received national recognition for its excellent series that deals with the needs of deaf children. Deaf actress Linda Bove has become as much a part of young children's lives as the Cookie Monster on Sesame Street.

At the secondary education level, National Technical Institute for the Deaf (NTID) is a leader in preparing students in this area. It offers a theatre program as a chance to gain confidence, improve communication skills, and develop abilities in those areas that will be of benefit to students in their chosen field of employment. If we, as educators, maintain that one of our goals in education is to prepare students for the real world, and we know that there is opportunity for employment in all aspects of theatre for the deaf, then our schools should take a careful look at the curriculum to ensure that the opportunity exists for those students whose talents lie in this area.

## ART

"It is still true that a thousand words scarcely exhaust the richness of a single image" (Bruner quoted in Silver, 1978).

The benefits of art in the education of the hearing impaired have been supported most strongly in two ways. The works of deaf painters, sculptors, and architects attest to the fact that many are truly gifted and compete readily with others in their field (Peterson, 1981). As mentioned previously, this may attest more to the fact that these people displayed a tenacity and perseverance in developing their talents, rather than to the existence of a supportive and encouraging educational system. A well-designed curricular focus on the arts in education may very well open many more avenues to many more talented hearing-impaired children.

In addition to these successful individuals, Silver's (1978) noteworthy research has provided a solid foundation for presenting a rationale for the inclusion of art in education. Silver's studies provide evidence that hearing-impaired children can be just as creative and just as expressive in art as hearing children, when given the opportunity to develop their potential. Children with hearing impairments are also just as appreciative of the visual arts and express an eagerness to learn. Art education and art therapy can go hand-in-hand.

It would be difficult, if not impossible, to find a time when art, in some form, was not included in schools for the deaf. However, curricula for all children were not common and few schools had ongoing programs. As mentioned earlier, both our knowledge of abilities of hearing-impaired individuals and teaching methods among art specialists and teachers have changed even in the last 20 years. It is difficult, however, to estimate the impact of these discoveries in schools for the deaf. It would appear that the impact has not been substantial despite a few innovative programs of note.

Silver's recommendation that art be used for assessment purposes is an exciting one. Its usefulness in this area has typically not been given the recognition it deserves. In art, one can find clues to the child's perceptions of himself and others, his or her interests or concerns and his or her level of development (Silver,1978). In addition, drawing procedures can assess and develop cognitive abilities—ordering sequentially, associating and representing concepts, and perceiving and representing spatial relationships.

The school situation in real life, however, remains somewhat discouraging. Broussard, Russell, & Rose (1985) informally surveyed 25 elementary school teachers of the hearing impaired and found that most were dissatisfied with the art curricula their schools provided. One had been in use, unchanged, for 20 years. Others were essentially uninspiring. Unfortunately, they also discovered that "what is frequently disguised as art education—is more likely to be arts and crafts." In an attempt to get away from this "egg carton art," they developed guidelines for teachers that outline the goals, and content areas for an art curriculum for the hearing impaired (Fig. 8-1).

A similar delineation of the content for an art curriculum (James & James, 1980), suggests that the art curriculum contain three parts: (1) fundamental exploratory experiences; (2) the opportunities for the development of motivation and ideas; and (3) technical help to assist children to develop their artistic skills.

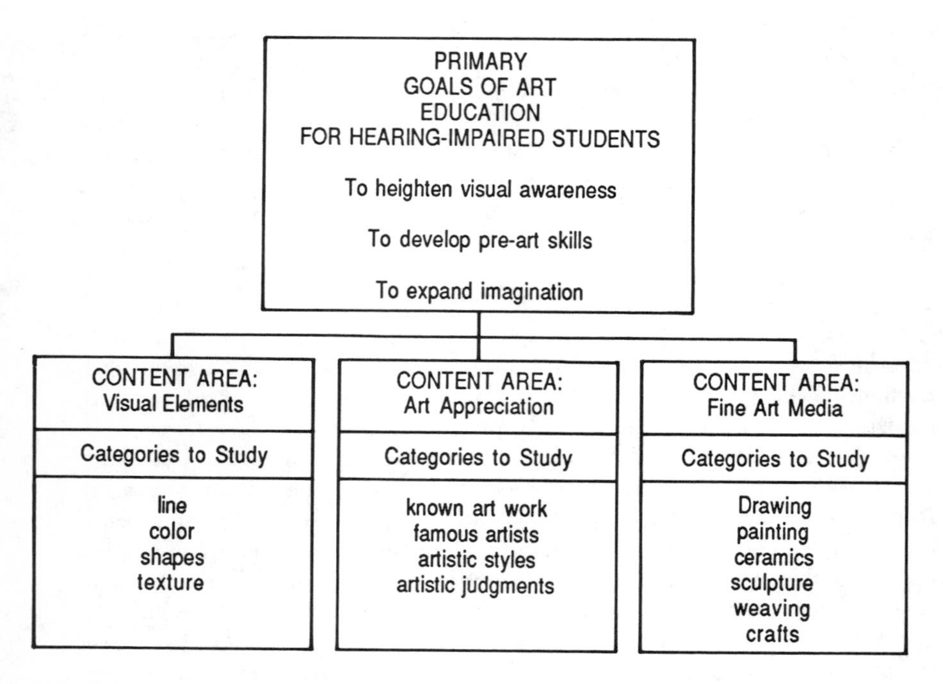


**Figure 8-1.** The goals of art education for hearing impaired students, the content areas, and the categories students should study to achieve those goals.

These suggestions closely parallel those suggested by Harrington & Silver (1968), which state that the essentials of a quality art program will include experiences in examining objects intensively, expressing ideas and feelings, and experimenting with art materials and processes.

In addition to looking at the specific content areas of an art curriculum, it is interesting to note the pervasive influence art can have on the overall educational setting when given a place of top priority within the curricular framework. The Rhode Island School uses the visual and performing arts as "a vital means of bringing understanding to all subjects in the students' world" (Geisser, 1985). For senior students, art becomes an important part of their life experiences when such subjects as art history become connected with politics, literature, math, science, dance and music. In fact, in an interesting twist to integration, Geisser states, the Senior Art Program has become "a model for humanities teaching in our community and has been offered to hearing high school students in our first reverse mainstream venture."

Research is beginning to reveal that learning styles and information processing may be very different for those people for whom the sense of hearing is impaired. Silver (1978) suggests that the role of art in the curriculum for the hearing impaired is very much underestimated; the potential for great learning and individual growth is there but not being tapped. Based on experiences in schools and from the literature, however, this writer suspects that there may be as much variation both in content and teaching philosophy in art as there are schools in North America. Art texts are readily accessible to all teachers and contain excellent suggestions for creative teaching. How these texts are used, however, will depend very much on the teachers own philosophy and expertise.

## DANCE

Although one of the first references to the use of dance with the deaf was by Lehmann in 1936, the main body of literature about dance does not appear until the 1970s. This focus was spearheaded by the work of Peter Wisher, originator and director of the Gallaudet College Modern Dance Group, formed in 1955. Since then, it has performed throughout North America and Europe. Influenced greatly by the development of American Sign Language, Wisher and his students created "a new art form" which, in essence, is "the transformation of signs to dance movement" (Wisher, 1978). Sherrill (1979) states:

> It is living proof that deaf persons can be creative, graceful in movement, and skillful in dance . . . For the hearing, dance can be considered as a supplementary vehicle in the learning process. For the deaf, it is an indispensible tool."

Deaf people throughout the world are becoming interested and involved in dance, both professionally and recreationally. Groups like the 18-member Kol Demama Modern Dance Company from Israel have been very well-received on world-wide tours; college level courses at Gallaudet and NTID in social and modern dance and the performing arts give deaf students opportunities to test and display their talents.

Although the aforementioned progress is true, and the talents of hearing-impaired dancers are applauded, as far as this author is aware, there are no specific curricular materials available in dance for working with hearing-impaired children. For the most part, programs emerge where the interests and abilities of staff enable the development of creative programs. A program in New York City, for example, developed in a formal way when the director and administrator of the Joffrey Ballet School agreed to work with a teacher of the deaf and 12 children from the New York Schools for the hearing impaired (Donniger & Evans 1979). "Ballet for Deaf Children" was highly successful for the children who worked with an interpreter and "hearing buddies." The program received a great deal of attention from both the dance and the deaf communities. "After two full years of operation, 'Ballet for Deaf Children' has succeeded in achieving its original goal of presenting young deaf children with classical ballet technique of a quality equal to the best available to hearing children" (Evans, 1980). Unfortunately such programs are rare.

Programs at schools for the deaf in which dance is taught have pursued a second important goal: "The child is encouraged to integrate these creative skills into meeting the language and objectives of the classroom. This is attained by finding the commonalities between this art form and basic learning skills . . . the approach is visual, tactile, kinesthetic, physical and, most of all, motivational" (Chamberlain-Rickard, 1982). Where dance is seen to have benefit for other subjects, as well as those for the discipline itself, greater acceptance may be anticipated.

There is a body of literature that discusses the merits of teaching dance to the hearing impaired, but apart from Silver (1970, 1977, 1978, 1983), Lubin & Sherrill (1980), and Reber & Sherrill (1981), little experimental research exists. The Reber-Sherrill study is noteworthy because, for the first time, a specific program of creative dance and movement was implemented to look at its effect on changes in creative thinking and dance movement skills. Creative thinking was measured by Torrance's (1974) *Thinking Creatively with Pictures, Figural Form B.* After 10 weeks of instruction with 10 students, aged 9 to 11, "the experimental group improved significantly in dance and movement skills, figural originality, figural elaboration, and composite score on thinking creatively" (Reber & Sherrill, 1981).

It is also interesting to note that the teaching methodology was creative rather than directive and minimized traditional teacher expectations; i.e., convergent productivity, imitation, and replication. "The significant improvement in the present study might be interpreted as evidence, not only of the growing ability to evolve details and expand ideas, but of security in the belief that one's ideas are worthy of acceptance, that classmates and teachers are interested in and willing to take the time for added details, and that one's own dance composition (and hence oneself) is important" (Reber & Sherrill, 1981). The authors concluded with a strong rationale to include "creative dance in the physical education instruction of young children . . ." (and) "to employ a dance specialist as one of the physical education teachers."

Dance and movement are beginning to gain recognition as therapeutic tools as well. "Body movement therapy, or dancy therapy, is the planned use of any aspect of dance, movement, and sensory experience to further the physical and psychic integration of the individual . . . movement therapy may also include some aspects of music therapy, the main difference being that the ultimate goal of the former is a movement experience rather than an auditory experience" (Weisbord, 1972).

In some schools for the hearing impaired, children will have access to a dance and movement therapist, one who has had special training in the use of dance or movement as the mode of intervention in therapy or change in personal growth. This specialist has training in movement observation and analysis and is able to plan programs to meet the specific needs and abilities of individual children. One form of movement therapy, *eurythmy* (Ogletree, 1976), is often confused with Dalcroze's *eurythmics* "a form of dance to melody." Created by Rudolf Steiner in 1912, it "differs from other arts of movement such as ballet, modern dance and mime which are generally confined to music or gesture interpretation. Instead, eurthmy is a disciplined art of movement of the arms and body that visibly expresses the vowels and consonants of speech and the tones and intervals of musical melody" (Donath, quoted in Ogletree, 1976). Innovative teachers of the hearing impaired should be encouraged to explore this technique.

Although Boorman (1973, 1982) writes for all children, not specifically those with special needs, her rationale for the significance of creative dance in the curriculum seems especially important for hearing-impaired children.

> There are ideas, images and feelings that can be expressed and communicated in dance that cannot be rendered in verbal language, be it spoken or written, music, the visual arts, or any other idiom . . . . The creative dance form . . . is conceptually based. The child is introduced to the language of concepts be they spatial: above, below, near, far; temporal: lingering, hastening, sparkling; motor: leaping, whirling, sinking, hopping; and he develops these concepts alone and in social situations with others. This conceptual base has the broadest and deepest 'language' potential for children's dance. When these concepts . . . are used in the richest possible way and then the added factor of social interrelationships is encompassed, the learning environment for the child becomes a "powerhouse" of articulation, expressions and communication.

## MUSIC AND RHYTHM

Music and rhythm have been soundly documented in the history of education of the hearing impaired. It is interesting to note that of all the four major areas—music, dance, art, and drama—the greatest number of articles was found to focus on the area of greatest disability. Music requires sound perception, and of course the variability within the hearing-impaired population is great. Hearing loss forces the teacher to look closely at the development and remediation of language, speech, and residual hearing; these are the areas in which music and rhythm have seemed to be most useful.

In 1984, Spitzer published survey results that reviewed the extent to which music was used in schools for the hearing impaired. Of 91 respondents, 57 percent incorporated music into their programs. Of the 52 schools involved, 13.5 percent used music for the sole purpose of speech improvement and curriculum enrichment only, and 36.5 percent used it for curriculum enrichment only. While 34 schools had a specially trained person for the subject, 18 schools used regular classroom teachers.

Hearing-imparied children are exposed to varying amounts of musical training determined largely by the philosophy of each school. The amount of structure within the program and the degree of emphasis placed on it varies widely. Programs planned with consistency and skill would seem to hold the greatest chance for success.

Numerous articles describe approaches which have been described by teachers interested in working with hearing-impaired children and music (Atkins & Donovan, 1984; Bang, 1980; Brick, 1973; Fahey & Birkenshaw, 1972; Kanter, 1984; Kelly, 1980; McDermott, 1971; Stern, 1975; Sullivan, 1982; Swaiko, 1974). The abilities of these children differ greatly. Many enjoy participation in school rhythm bands; some profoundly deaf individuals have learned to play solo instruments in ways which are equivalent to musical hearing children (Robbins, Robbins, & Boothroyd, 1980).

Early uses of music with deaf children in some formal sense were recorded by Itard in 1802 (Hummel, 1971). In North America, in 1877, first records indicate the use of the drums at the New York School for the Deaf in their military training classes (Korduba, 1975). Numerous authors have written about the benefits of musical and rhythmical activity for the hearing impaired; as with the other areas in the arts, few have been scientifically investigated. Literature in both the areas of sound perception and importance of rhythm in speech development relate well to the use of music, and findings in these areas can aid very much in program planning and individualizing instruction.

There is some research evidence that the rhythmic responses of hearing-impaired children are unrelated to factors such as intelligence, home environment, and musical background. Although slower to respond, deaf children's responses to rhythmic patterns appeared equivalent to hearing children (Blatt, 1964; Rileigh, 1971). Korduba (1975) found that the deaf averaged fewer errors in both beat and rhythm scores, and, in some cases, did better. It was hypothesized that the deaf students were able to make better use of their attending and imitating strategies.

Other research has shown that, with training, deaf children who have a loss greater than 90 dB can hear differences between two notes that are a tone or semitone apart, a 6 percent change in pitch, and that with suitable hearing aids, most deaf children can hear not only the fundamental frequency, but also most of the overtones of the majority of the instruments (Robbins, Robbins, & Boothroyd, 1980). The use of music to indirectly train the basic functions of speech and language has also been investigated (Bang, 1980). Little doubt exists that hearing-impaired students can participate in music and rhythm activities if given the opportunity.

There is, in this area of the arts, also, a body of literature that describes programs of the foremost proponents of music use in the education of the hearing impaired. These programs have become the basis of curricular content in schools in which music and rhythm have been used. This chapter can provide only a brief introduction to the major components of the programs; the reader is encouraged to refer to the references for further reading. In the following section, the works of Orff, Van Uden, Birkenshaw, and Guberina will be briefly reviewed.

Orff, a German composer and musician well known for his choral works such as the magnificient *Carmina Burana*, has been influential in the development of music programs for hearing-impaired children. His "Schulwerk" (Hall, 1960; Orff, 1955), the collective name for publications of 5 volumes of *Music for Children*, was designed to introduce children to music in the way primitive man is thought to have discovered it: first through rhythm, then melody, later harmony, and, still later, through form. Orff believed that the child must learn to feel music inwardly before studying of notes and other formal attributes. To achieve this aim, movement, melody, and rhythm should be rejoined. His work entails the blending of the two basic sources of rhythm—movement (e.g., walking and running) and speech (Birkenshaw, 1965).

The blending of body movement with speech in a rhythmical sense is the general focus for children with hearing impairments. Teachers use Orff's music in one of three ways:

1. as a method, using the printed work without making changes in rhythm, melody or instrumentation, or by adapting the material to the specific needs of a specific group of children
2. as a model, treating the publications as a collection of examples showing one of several ways in which certain aims may be realized
3. as an approach, basing it on the theory inherent in *Music for Children* (Sandvoss, 1970).

Orff's work is characterized by the use of improvisation and incorporates the use of specially designed instruments that are extremely important to teachers of the deaf because of their low frequency vibrations and extremely pleasant tonal quality. Relaxation, rhythmic movement, listening, echo clapping, notation, songs, and instrumental work form the basis of Orff's program. The joy of creating and making music with others is also emphasized.

The work of Van Uden in Holland, is perhaps best known (Van Uden, 1953, 1960, 1963, 1965, 1970, 1981, 1983). He and his colleagues have been responsible for a large body of research and writing that investigates the rhythm of language and speech, motor development, and the effect of music and rhythm programs on the development of children with hearing impairment. Van Uden's work has been influential in many areas of education of the deaf, notably that of the development of oral speaking skills and language development. The reader is encouraged to become familiar with his works.

Van Uden's sound perception method, in combination with music, expressive movement, and dance, have been adopted fully and integrated into the entire teaching philosophy of Sint Michielsgestel School in Holland. Van Uden's method looks carefully into the communication aspects of developing language and what he calls the conversational method. Emphasis is placed on sound perception with the use of special organs, instruments, and loud speakers; on breathing and breath control; on the sense of rhythm that moves from body movement to speech to language and culminates in what he calls the "play song." As Van Uden states "In my opinion an intense training in rhythm of the whole body, of breathing and speech, integrated with sound perception, auditory remnants and vibration feeling is a must in schools for the deaf" (Van Uden, 1970).

Birkenshaw has been one of the foremost North American music educators working with hearing-impaired children. Basing her work on Orff's methods, she has developed a tremendous understanding of the needs of children with disabilities and especially those with hearing impairments. Her book, *Music for Fun: Music for Learning* (1982) is a treasure of ideas for both music specialists and classroom teachers and is easily translated into practice by those with little or no musical training (see Fig. 8-2).

In addition to those already mentioned, Guberina has developed what is called the *Verbotonal Method*, one which "creates speech structures based on the rhythm of nursery rhymes and the rhythm of body movements" (Hummel, 1971). His method requires the use of highly specialized expensive and sensitive equipment and perhaps for this reason has not been widely implemented in classes for the hearing impaired. His program also depends on the amplification of an extremely low frequency range of sound "down to one cycle i.e., infra sound" and has been questioned on a theoretical basis by educators and audiologists. Nevertheless the emphasis on rhythm and sound perception together has contributed well to the area.

The name *eurythmics* occurs, too, in the titles of articles that describe programs for deaf children. It is a system of education in the arts originated by Dalcroze, a Swiss composer and music teacher (Swaiko, 1974). Because of the combination of creative movement, vibration, vocalization, sound

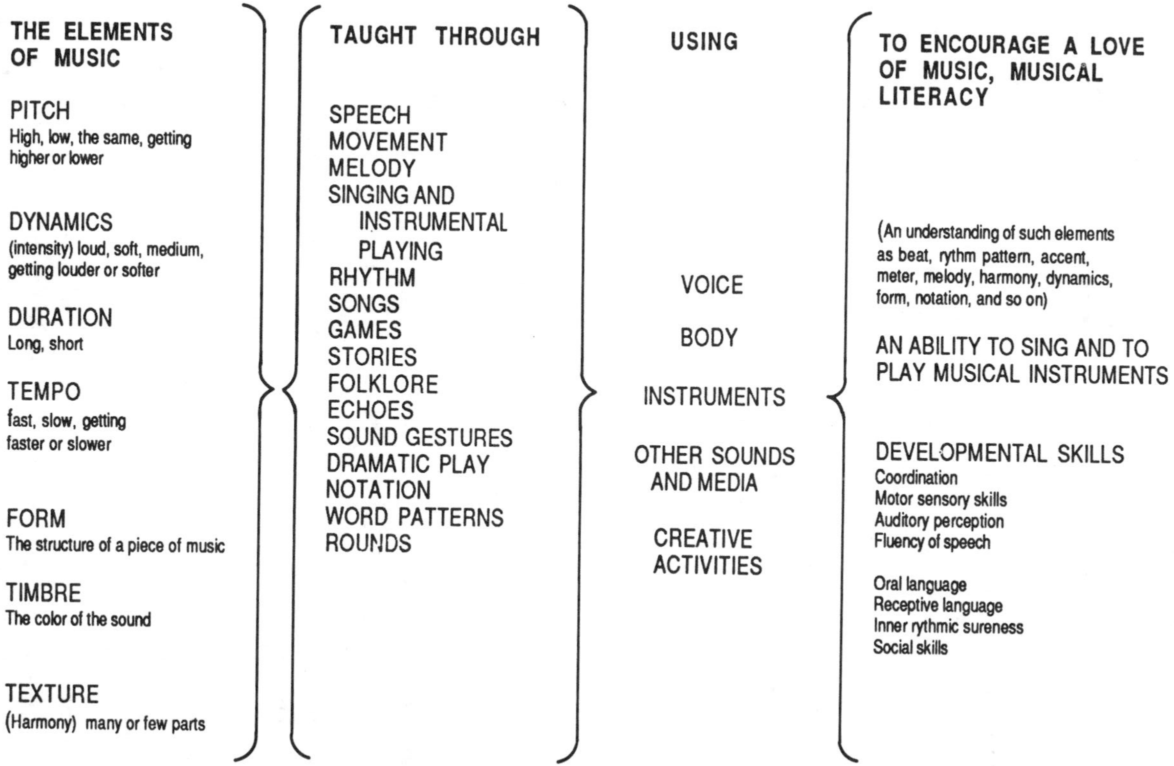

THE ELEMENTS OF MUSIC

PITCH
High, low, the same, getting higher or lower

DYNAMICS
(intensity) loud, soft, medium, getting louder or softer

DURATION
Long, short

TEMPO
fast, slow, getting faster or slower

FORM
The structure of a piece of music

TIMBRE
The color of the sound

TEXTURE
(Harmony) many or few parts

TAUGHT THROUGH

SPEECH
MOVEMENT
MELODY
SINGING AND INSTRUMENTAL PLAYING
RHYTHM
SONGS
GAMES
STORIES
FOLKLORE
ECHOES
SOUND GESTURES
DRAMATIC PLAY
NOTATION
WORD PATTERNS
ROUNDS

USING

VOICE
BODY
INSTRUMENTS
OTHER SOUNDS AND MEDIA
CREATIVE ACTIVITIES

TO ENCOURAGE A LOVE OF MUSIC, MUSICAL LITERACY

(An understanding of such elements as beat, rythm pattern, accent, meter, melody, harmony, dynamics, form, notation, and so on)

AN ABILITY TO SING AND TO PLAY MUSICAL INSTRUMENTS

DEVELOPMENTAL SKILLS
Coordination
Motor sensory skills
Auditory perception
Fluency of speech

Oral language
Receptive language
Inner rythmic sureness
Social skills

**Figure 8-2.** From L. Birkenshaw. (1982). *Music for fun: Music for learning*, Toronto, Ontario: Holt, Rinehart and Winston. Reprinted by permission.

perception, and simple orchestration, it also becomes a useful and expressive tool for developing musical awareness in children. "Intended for teaching music, it also has proved effective as a general method of using rhythm as a co-ordinating factor in all of the arts."

In addition to the above, the influence of music therapy is being seen in educational fields. The aims for therapy are centered on the client and do not start from the music. The music therapist must first have a diagnosis that works toward developing expanding communication. Music therapy "is the controlled application of specially organized music activities with the intention of furthering the development and cure during the treatment, education and rehabilitation of children and adults who have motor, sensory or emotional handicaps" (Bang, 1981). Though little used with hearing-impaired students to date, music therapy should not be ignored by curriculum designers. There is a place for the use of music and rhythm in the curriculum for hearing-impaired children. To the extent that hearing-impaired children can benefit from a musical education and, more importantly, to the extent that they can enjoy their experiences, "music for every child" can become a reality.

## SUMMARY

In this chapter, the arts in the education of the hearing impaired has been examined. Issues that concern educators: those dealing with the priority of the arts in education, staffing, teaching style, training and research, were outlined in an attempt to provide a broad background to specific educational problems.

The need to teach to the inherent strengths of hearing-impaired students was also addressed. The abilities of many children, in most respects equivalent to their hearing peers, have yet to be tapped. The enormous successes that have already been achieved by many individuals in spite of a system that largely ignores creative endeavor, attests to the dedication and perseverance of these individuals. The goals for and benefits of an arts curriculum were also summarized.

Looking at both curricula for the mainstreamed student, and the student in self-contained classes, the chapter examined in depth the areas of art, drama and theatre, dance, and music and rhythm. Examples of some school programs already in existence, and concerns specifically related to each area were addressed.

It is worthwhile noting that in some areas, at least, there seems to be little disagreement. A focus on the arts in education is becoming apparent at all levels of concern. Curriculum planners can no longer afford to exclude them from the curriculum. Formal planning is essential. In an age in which educators are trying to meet the needs of children by offering choices and alternatives, the arts can indeed present exciting and challenging options.

A recent survey of provincial curricula in the arts in Canadian schools (Council of Ministers of Education, 1983), indicates that there is a positive and active "trend toward the acceptance of aesthetic values as being central to education." Ministries of Education are making provision for teachers to receive retraining and upgrading in the arts; school divisions are employing arts consultants or coordinators; some schools have visiting artist programs.

The arts in education of the hearing impaired should be no different. Teachers are constantly looking for ways to help create positive, enriching and stimulating learning environments. Music, dance, drama, and art may indeed provide ways to achieve this end.

## TYPE ART RESOURCES IN REVIEW

*Introduction to Painting (Program)* and *Communication Activities for Introduction to Painting* (Program) Model Secondary School for the Deaf (1977)

*Music for Fun: Music for Learning* (Activities) L. Birkenshaw (1982)

*Music for the Hearing Impaired and Other Special Groups* (Curriculum) C. Robbins, C. Robbins, and A. Boothroyd (1980)

## *INTRODUCTION TO PAINTING* AND *COMMUNICATION ACTIVITIES FOR INTRODUCTION TO PAINTING*

### Model Secondary School for the Deaf

*Publisher*:
The Model Secondary School for the Deaf
Gallaudet College
Washington, D.C.

*Skills taught*: Classification of Paintings, Watercolor Painting, Acrylic Painting and Oil Painting

*Age/grade range*: 14–20 years of age, reading at a 3.5 grade level or higher

*Group size*: Suggested five students maximum per class

**THEORY:** This course in painting is one of a series of courses that have been developed by the Pre-college Programs at Gallaudet College. Others in the series include courses in the Elements of Art, Sculpture, Drawing, Ceramics, Photography, Printmaking and Music. A complete list can be obtained from the college.

Because of the commitment of the Programs to serve the profession at large, these course guides are available to interested schools. Although their effectiveness has not been scientifically validated, they have been used successfully by experienced teachers and are offered as guidelines that can be easily adapted to meet the needs of students and teachers.

**DESCRIPTION:** The course guide is intended primarily for use with hearing-impaired students but could easily be adapted to fit the needs of hearing students as well. Each unit contains specific "Terminal Performance Objectives", and smaller more precise ones called "Enabling Objectives." In addition, the authors include relevant learning activities and tests designed to enhance and meet these objectives. Students are encouraged to proceed at their own pace and each course contains an estimated time for completion. In painting, for example, a fast student may take approximately 21 weeks given 3 hours per week of class; a slower student may take as long as 49 weeks to complete it.

Each overview contains a rationale, description of the student population, necessary prerequisite skills and concepts (e.g., how to mat flat art, kinds of lines—their directions and characteristics), a list of supplies and materials, and a bibliography.

The lessons themselves contain the objectives, teacher preparations, in-class preliminaries and learning activities. The text for the activities carefully defines the language and specific concepts being introduced and gives the teacher a clear example of how to explain the new work.

In addition to the course guide itself, individual studies are also made available to the student. These studies list possible projects for an individual who is then required to contract for *X* number of projects. This enables the student and the instructor to focus on specific areas of weakness and strength and interest.

The Course Guide is also strengthened and enhanced for deaf students through use of a supplementary communication activities guide. This supplement "is intended to provide practice in all communication modalities available to students, but particularly stresses attending, listening and speechreading skills." All activities incorporate the subject matter of the Introduction to Painting Course and are designed to be used as part of that course.

Many of the activities are designed to be used with a Language Master or similar audiocard readers and contain both the materials to be used in preparation of the cards and student worksheets. Illustrations of all the vocabulary and concepts are also provided.

**EVALUATION:** This series is unique in its thoroughness. Any teacher who values the idea of enhancing communication skills through the use of meaningful and relevant materials will appreciate the detail of these guides.

The Introduction to Painting course itself is fairly advanced, and necessitates some background and experience on the part of the students. In addition, the teacher must have some artistic knowledge and experience and should be able to achieve "some professional judgement of the artistic merit of student productions." However, the clear listing of behavioral objectives and the provision for individualized instruction are among the guides' foremost strengths. The attention given to the language level and clarity of vocabulary is also of great benefit to prospective users of this guide.

### *MUSIC FOR FUN, MUSIC FOR LEARNING*

**L. Birkenshaw**

*Publisher*:
Holt, Rinehart and Winston Ltd.
55 Horner Avenue
Toronto, Ontario
M8Z 4X6

*Skills taught:* The activities are designed to help the child attain motor, auditory, and rhythmic skills through games, songs, dances, rhythmic activities, and speech activities.

*Age/grade range*: All ages, developed especially for children with handicaps

*Group size*: Small class or individual

**THEORY:** This book presents fun and simple activities that have been used with handicapped as well as with other children. Birkenshaw has incorporated the philosophical approach of Carl Orff into her work, but because the book has been prepared for the regular classroom teacher, who has little or no music background, all activities and explanations have been kept simple. "No great skill is necessary to use them — all you need is enthusiasm" (Birkenshaw, 1982).

**DESCRIPTION:** The book is wonderfully easy to read and to use. It begins with a rationale for music in special education, gives hints as to how to most effectively use the book, and explains some unfamiliar terms.

The activities are grouped under chapter headings such as "Let's Sing," "Relaxation," "Coordination," "Spatial Relationship and Body Rhythm," and "Painless Learning with Songs, Poetry and Movement." The ideas are numbered for easy reference, and cross referencing allows for expansion of a specific idea or skill. Some sections may be taught in a progressive manner; others may be selected for fun and interest. Sample lesson plans, in fact, encourage the teacher to pick and choose ideas from a variety of spots so as to include different sections for presentation. A lesson plan using a transportation theme, for example, includes ideas covering warm up, let's move, let's listen, speech, song, notation, and instruments.

Most of the games, activities, and poems have one or more side headings adjacent to the main text. These headings (e.g., directionality, auditory sequencing, coordination, group participation, visual discrimination) indicate the concepts the activity promotes. In addition, simple melody lines are provided for various activities and the text is abundant with the names of additional songs, poems, books, and records that may be used.

**EVALUATION:** Birkenshaw notes in the introduction: "I hope that the use of the ideas presented will help make your music time more relaxed and happy." I believe that she has presented her material in such a way as to allow this to happen. The content, as well, is delightful and it becomes increasingly easier for the teacher to incorporate these activities into the daily routine, i.e., singing while waiting for the bus.

The teacher working with hearing-impaired children must adapt the presentation of these materials to the special needs of these children. This requires little effort however as the ideas themselves are simply presented and visually emphasized; very often special speech and language considerations have already been incorporated. A creative and enthusiastic teacher will enjoy this text immensely.

## *MUSIC FOR THE HEARING IMPAIRED*

### C. Robbins and C. Robbins (with an audiological Introduction by A. Boothroyd)

*Publisher*:
Magnamusic—Baton
10370 Page Industrial Boulevard,
St. Louis, Missouri 63132

*Skills taught*: Classroom Instrumental Work, Music Knowledge, Music Reading, Singing, Musical Auditory Training, Plays and Stories with Music, Movement and Dance

*Age/grade range*: Ages 3 to 16

*Group size*: Class group or individual

**THEORY:** *Music for the Hearing Impaired* was developed for children with severe-to-profound hearing losses and is a product of a 4-year developmental music program at the New York State School for the Deaf, in Rome, N.Y. The philosophical approach stems from the Robbins' belief that musicality is inborn in all children, including the deaf. As the program unfolded, they discovered that, indeed, there was a continuum of abilities and interests among these children—from those who were profoundly deaf and musically gifted, to those who had more hearing but less interest and motivation.

The Robbins have attempted to maintain the program as a *music* program, so that "its own musical purposes would be fulfilled." At the same time, they are able to recognize the contribution of their program to other areas of the students' development: social awareness, speech and language development, and auditory training. They maintain that the curriculum itself should not be self-serving. "It was not a question of the students fulfilling the curriculum, but of the curriculum fulfilling the students."

The authors have attempted to blend within this framework, the philosophical awareness and practical techniques from several well-known musical programs for hearing people. Although some work from both Orff and Kodaly appears in the curriculum, most of the writing developed as a result of the integration of the instructors' personal and theoretical backgrounds in order to meet the needs of the hearing-impaired students. The authors themselves recognize the unique quality of their own program and the contribution of other musicologists to the field. They encourage music teachers to incorporate different areas of expertise into their programs. This curriculum is meant to serve "as a reference, a source of useful materials, and a guide."

**DESCRIPTION:** The Resource Manual and Curriculum Guide covers eight major areas of the music program: singing, classroom instruments, music reading, musical auditory training, instrumental instruction, movement and dance, and music knowledge. Each of these areas can be taught in a separate manner, or may also "combine productively with each of the others."

The book opens with an Introduction by Arthur Boothroyd on the "Audiological Considerations in Music with the Deaf." Boothroyd uses a question and answer format to clearly explain the relationship between musical perception and hearing loss. Included are audiometric configurations that show the measurements of the frequencies and decibel levels of the sounds put out by various instruments.

Each chapter is introduced by writing that gives the reader a rationale for the activities and the background information needed to pursue the goals for that section. Each activity is then described in detail, with appropriate directions and suggestions for the teacher. In addition, musical scores accompany each activity, and include suggestions for further use and development. Although the activities were developed for a leader working with an accompanist, suggestions are given for adaptation by a teacher who works alone.

Each item in a chapter has been given both progressive and suitability gradings. A progressive grading indicates the ages that will benefit most by incorporating the piece into a developing curriculum. The piece, however, can still be effective with older students who have had little or no experience; it is called the suitability grading.

The appendices also contain sample Individual Educational Programs (IEP), an introduction to pentatonic piano improvisation, application of the program to other special groups and suggestions for further research.

**EVALUATION:** *Music for the Hearing Impaired* is a thorough compilation of activities and ideas that are essential to the development of any musical program for hearing-impaired children. In fact, it is the only music curriculum of its kind that has been produced directly from experiences in working with this population. Both the varied content and the specificity of directions are the strengths of the writing.

It has been intended as a guide for people who have some musical training and as such it is invaluable. The program is seen as worthwhile in and by itself and there has been no attempt made to incorporate musical activities into the regular classroom time. For those schools with the financial backing to both develop music programs and hire music teachers, this curriculum will be of great interest. Any music teacher of hearing children, who is trying to meet the needs of a hearing-impaired child in an integrated setting, will also benefit greatly from the special suggestions offered.

The author would also like to suggest however, that there is a wealth of information and ideas available as well, for the teacher who has very little musical background. The sections on singing, auditory training, and movement and dance can be incorporated into daily classroom experiences and therefore it is hoped that the inexperienced teacher will not be put off by the rather overwhelming appearance of musical text and photographs of exciting, though formal, music classes. For teachers interested in providing challenging educational and socially satisfying experiences, the Robbins have contributed a great deal.

## REFERENCES


Anderson, F.E. (1978). *Art for all the children: A creative sourcebook for the impaired child*. Springfield, IL: Charles C. Thomas.

Arnheim, D.D. (1973). *Principles and methods of adapted physical education* (2nd ed.). St. Louis: C.V. Mosby.

Arnold, B. (1980). Teaching deaf children rhythm-ballet-pantomime. In J.G.Verlag (Ed.), *Proceedings of the International Congress on Education of the Deaf* (Vols. 1, 2, 3). Hamburg.

Atkins, W., & Donovan, M. (1984). A workable music education program for the hearing-impaired. *Volta Review 86*(1), 41-44.

Auxter, D. (1971). Learning disabilities among deaf population. *Exceptional Children, 37*(8), 573-577.

Bang, C. (1980). A world of sound and music. *Teacher of the Deaf 4*(4), 106-115.

Bang, C. (1981). A world of sound and music for hearing impaired and multiply handicapped children. In Somerset Education Authority (coordinator), *Ways and means 3*. Hampshire, England: Globe Education.

Birkenshaw, L. (1965). Teaching music to deaf children: An application of Carl Orff's music for children. *Volta Review 67*,(5), 352-358, 387.

Birkenshaw, L. (1967). A suggested program for using music in teaching deaf children. In *Proceedings of the International Congress on Oral Education of the Deaf*, (Vol.2). Washington, DC: Alexander Graham Bell Association for the Deaf.

Birkenshaw, L. (1982). *Music for fun: Music for learning* (3rd ed.). Toronto: Holt, Rinehart and Winston of Canada.

Blatt, A. (1964). Rhythmic responsiveness of normal elementary school children. *Dissertation Abstract, 25* (2), 1315.

Boorman, J. (1973). *Dance and language experience with children*. Don Mills, Ontario, Academic Press Canada.

Boorman, J. (1982). Movement education. *Elements: Translating theory into practice*, (Vol. *13*, No. 8). Edmonton: University of Alberta, Department of Elementary Education.

Booth, D., & Reynolds, H. (1983). *ARTS: a survey of provincial curricula at the elementary and secondary levels* Council of Ministers of Education, Canada.

Bragg, B. (1972). The human potential of human potential—art and the deaf. *American Annals of the Deaf, 117*(5), 508-511.

Brick, R.M. (1973). Eurythmics: One aspect of audition. *Volta Review, 75*, 155-160.

Broussard, B.L., Russell, C.L., & Rose, S. (1985). Art education or arts and crafts... Which one are we providing students? *Perspectives for Teachers of the Hearing-Impaired, 3*(4) 10-13.

Cayton, H. (1981). The contribution of drama to the education of deaf children. *Teacher of the Deaf 5*(2), 49-54.

Chamberlain-Rickard, P. (1982). The use of creative movement, dramatics, and dance to teach learning objective to the hearing-impaired child. *American Annals of the Deaf, 127*(3), 369-373.

Clements, C.B. & Clements, R.D. (1984). *Art and mainstreaming: Art instruction for exceptional children in regular school classes.* Springfield, IL: C.C. Thomas.

Council of Ministers of Education. (1983). *Arts: A survey of provincial curricula at the elementary and secondary levels.* Toronto, Ontario: Author.

Craig, W., & Collins, J. (1970). Communication patterns in classes for deaf children. *Exceptional Children, 37,* 238-239.

Crandall, K., & Albertini, J. (1980). An investigation of variables of instruction and their relation to rate of English language learning. *American Annals of the Deaf, 125,* 427-434.

Davies, D.G. (1984). Utilization of creative drama with hearing-impaired youth. *Volta Review, 96*(2), 106-113.

Denis, T.B., (1966). Repertory theatre for the deaf. *The Deaf American, 19*(4), 26-27.

Donniger, M. & Evans, J. (1979). Ballet for deaf children. *Deaf American, 31*(7), 3-7.

Evans, J.F. (1980). Ballet instruction for deaf children. In J.G. Verlag, (ed.), *Proceedings of the International Congress on Education of the Deaf Hamburg, (p. 447).*

*Fahey, J.D., & Birkenshaw, L. (1972, April). Bypassing the ear: The perception of music by feeling and touching. Music Educators Journal, 58*(8), 44-49, 127-128.

Furth, H.G. (1966). *Thinking without language. Psychological implications of deafness.* New York: The Free Press.

Furth, G., & Wachs, H. (1975). *Thinking goes to school.* Toronto, Ontario: Oxford University Press.

Furth, H. (1970). A review and perspective on the thinking of deaf people. In J. Hellmuth (Ed.), *Cognitive studies: Vol. 1,* pp. 291-238. New York, NY: Brunner-Mal Publishers.

Gaffney, J.P., Jr. (1952). Creative dramatics for hard of hearing children. *Volta Review, 54,* 40.

Geisser, P.J. (1985). *Art history: More than a cut-paste lesson for deaf education.* Paper presented at the International Congress on Education of the Deaf, University of Manchester, England.

Gerits, B. (1980). Expressive movement and dance in the education of the deaf. In J.G. Verlag (Ed.), *Proceedings of the International Congress on Education of the Deaf,* Hamburg.

Gould, D.G. (1983). Nurturing expression via creative dramatics. *Perspectives for Teachers of the Hearing Impaired, 1*(3), 4-7.

Hadary, D.E. & Cohen, S.H. (1978). *Laboratory science and art for blind, deaf and emotionally disturbed children: A mainstreaming approach.* Baltimore: UP Press.

Hall, D. (1960). *Teachers manual. Orff-Schulwerke. Music for Children* Mainz: B. Schott's Sohne.

Harrington, J.D., & Silver, R.A. (1968). Art education and the education of deaf students. In H. Kopp (Ed.), *Curriculum, cognition and content* [Monograph]. Washington, D.C.: Alexander Graham Bell Association for the Deaf.

House, E. (1979). Careers in the theatre for the skilled. In A.M. Shaw & C.J. Stevens (Eds.), *Drama, theatre and the handicapped.* New York: The American Theatre Association, (pp. 31-34).

Hummel, C.J.M. (1971). The value of music in teaching deaf students. *Volta Review, 73*(4), 155.

James, P. & James, C. (1980). The benefits of art for mainstreamed hearing-impaired children. *Volta Review, 82*(2), 103-108.

Johnston, J., & Kral, B. (1979). Programs and projects in progress, In A. Shaw & C.J. Stevens (Eds.), *Drama theatre and the handicapped.* Washington, D.C.: American Theatre Association.

Jones, T. (1981). Language for and through gymnastics. In Somerset Education Authority

(Coordinator), *Ways and means 3*. Hampshire England: Globe Education.

Kanter, A. (1984) The N.T.I.D. combo. *NTID Focus*, Rochester, NY: National Technical Institute for the Deaf.

Kelly, J. (1980). Something to sing about. *Volta Review, 82*(5), 289-293.

Korduba, O.M. (1975). Duplicated rhythmic patterns between deaf and normal hearing children. *Journal of Music Therapy, 12*(3), 136-146.

Kretschmer, R.R., & Kretschmer, L.W. (1978). *Language development and intervention with the hearing impaired*. Baltimore: University Park Press.

Latimer, G., & Vollmar, S. (1982). Using puppets to develop language, creativity, and speech skills with hearing-impaired pupils. *Teacher of the Deaf, 6*(4), 106-111.

Lawson, J.C. (1967). Physical education and deaf children. *Teacher of the Deaf, 65*, 189-193.

Leaf, L. (1979a). Drama, theatre and the handicapped: A review of the literature. In A.M. Shaw & C. Stevens (Eds.), *Drama, theatre and the handicapped*. Washington, DC: American Theatre Association.

Leaf, L. (1979b). Drama theatre and the handicapped: A selected and annotated bibliography. In A.M. Shaw & C. Stevens (Eds.), *Drama, theatre, and the handicapped*. Washington, D.C.: American Theatre Association.

Lehmann, E.M. (1936). *A study of rhythms and dancing for the feeble minded, the blind, and the deaf*. Masters Thesis, Ohio State University, Columbus.

Lindsay, D., & O'Neal, J. (1976). Static and dynamic balance skills of eight year old deaf and hearing children. *A.A.D., 121*(1), 49-55.

Lubin, E., & Sherril, C. (1980). Motor creativity of preschool deaf children. *A.A.D., 125*(4), 460-466.

McCaslin, N. (1984). *Creative drama for the special child*. New York: Longman.

McDermott, E.P. (1971, April). Music and rhythms: From movement to lipreading and speech. *Volta Review, 73*(4), 229-232.

Model Secondary School for the Deaf. (1977a). *Introduction to painting*. Washington, DC: Gallaudet College.

Model Secondary School for the Deaf. (1977b). *Communication activities for introduction to painting*. Washington, DC: Gallaudet College.

Myklebust, H.R. (1964). The *psychology of deafness* (2nd ed.). New York: Grune and Stratton.

Nocera, S.D. (1979). *Reaching the special learner through music*. Morristown, NJ: Silver Burdett Co.

Nordoff, P., & Robbins, C. (1971). *Therapy in music for handicapped children*. Suffolk, England: St. Edmundsburg Press, Bury St. Edmunds.

Ogletree, E.J. (1976). Eurythmy: A therapeutic art of movement. *Journal of Special Education, 10*(3), 305-319.

Olson, J.R. & Horland, C. (1972). The Montana State University Theatre of Silence. *American Annals of the Deaf, 117*(6), 620-625.

Orff, C., & Keetman, G. (1955). *Music for Children* (Book 1) Mainz: B. Schott's Sohne.

Panara, R.F. (1980, May). Cultural arts among the deaf. *The Deaf American*, p. 9.

Perks, W., Shaw, A., & Stevens, C.J. (Eds.). (1981). *Perspectives: A handbook in drama and theatre by, with and for handicapped individuals*. Washington, D.C.: American Theatre Association.

Petersen, G. (1981). William Sparks: Portrait Painter. *The Deaf American, 33*(9), 5-7.

Pintner, R. (1941). Artistic appreciation among deaf children. *A.A.D., 86*, 218-223.

Reber, R., & Sherrill, C. (1981). Creative thinking and dance/movement skills of hearing-impaired youth: An experimental study. *American Annals of the Deaf, 126*(9), 1004-1009.

Repp, W. (1980). 200 Deaf students learn to play musical instruments. *NTID Focus*, Rochester, N.Y.

Rileigh, K. (1971). Perception of rhythm by subjects with normal and deaf hearing. *Dissertation Abstracts International, 32*(2BO), 1256-1257.

Rios, Charlotte R. (1979, January). Poetry in the palm of your hand. *The Deaf American*, pp. 9, 11, 13.

Robbins, C., Robbins, C., & Boothroyd, A. (1980) *Music for the Hearing Impaired and other special groups*. St. Louis, Missouri: Magnamusic-Baton.

Robertson, C.W. (1979). Creating a children's theatre for the deaf. In C. Sherrill (Ed.), *Creative arts for the Severely handicapped*. Springfield, IL: Charles C. Thomas, p. 125.

Sandvoss, J. (1970). *Orff*. Unpublished paper, St. Michielsgestel, Holland.

Seeley, A., & Camus, J. (1983). Developing an approach to drama with hearing-impaired children. *Teacher of the Deaf, 7*(2), 30-34.

Sherrill, C. (Ed.). (1979). *Creative arts for the severely handicapped* (2nd ed.). Springfield, IL: Charles C. Thomas.

Silver, R. (1977). The question of imagination, originality, and abstract thinking by deaf children. *American Annals of the Deaf, 122*(3), 349-354.

Silver, R.A. (1966). The role of art in the conceptual thinking, adjustment and aptitude of deaf and aphasic children. In F. Anderson (Ed.), *Art for all the children: A creative sourcebook for the impaired child*. Springfield, IL; Charles C. Thomas.

Silver, R.A. (1970). Art and the deaf. *American Journal of Art Therapy, 9*(2), 63-77.

Silver, R.A. (1978). *Developing cognitive and creative skills through art: Programs for children with communication disorders or learning disabilities*. Baltimore: University Part Press.

Silver, R.A. (Ed.). (1983). Cognitive skills development through art experiences: An educational program for language and hearing impaired and asphasic children. *Rehabilitation Literature, 34*,10.

Smith, S.L. (1979). Teaching academic skills through drama to learning disabled students. In A.M. Shaw & C.J. Stevens (Eds.), *Drama, theater, and the handicapped*. New York: The American Theatre Association.

Spitzer, M. (1984). Programs in action: A survey of the use of music in schools for the hearing-impaired. *Volta Review, 86*(7), 362-363.

Stern, V. (1975). They shall have music. *Volta Review, 77*(8), 495-500.

Sullivan, K. (1982, spring). Getting the jump on Beethoven. *NTID Focus*, Rochester, NY.

Swaiko, N.(1974, June). The role and value of an Eurhythmics program in a curriculum for deaf children. *American Annals of the Deaf, 119*(3), 321-324.

Timms, M.L. (1985). Roleplaying and creative drama: a language arts curriculum for deaf students. Unpublished doctoral dissertation.

Tomlinson-Keasey, C., & Kelly, R. (1978). The deaf child's symbolic world. *American Annals of the Deaf, 123*(4), 452-459.

Tomlinson, R. (1982). *Disability, theatre and education*. Bloomington: Indiana University Press.

Lexington, MA: Ginn and Co.

Truax, R. (1978). Reading and language. In. R.R. Kretschmer and L. Kretschmer (Eds.),

Torrance, E.P. (1974). Torrance tests of creative thinking: Norms-technical manual. *Language development and intervention with the hearing impaired.* Baltimore, MD: University Park Press.

Uhlin, D.M., & De Chiara, E. (1984). *Art for exceptional children* (3rd ed.). Dubuque, IA: W.C. Brown.

van Uden, A. (1953). An electrical wind instrument for severely or totally deaf children. *Volta Review,* 55, 241.

van Uden, A. (1960). A sound-perceptive method. In A. Ewing (Ed.), *The modern educational treatment of deafness.* Manchester, Eng: University Press.

van Uden, A. (1963. Instructing prelingually deaf children by rhythms of bodily movements and sounds by aural mime and general bodily expressions: Its possibilities and difficulties. *Report on the Proceedings of the International Congress on Education of the Deaf and the 41st Meeting of the Convention of American Instructors of the Deaf,* 852-873.

van Uden, A. (1965). The physical education of prelingually deaf children. *Teacher of the Deaf, 63,* 307-314.

van Uden, A. (1970). *A world of language for deaf children: Part 1, basic principles.* Rotterdam, Holland: University of Rotterdam Press.

van Uden, A. (1981). Music and dance for the prelingually profound deaf child. In Somerset Education Authority (Coordinator), *Ways and means 3.* Hampshire, Eng: Globe Education.

van Uden, A. (1983). *Diagnostic testing of deaf children: The syndrome of dyspraxia.* Lewiston, NY: C.J. Hogrefe.

Volpe, M.H. (1979). A summer arts program for the hearing-impaired. *A.A.D., 124*(1), 34-37.

Weisbord, J.A. (1972). Shaping a body image through movement therapy. *Music Educators Journal, 58*(8), 66-69.

Wisher, P. (1974). Therapeutic values of dance education for the deaf. In K. Mason (Ed.), *Dance therapy: Focus on dance VII.* Washington, D.C.: American Alliance for Health, Physical Education, and Recreation.

Wisher, P. (1978). Dance and the deaf. In D. Fallon (Ed.), *Encores for dance.* Washington, D.C.: American Alliance for Health, Physical Education, and Recreation.

Wood, D., Griffiths, D., Howarth, S., & Howarth, C. (1982). The structure of conservation with 6-to 10-year old children. *Journal of Child Psychology and Psychiatry and Allied Disciplines, 23,* 295-308.

## CHAPTER 9

# *Curricula and the Mainstreamed Student*

Curricular concerns in the area of mainstreaming differ from those in other areas of education of the hearing impaired. Mainstreamed students use curricula designed for their hearing peers or, as necessary in support situations, those developed for hearing-impaired students. For many, regular curricula need only be minimally modified to meet particular needs. For others, although routine curricula are employed without change, the pace of progress through curricula is altered. However, these modifications and alterations do not solve all problems. Major concerns related to curricular content and progress in school remain and must be considered by responsible educators. Among these concerns are the type and degree of mainstreaming best for the student, the advantages and disadvantages of mainstreaming, mainstreaming criteria, predictors for success, the relationship between the specialist teacher of the hearing impaired and the regular classroom teacher, program coordination, approaches to curricula, and decision-making in mainstreaming.

### TYPE AND DEGREE OF MAINSTREAMING

Contemporary educational philosophy assents that exceptional individuals should have the right to education under the same conditions as their nonexceptional peers. Bitter (1976) placed the argument in a constitutional framework affirming "that unnecessary segregation and labeling violate the rights of exceptional children to equal educational and social opportunities." Leslie (1976) placed it in a legal framework noting "the court's decision is clear.

Hearing-impaired children have the right to a mainstream education—regardless of expense." Interpretations of legislation in the United States and in Canada have left us in no doubt that the hearing-impaired student has the right to appropriate education, and that the mainstreamed situation may be deemed appropriate for many.

What does *mainstreamed* mean? The term is bandied about loosely as is *integration*. At times they are viewed as interchangeable; at others, as possessing distinctly different meanings. The distinction between them is not merely semantic. Most authorities would agree that *mainstreaming* connotes the actual presence of a student in a classroom with normally hearing peers. The mainstreaming may be for all subjects or for selected subjects only. *Integration* may bear this meaning but, may also mean education in the same building as normally hearing peers, but in a separate classroom. For the purposes of this discussion *mainstreamed* will be used to indicate full-time education in classrooms with normally hearing peers as well as placement with normally hearing peers for specified subjects only.

A third term about which discussion may take place is *assimilation*. Ross (1976) referred to assimilation as "the hearing-impaired child's ability to function and profit from the normal school environment much as his normally hearing peers do—although certainly some supportive help is not precluded." Nix (1976) observed that some hearing-impaired students are assimilated to such a degree that they are not reported in educational surveys of the hearing-impaired population, and are not recorded as being in any type of special program. An *assimilated* hearing-impaired student, by general definition, is one whose academic and social skills do not set him apart from his normally hearing peers. As Ross (1978) has noted, even when this student does not respond well to auditory signals, such response is put down to lack of attention or misbehavior by the teacher rather than to hearing impairment. The student is not regarded as hearing impaired. This level of achievement and acceptance is considered to be the pinnacle of mainstreaming. Maximum success is won with minimal need for intervention by a specialist teacher of the hearing impaired. No significant change to the routine curricula of the class is required.

Not all students mainstreamed full-time are assimilated and make acceptable academic and social progress. A number are able to cope with the academic aspect of school life successfully, but do not fare well socially. This is especially true of both those with limited oral communication skills and those with minimal interpersonal skills. Conversely some hearing-impaired individuals are strong socially, but encounter significant difficulty with the academic requirements of the mainstreamed situation. Antia (1982, 1985) and Ross (1978) have noted a tendency among those with limited communication skill to socialize with others like themselves rather than their hearing peers. This is of import if a curricular emphasis is socialization with nonhearing impaired peers. On the academic side, Nix (1976) and Ross (1976) have emphasized that the student who does not achieve may be receiving concurrent education, but that simple physical presence in a class should not be misconstrued as mainstream education. For these students specific alterations to regular curricula, or the pace at which regular curricula are covered, are necessary.

The standard method of dealing with less than successful mainstreaming is to arrange for out-of-mainstream class support. This may range from a short, regular period of withdrawal for supportive academic work to placement in a special class or resource room situation for the major part of the school day (Brill, 1978). The time spent in the support situation and the subjects selected for mainstreaming should be determined on the bases of child need and ability. In the regular classroom the curricula of that classroom, with appropriate modification, is to be used. In the support situation, specialized curricula may be required.

However, what should be and what actually occurs are different at times. Various dynamics affect the appropriate placement and support of many students. Among these are lack of sufficient time for specialist staff to support mainstreaming adequately, lack of acceptance by regular class teachers, lack of support by administrators, lack of interpreters for mainstream support, difficulty in accurately monitoring and reporting progress, and differences of opinion among responsible parties. Those planning for the mainstreaming of hearing-impaired children must deal with these factors directly and sensitively. How they are handled will relate significantly to the curricula offered the child and the degree of success met in the mainstream classroom.

## PURPOSES AND LIMITATIONS OF MAINSTREAMING

Mainstreaming is regarded by many parents, teachers, and others as advantageous for hearing-impaired students. It is not altogether clear, however, whether the primary advantage falls on the side of academic achievement or that of socialization with normally hearing peers. The ultimate purpose of experiencing education with and as nonimpaired peers combines both advantages. The difficulty is achieving a balance.

According to Ling and Ling (1978) "the longer a hearing-impaired child gainfully attends a regular school, the better are his prospects of integrating fully into society at large." This statement appears to presuppose that both academic and social benefits will accrue from attendance in a regular school. A qualifier is included, however, in the word *gainfully*. Attendance must not be simply for the purpose of attendance in a school close to the home, or for other children to see and accept the presence of hearing-impaired individuals in society, or any other such nebulous reasons. Most professionals would agree with Ross (1976) that the student "must be there for a purpose, and that purpose must be demonstrated superior academic and personal performance than that achievable in a special school or class setting," and Bitter (1976) who asserted "the final determiner of whether mainstreaming is successful or not is dependent upon what happens socially, academically, emotionally, and vocationally to the individual."

The hearing-impaired student must be regarded as a rounded individual, a person with both social and academic sides. Teachers, regular classroom, resource room, or itinerant, achieve this objective through curricula. These are the tools through which they work. For mainstreamed students, the specific educational purposes to be achieved are those outlined in the various cognitive and affective curricula of the regular classroom in which they are placed. They must be able to achieve as do their normally hearing counterparts or the mainstream decision must be questioned. If the student cannot deal with the cognitive or affective curricula of the class, curricula that can be dealt with must be offered. To require a student to deal with academic and social tasks that are known to be overly challenging, is to discard the basic tenets of education and to accept the concept of mainstreaming for mainstreaming's sake alone. However, at times, it may be deemed that mainstreaming should proceed even if a student cannot deal effectively with either the social or academic work of the class. In this case obvious difficulties will be met. This does not mean that such mainstreaming decisions should not be made. It does mean that those making the decision must know what their purposes are, and must be prepared to offer curricula that will promote these purposes while, at the same time, supporting other aspects of the student's class life in appropriate fashion.

That not all consider academics and socialization to be of equal importance is apparent in McGee's (1976) statement that "the purpose of mainstreaming is the promotion of natural contact and meaningful communication among hearing impaired and normally hearing children in age appropriate peer groups. A secondary purpose is to heighten the expectation levels of achievement for and by hearing-impaired students." If socialization is to be paramount, a curriculum designed to encourage and achieve socialization is necessary. If academics are to be secondary, and the primary concern is not to achieve at the level of the class, academic curricula appropriate to the student's level of functioning are necessary. The same need holds if socialization is to be secondary and academics primary. This thought cannot be stressed enough. Responsible professionals must know *why* a hearing-impaired individual is mainstreamed. Next they must bring appropriate curricula to bear to achieve these purposes.

The choice of appropriate curricula is a major task. For a limited number of hearing-impaired individuals, the social and academic curricula of the regular class are fine and there is no problem. For many other students the curricula are almost appropriate and with certain modifications, they, too, will be fine. For still others, specific curricula are acceptable with minimal modifications, but other curricula are inappropriate or require major modification. An observant professional will note these variations and come to conclusions regarding the appropriateness of curricula.

Modifying curricula and substituting appropriate ones for the inappropriate is another task, however. Most teachers are not well trained in curriculum modification and design. While able to recognize a curricular problem, they are unable to act with certainty and accuracy to deal with it. One of the most significant challenges for the regular class teacher and the specialist teacher is the provision of curricula in forms and at levels to meet the abilities of hearing-impaired students. This point was highlighted by French and MacDonnell (1985) who surveyed regular class teachers to determine questions they would pose to specialist teachers of the hearing impaired regarding their mainstreamed children. Of the 113 responses in 18 categories, approximately 74 were questions related to dealing with content curricular matters and 11 related to socialization. Difficulty in dealing with academic and social curricula is a major limitation in mainstreaming.

Other limitations of a curricular nature are perceived by a number of professionals. Among these are:

1. A mainstreamed hearing-impaired student added to an already sizeable class strains teacher time (Freeman, Carbin, & Boese, 1981).
2. Students may have a restricted choice of subjects (DeSalle & Ptasnik, 1976; Kindred, 1976).
3. Students often must give up free time for additional study and assistance (Kindred, 1976).
4. Limited language and reading skills create a need for tutoring (Kindred, 1976).
5. Close, frequent contact between specialist staff and regular class teachers is necessary.
6. Administrators, who must support the program, frequently are unversed in any aspect of hearing impairment.
7. Communication among students may be difficult.
8. The hearing-impaired student misses much routine teacher-students interchange that other students pick up (Mathis & Merrill, 1978).
9. Support staff knowledgeable in curriculum and hearing impairment are limited.

The major weapon teachers and administrators may wield against limitations such as these is accurate selection of candidates for mainstreaming. Certain students will be good candidates for the experience. Others will not. It would appear sensible to define criteria for placement in mainstream programs as clearly as possible to maximize the opportunity for students who will benefit from mainstreaming to be selected, and to minimize the possibility of accepting students for whom mainstreaming would be a negative experience. Accurate selection and its logical consequence, accurate monitoring of progress, are complex tasks, however. As Nix (1976) rightly noted, "One of the most difficult problems encountered in the implementation of a mainstream program is the determination of which children are to be considered candidates for a regular class placement. Instrumentation and selection procedures need further development."

## CRITICAL PREDICTORS OF MAINSTREAMING

A number of predictors for mainstreaming selection and success emerges from any review of the literature, or from any discussion on the topic with knowledgeable professionals. Garstecki (1977) suggested that these include "the child's internal motivation, personality, cognitive and communicative skills, academic skills, degree of support from home, creativity and competence in the teaching staff, and attitude of the school population." Northcott (1976) and Mathis and Merrill (1978) reiterated these themes as did the members of a Task Force on Childhood Hearing Impairment (Department of National Health and Welfare, 1985) in Canada. In general, writers on this topic include in their sets of predictors or criteria a wide range of items. Some relate to academic functioning in school, some to communicative functioning, cognitive abilities, social functioning, and parental support; others relate to the creativity and ability of teachers, classroom management, and peer attitudes. The very diversity of predictors makes the task of accurate prediction difficult.

From among the variables related to mainstreaming, however, a limited number are believed to relate more directly to success than others. As is so frequently the case in hearing impairment, such belief is based primarily on subjective opinion rather than empirical evidence. Be that as it may, opinion does agree on a subset of critical predictors, which may be discerned from among those included in integration guides and rating systems developed by Rudy and Nace (1973), Blumberg (1973), Hinkle and White (1979), Peck and Keller (1981), Beswick and French (1983), and Bunch (1977, 1986). (See Table 9-1.)

Academic skills receive most frequent mention with such language-related skills as vocabulary, reading, spelling, and language in general that stands out as a subgrouping. Other variables in order of frequency of mention are communication skills (hearing acuity, hearing usage, speech reading, and speech intelligibility), social skills, parental support, and intellectual potential. The primacy of language and communication skills in the appreciation of those working on mainstreaming instruments is obvious.

This appreciation, however, as noted earlier, does not rest on a firm bed of research evidence. Pflaster (1980, 1981) has contributed most in terms of empirical research. She studied factors related to success in mainstreaming among 182 hearing-impaired children from 6 years and 6 months to 19 years and 8 months of age. Reading ability was used as a dependent variable against

**Table 9-1.** Primary Variables of Concern for Mainstreaming Hearing-Impaired Students Based on Selected Mainstreaming Instruments and Guidelines

| Variable | Rudy and Nace (1973) | Blumberg (1973) | Peck & Keller (1981) | Hinkle & White (1979) | Beswick & French (1983) | Bunch (1986) |
|---|---|---|---|---|---|---|
| Communication skills | | | | | | |
| hearing acuity | × | | | × | × | × |
| hearing usage | | × | × | | × | × |
| speechreading | | × | | × | × | × |
| speech intelligibility | | × | | × | × | × |
| Social skills | × | × | × | × | × | × |
| Parental support | | × | × | × | × | × |
| Academic skills | | | | | | |
| general | | × | × | | | |
| reading | × | × | | × | × | × |
| spelling | × | | | | × | × |
| arithmetic | × | × | | | × | × |
| science | × | | | | × | × |
| social science | × | | | | × | × |
| vocabulary | × | | | | × | × |
| language | × | | | × | × | × |
| Intellectual potential | × | | × | × | × | × |

which 64 independent variables were correlated. Eleven groups of factors were found and listed by percentage of contribution to the variance found. These groups were:

1. Suprasegmentals (20.4 percent)
2. Expressive language (16.2 percent)
3. Motivation (15.4 percent)
4. Receptive language (13.0 percent)
5. Speech reading skills (9.4 percent)
6. Interpersonal behavior (7.4 percent)
7. Communicative attitude (6.3 percent).
8. Personal adjustment (4.2 percent)
9. Sibling constellation (2.7 percent)
10. Auditory attitude (2.5 percent)
11. Classroom communication (2.4 percent)

The *Integration Rating Guide* (IRG) developed by Bunch (1985, 1987) combines conventional wisdom and the minimal research evidence available. The IRG is an instrument designed to assist teachers, consultants, and administrators in determining the probable success of individual hearing-impaired students in the mainstream situation, and the amount of specialist-teacher support needed to support a student appropriately. The IRG evaluates functional levels in the areas of language arts, communication, subject achievement, socialization, and parental support. These variables are given weighted values based on their perceived contribution to mainstream success. The IRG may be employed to select candidates for mainstreaming or to monitor the progress of already mainstreamed students and has been found to be a useful instrument. A completed IRG may be found in Appendix A.

The purposes of rating scales and guides is to predict candidates who will do well in the mainstreamed situation, and to monitor the progress of those already mainstreamed. In other words, these instruments suggest which students will be able to deal with regular curricula and evaluate their success in doing so. If a student is successful when challenged by any particular curriculum, the specialist teacher and the regular class teacher need to document the degree of success to appropriately select future curricula and levels of support. Conversely they must be aware of degree of difficulty for those meeting less than desired levels of support. A useful guide can contribute considerably to the joint efforts of both teachers.

## WORKING WITH THE REGULAR CLASS TEACHER

The regular class teacher is the central ingredient in successful mainstreaming. Instruments such as Bunch's *Integration Rating Guide* are useful only to the degree that the regular class teacher is able to understand and use them. Purposes and limitations of mainstreaming become meaningful only to the degree that the regular class teacher supports or does not support the hearing-impaired student. It is through this teacher that curricula are delivered. Although a specialist teacher may assist in adopting curricula, it is the regular class teacher who must deliver them. Similarly, if a student requires extra time and attention in class, it is the regular class teacher who must provide them.

While the preceding comments are true, it is not true that the regular class teacher has any extensive concept of what a hearing-impaired student may achieve, or what difficulties the student faces. It is the responsibility of the specialist teacher to provide guidance and assistance, especially in the period prior to placement of an impaired student, and during the early stages of mainstreaming. A carefully conceived plan must be prepared to inform both teachers and normally hearing students about hearing impairment and how to deal effectively with it. Ideas and materials for such plans are readily available (Anderson, 1977; Brock, Friedlander, Gemmell, Hughes, & Staley, 1986; Culhane &

Mothersell, 1979; Germain, 1973; Gildston, 1973; Greco, Mathias, Peterka, Sheldon, Strazewski, & Theoharis, 1983; Northwestern Illinois Association, 1980; Lamont, 1986; Nober, 1975). The challenge is to organize a program, deliver it effectively, and monitor it into the future. That this challenge is often not met was commented on by Brill (1978) who noted that "probably more than half of the programs give 'lip service' to the importance of orientation. In fact, such orientation often consisted of the special teacher or resource teacher talking briefly with the receiving teacher about the particular child who was going into the hearing class." Much more than this must be done if curricular matters are to be approached appropriately and effectively.

Basic to the various suggestions is the position that the specialist teacher must build in the regular class teacher a feeling of competence and the knowledge that assistance can be obtained as required. The specialist teacher must avoid at all costs creating the image that only a trained teacher of the hearing impaired can really do the job required. Golf (1976) correctly warned "the resource teacher should be very careful not to say to the regular teachers 'I am the expert. I will take these children out of the classroom, work with them, fix them up and then bring them back to you.'"

The following suggestions focussed on the curriculum will assist the specialist teacher in preparing and supporting the regular class teacher charged with mainstreaming responsibilities.

1. Explain in simple terms how hearing loss interferes with learning. Emphasize effect on communication, language acquisition, and vocabulary development. It will be necessary to explain this in advance and to return to the topic frequently until the regular teacher appreciates this point in terms of curriculum.
2. Discuss the fact that most hearing-impaired students do not have a wide range of incidental knowledge. Use curricular examples to point out how much background information is assumed with regular students.
3. Outline the general academic expectations you have in particular areas. Explain the basis for your expectations.
4. Present clearly and concisely the role you will play in providing support for the classroom teacher and the mainstreamed student.
5. As the program is implemented, work with the teacher to show how program modifications may be made to best support the hearing-impaired student, teach desired content to all students, and remain sane.
6. Advise the teacher of curricular support materials suitable for the hearing-impaired student specifically and for both hearing impaired and normally hearing students generally.
7. Work with the teacher in evaluating work samples fairly despite the overlaid problems of language, speech, and hearing limitations.
8. Suggest when individual instruction is typically required. Go on to indicate how you will assist in this area and how to use parents, teacher aids, fellow students, and older students to meet individual teaching needs.

9. Assist the teacher in establishing and improving two-way communication with the mainstreamed student.
10. Show the regular teacher that handling the curriculum is a shared responsibility and that together the specialist and regular teacher can do the best possible job.

These suggestions require a great deal of work of a specialist teacher with a finite amount of time. Not all need to be done in detail before the student enters the classroom. Some matters can be broached in general terms during the school orientation sessions or during preliminary discussions. Others may be approached as the student works within the class and opportunities arise for teacher-to-teacher consultation. It is much more effective to provide assistance and clarification based on a real situation than on a hypothetical future event. What is essential is that the specialist teacher plan what to accomplish at the various stages of mainstreaming and that the regular class teacher develop increasing confidence in the specialist teacher and in personal competence. As Reich, Hambleton, and Houldin (1977) stated, "the most important function of the itinerant teacher seems to be interacting with the regular classroom teacher to help improve the programming for the child. Itinerant teachers often have to take an active role in this process." It is the specialist who must lead. A well-thought-out curricularly oriented plan for gradual education of the regular class teacher provides the framework for this leadership.

## APPROACHING THE CURRICULUM

Little evidence is available that educators have put forth substantial effort in writing, rewriting, or modifying regular curricula for mainstreamed hearing-impaired students. The assumption appears to be that students will learn the regular curriculum and that the regular class teacher, with some assistance from a specialist teacher, will be able to modify the curriculum appropriately. What is available to support the actual work is a series of mentions of the general problem, global teaching ideas, and a few relatively short examinations of curricular concerns. Hinkle and White (1979) stressed that flexibility will be needed to blend the special needs of the hearing impaired into the regular curricula, that an individualized teaching style may be best, and that past, present, and future curricula must be rationalized. Kolzack (1983) noted that mainstream modifications in a number of areas, including curricula, will be necessary. Culhane and Mothersell (1979) suggested useful, general ideas for the development of material and media. Modifications such as careful enunciation, additional tutoring, specific seating, and assigning a buddy were suggested by Reich, Hambleton, and Klein (1975). Methods for promoting social communication skills and interaction skills in support of the social curriculum were outlined by Antia (1982, 1985). Mathis and Merrill (1978) provided a list of eighteen points delineating a guideline for consideration of curriculum and program philosophy. Such varied and sketchy mentions of curriculum and the mainstreamed hearing-impaired students are characteristic of this area of education. It is obvious that teachers desire more information on curricula and how to approach them in the mainstream situation.

In an attempt to define curricular concerns, and to explore teacher responses to these concerns, Bunch (1986) designed and distributed a questionnaire addressing various aspects of curriculum. Respondents were practicing itinerant teachers of hearing-impaired students covering the elementary and secondary grades. Questions and summaries of responses are noted below.

**HOW DID YOU BECOME FAMILIAR WITH THE CURRICULAR NEEDS OF MAINSTREAMED STUDENTS?** The routine response was that knowledge was gained primarily through experience with mainstreamed students. The majority of itinerant teachers first considered the problem when they were faced with it. Once aware of the necessity to meet specific needs a variety of techniques, such as reviewing regular curricula for problem areas, informal observation of students in the regular classroom, attending workshops on regular curricula, and formal testing to establish functional levels, were used. No teacher noted that the topic had been addressed during their specialist training.

**DO YOUR STUDENTS FOLLOW THE REGULAR CURRICULA FOR THE CLASSROOM INTO WHICH THEY ARE MAINSTREAMED? PLEASE NAME CURRICULA AND TEXTS.** All teachers indicated that regular curricula were followed. A number qualified their responses with terms such as, "as closely as possible" and noted that some curricula were "very difficult." When noting actual curricula and texts, teachers focussed on those in mathematics. A limited number mentioned basal reader series and novel study. A significant minority noted that some students were on individual programs and followed curricula other than those used for most students. Texts and curricula named were clustered at the lower elementary levels for the most part.

**DO YOU USE CURRICULA FOR THE HEARING IMPAIRED TO SUPPORT YOUR MAINSTREAMED STUDENTS? IF SO, HOW?** Auditory training curricula were used by most itinerant teachers to work on the listening skills of their students. To a lesser degree speech curricula and language curricula for the hearing impaired were employed. Some teachers drew on the resources of nearby residential schools for additional, specially designed support materials such as high interest-low vocabulary books. A number observed that curricula and materials specifically designed for the hearing impaired were too limiting for their students. A withdrawal system was routinely used where special curricula were employed.

**DO MAINSTREAMED CHILDREN NEED SPECIAL CURRICULA? IF SO, TO WHAT DEGREE?** This question obtained a variety of responses. Rather than answering the question directly, most teachers noted that it depended on the individual ability and communication skills of the student. A number noted that some children were not mainstreamed for all subjects and, when not mainstreamed, required special curricula. Indications of greater need for special curricula at the high school level and for children experiencing problems were given. A general preference for a slower pace through the regular curriculum rather than a special curriculum was obvious.

**TO WHAT DEGREE DOES THE REGULAR CLASSROOM TEACHER ACCEPT RESPONSIBILITY FOR CURRICULUM MODIFICATION?** Respondents routinely noted that the acceptance of responsibility for curriculum modifications varied from teacher to teacher. Few accepted complete responsibility. The majority shared responsibility with the itinerant teacher and a significant minority saw no reason to alter the regular curriculum or depended completely on the itinerant teacher.

**HOW DO YOU HANDLE THE LANGUAGE-READING NEEDS OF YOUR STUDENTS WHEN THEY MUST READ ASSIGNED REGULAR TEXTS?** Responses to this query fell into two main categories. One involved preteaching vocabulary to reduce difficulty when a regular text was required. Suggestions such as using parents in this process, placing vocabulary in an appropriate context, reviewing whole passages, and highlighting key vocabulary were given. The second major system was to rewrite material and teach it in advance of a lesson. Suggestions here included paraphrasing, summarizing, providing a glossary or thesaurus, and using parents as assistants.

**WHAT ARE THE MOST SIGNIFICANT CURRICULAR DIFFICULTIES YOU FACE IN YOUR WORK?** Teaching at a slower pace to ensure understanding while simultaneously keeping up with the class was the primary difficulty noted by itinerant teachers. Related to this central point were the necessity to become familiar with a wide range of regular curricula, avoidance of overloading the student, and preteaching needs.

**WHAT ARE THE MOST SIGNIFICANT CURRICULAR BENEFITS YOU FIND IN YOUR WORK?** This item typically called forth responses that indicated the satisfaction found in assisting a hearing-impaired student to keep pace in a regular classroom. The ability of a hearing-impaired youngster to be "normal" in an important aspect of life was valued.

**WHAT ARE THE MAJOR CURRICULAR ADJUSTMENTS YOU AND YOUR STUDENTS MUST MAKE?** Language and reading demands and the amount of content to be covered created the greatest need for adjustments. These called for adjustment of personal timetables or adjustment to the pace of the timetable. Particular mention was made of the demands experienced at the secondary level. Confounding the general situation was lack of time to spend thinking about topics, or to ask enough questions, and inadequacy in background information expected of regular students.

**AT WHAT GRADE LEVELS ARE REGULAR CURRICULA MOST SATISFACTORY OR MOST UNSATISFACTORY?** Responses almost uniformly concurred that regular curricula are most suitable and manageable at the primary levels, become somewhat awkward at the mid-elementary level, become quite difficult for many students at the upper elementary level, and present severe challenges for the most students at the secondary level. Difficulties varied from student to student but, as reading and language needs increased, all experienced need for increased intervention by regular class teachers and itinerant teachers.

**FOR WHICH SUBJECTS ARE REGULAR CURRICULA MOST SATISFACTORY OR UNSATISFACTORY FOR YOUR STUDENTS?** Mathematics, art and spelling were noted as most satisfactory, especially at the lower levels, as were family studies, environmental studies, and physical education. History and geography were noted as particulary unsatisfactory, with language and reading mentioned as well. There was general growth away from satisfactory for most curricula as grade levels progressed.

A number of general points emerge from this information:

1. Teachers of the hearing impaired do not feel that their training dealt sufficiently with the topic of curriculum and the mainstreamed student.
2. As much as possible regular curricula should be utilized even though they may be too difficult for the student. When curricula are too difficult specific responses are helpful:
   (1) slow down the pace of instruction;
   (2) preteach vocabulary and language;
   (3) rewrite lessons using paraphrasing and summarizing; and
   (4) use parents or other aides to preview material.
3. Primary grade regular curricula call for the least change. As the student goes through the grades curricula are less and less suitable. Unsuitability relates primarily to language and vocabulary levels.
4. Mathematics, art, and spelling are the most satisfactory areas for mainstreaming. History and geography are the least satisfactory.
5. Curricular materials and approaches designed specifically for hearing-impaired students are too limiting for mainstreamed students. Only aural habilitation curricula appear appropriate for the majority.
6. Mainstreamed hearing-impaired students require the support of specialist personnel. A major function of the specialist is explaining the needs of the student to the regular teacher so that teacher can accept responsibility for instructing the child.

Information such as the above will not surprise most itinerant teachers. While they may not have structured it in their minds, they are familiar with the general advantages and difficulties of dealing with curricula and the mainstreamed child. However, it is useful to document such points. Emphasizing central concerns will focus our attention and enable us to deal more expeditiously with these concerns. Dissemination of the information will make it easier to advise regular class teachers and administrators of general difficulties and approaches in this area of education. Lastly it may impress on those professionals responsible for teacher preparation in hearing impairment that specific attention must be paid to curriculum and the mainstreamed student.

## SUMMARY

The established position in mainstreaming of hearing-impaired students is that regular curricula are to be used whenever possible, and in the same fashion as for normally hearing students. When this is not possible, and it appears not to be in the majority of cases, modifications of the curricula are appropriate. These modifications may be in the pace at which a curriculum is covered or in the support techniques employed by the classroom teacher or the specialist teacher. When a change in pace is employed, the student falls behind his chronological peers. When other support techniques are used, they tend to focus on preteaching language and vocabulary and rewriting material. Even when these techniques are used, students, especially those in the higher grades, continue to encounter difficulty keeping pace.

Educators attempt to minimize the difficulties frequently encountered in mainstreaming by accurate selection of candidates and by constant support of the regular classroom teacher. A number of integration rating scales and guides have been devised and employed to various extents. Unfortunately, little research has been done in this area and the critical predictors for mainstreaming success have not been exactly laid out. What research is available, however, agrees that certain predictors suggested by experience stand out in importance. These are academic ability, especially in language and reading, communicative skill, social ability, parental support, and intellectual potential. Difficulties remain in determining the degree to which each of these contributes to successful mainstreaming, and in their accurate measurement.

Support of the student by the regular classroom teacher is important. It is the responsibility of the specialist teacher to advise the regular teacher of educational aspects of hearing impairment, to suggest workable teaching techniques, and to directly teach the student as necessary. Simply placing a student in a class and providing minimal support is regarded as inappropriate. A carefully laid-out and implemented plan of support for the classroom teacher is necessary if the student is to have a fair chance at mastering the curricula of the classroom.

Curricular knowledge and planning is not a particularly strong aspect of the average specialist teacher's array of skills. They tend to learn on the job rather than during their training. The result is some discomfort in assisting regular classroom teachers with curriculum modification. The mismatch of student and curricula increases as higher grades are reached and more and more difficulty is encountered both by students and teachers. There appears to be a need to focus on this aspect of teacher preparation in hearing impairment both in initial preparation and in-service training.

Despite the various challenges noted above, considerable progress in matching children and curricula is obvious. The numbers both of mainstreamed children and successfully mainstreamed children is increasing. Progress will continue if constant attention is paid to accurate selection of candidates, support of the regular classroom teacher, and careful analysis of curricular needs and methods.

## REFERENCES

Anderson, J. (Ed.). (1977). *The hearing-impaired student in the regular classroom.* Victoria, B.C.: Ministry of Education, Special Programs Branch.

Antia, S. (1982). Social interaction of partially mainstreamed hearing-impaired children. *American Annals of the Deaf, 127,* 18-25.

Antia, S. (1985). Social integration of hearing-impaired children. *Volta Review, 87,* 279-289.

Beswick, J., & French, D.B. (1983, June). *Assessment of integration potential of hearing-impaired students: A preliminary report.* Paper presented at the joint meeting of the Association of Canadian Educators of the Hearing Impaired and the Convention of American Instructors of the Deaf, Winnipeg, Manitoba, Canada.

Bitter, G.B. (1976). Maximum cultural involvement for the hearing impaired: Environmental impact. In G.W. Nix (Ed.), *Mainstream education for hearing-impaired children and youth* New York: Grune & Stratton, pp. 87-100.

Blumberg, C. (1973). A school for the deaf facilitates integration. In W.H. Northcott (Ed.), *The hearing-impaired child in a regular classroom* Washington, DC: Alexander Graham Bell Association, pp. 169-176.

Brill, R.G. (1978). *Mainstreaming the prelingually deaf child.* Washington, DC: Gallaudet College Press.

Brock, M., Friedlander, A., Gemmell, L., Hughes, P., & Staley, J. (1986) *Information for teachers and parents of hearing-impaired children.* Mississauga, Ont.: Dufferin-Peel Roman Catholic Separate School Board, Speech/Language Services.

Bunch, G.O. (1977). Mainstreaming and the hearing-impaired child: Decision making. *B.C. Journal of Special Education, 1,* 11-17.

Bunch, G.O. (1985). *Integration Rating Guide.* Toronto, Ont.: G.B. Services.

Bunch, G.O. (1986) *Mainstreaming and curricula.* Unpublished questionnaire.

Bunch, G.O. (1987) Designing an integration rating guide. *Volta Review, 89,* 46-56.

Culhane, B.R., & Mothersell, L.L.(1979) Suggestions for the regular classroom teacher. In M.E. Bishop (Ed ), *Mainstreaming: Practical ideas for educating hearing impaired students* (pp. 98-119). Washington, DC: Alexander Graham Bell Association.

DeSalle, J.M., & Ptasnik, J. (1976). Some problems and solutions: High school mainstreaming of the hearing impaired. *American Annals of the Deaf, 121,* 533-536.

Department of National Health and Welfare. (1985). *Childhood hearing impairment* (Catalogue No. 839-81/1985E). Ottawa, Ont.: Health Services Directorate.

Freeman, R.D., Carbin, C., & Boese, R.J. (1981). *Can't your child hear?* Baltimore, MD: University Park Press.

French, D.B., & MacDonnell, B.M. (1985). A survey of questions posed by regular classroom teachers integrating hearing impaired students in Nova Scotia and New Brunswick. *ACEHI Journal, 11,* 12-23.

Garstecki, D.C. (1977). *The mainstreamed hearing impaired child* (ERIC Document Reproduction Service No. 139 156).

Germain, L.B. (1973). In-service training: Mini-model: Educating the hearing to educate the hearing impaired. In W.H. Northcott (Ed.), *The hearing impaired child in a regular classroom: Preschool, elementary, and secondary years* Washington, DC: Alexander Graham Bell Association, pp. 114-119.

Gildston, P. (1973). The hearing impaired child in the classroom: A guide for the classroom teacher. In W.H. Northcott (Ed.), *The hearing impaired child in a regular classroom: Preschool, elementary, and secondary years* Washington, DC: Alexander Graham Bell Association, pp. 37-43.

Golf, H.R. (1976). What do you do if the mainstreamed hearing impaired child fails? On mainstreaming: Sink or swim. In G.W. Nix (Ed.), *Mainstream education for hearing impaired children and youth* New York: Grune & Stratton, pp. 169-178.

Greco, R., Mathias, M., Peterka, B., Sheldon, B., Strazewski, L., & Theoharis, A. (1983). Mainstreaming hearing impaired children: Understanding is the answer. *Volta Review, 85,* 360-363.

Hinkle, W., & White, K.R. (1979). Assessment and educational placement. In M.E. Bishop (Ed.), *Mainstreaming* (pp. 74-97). Washington, DC: Alexander Graham Bell Association.

Kindred, E.M. (1976). Integration at the secondary school level. *Volta Review, 78,* 35-43.

Kolzak, J. (1983). The impact of child language studies on mainstreaming decisions. *Volta Review, 85,* 129-137.

Lamont, M. (1986). *In-class observation: A useful tool for determining the success of an integrated student.* Unpublished manuscript.

Leslie, P.T. (1976). A rationale for a mainstream education. In G.W. Nix (Ed.), *Mainstream education for hearing impaired children and youth* (pp. 23-37). New York: Grune & Stratton.

Ling, D., & Ling, A.H. (1978). *Aural habilitation.* Washington, DC: The Alexander Graham Bell Association.

Mathis, S.L., & Merrill, E.C. (1978). *The deaf child in the public schools.* Danville, IL: Interstate Printers.

McGee, D.I. (1976). Mainstreaming problems and procedures. In G.W. Nix (Ed.), *Mainstream education for hearing impaired children and youth* New York: Grune & Stratton, pp. 135-145.

Nix, G.W. (Ed.). (1976). *Mainstream education for hearing impaired children and youth.* New York: Grune & Stratton.

Nix, G.W. (1977). Mainstream placement/check list. *Volta Review, 79,* 345-346.

Nober, L.W. (1975). An in-service program for integrating hearing impaired children. *Volta Review, 77,* 173-175.

Northcott, W.H. (1976). Mainstreaming the pre-primary hearing impaired child. In G.W. Nix (Ed.), *Mainstream education for hearing impaired children and youth* New York: Grune & Stratton, pp. 111-133.

Northwestern Illinois Association. (1980). *Hearing itinerant manual.* Northwestern IL: Author.

Peck, B.J., & Keller, L. (1981). Guidelines for determining the most appropriate placement of hearing impaired children in Oregon. In G. Propp (Ed.), *1980's schools . . . Portals to century XXI* Silver Spring, MD: Convention of American Instructors of the Deaf, pp. 79-84.

Pflaster, G. (1980). A factor analysis of variables related to academic performance of hearing impaired children in regular classes. *Volta Review, 82,* 71-84.

Pflaster, G. (1981). A second analysis of factors related to the academic performance of hearing impaired children in the mainstream. *Volta Review, 83,* 71-80.

Reich, C., Hambleton, D., & Houldin, B. (1977). The integration of hearing impaired children in regular classrooms. *American Annals of the Deaf, 122,* 534-543.

Reich, C., Hambleton, D., & Klein, B. (1975). *The integration of hearing impaired children in regular classrooms* (Report No. 142). Toronto, Ont.: Board of Education.

Ross, M. (1976). Assessment of the hearing impaired prior to mainstreaming. In G.W. Nix (Ed.), *Mainstream education for hearing impaired children and youth* (pp. 101-108). New York: Grune & Stratton.

Ross, M. (1978). Mainstreaming: Some social considerations. *Volta Review, 80,* 21-30.

Rudy, J.P., & Nace, J.G. (1973). A transitional instrument for selection of hearing impaired students for integration. In W.H. Northcott (Ed.), *The hearing impaired child in a regular classroom* (pp. 128-133. Washington, DC: Alexander Graham Bell Association.

# APPENDIX A.

## Integration Rating Guide

Name: ______________________ Grade: ____________ Sex: M F

Date: ____ ____ ____ Date of Birth: ____ ____ ____ Age: ____ years ____ months

School: ______________________ Teacher: ______________________

| Line | RATING SUMMARIES | |
|---|---|---|
| | Integration Success Points | Integration Support Points |
| 1 | Language Arts ________ of 75 | Language Arts ________ of 75 |
| 2 | Communication ________ of 40 | Communication ________ of 40 |
| 3 | Subject Achievement ________ of 30 | |
| 4 | Intellectual Potential ________ of 20 | |
| 5 | Socialization ________ of 25 | |
| 6 | Parental Support ________ of 25 | |
| 7 | Integration Success Points Total ________ of 215 | Integration Support Points Total ________ of 115 |

### INTEGRATION SUCCESS RATINGS

| Score Range | Rating | Implication |
|---|---|---|
| 150 to 215 | High | Should succeed in all subjects with relatively minimal difficulty. |
| 100 to 149 | Acceptable | Should obtain passing grades with recommended level of support. |
| 50 to 99 | Slender | Academic success will be limited even with recommended levels of support. Key subjects must be the responsibility of a teacher of the hearing impaired. |
| 0 to 49 | Nil | Integration is for other than academic reasons. |

### INTEGRATION SUPPORT RATINGS

| Score Range | Rating | Implication |
|---|---|---|
| 99 to 115 | Level I | Complete integration with consultive support by a teacher of the hearing impaired. |
| 84 to 98 | Level II | Complete integration but with teacher of the hearing impaired support on a regular basis. |
| 69 to 83 | Level III | Integration for most subjects with teacher of the hearing impaired instruction for key subject areas. |
| 0 to 68 | Level IV | Integration for selected subjects with full-time instruction in a class for hearing impaired students. |

| Line | RATING AREA | RATING SOURCE | | RATING POINTS | | | |
|---|---|---|---|---|---|---|---|
| | | | Grade/Score | Top 25% | 2nd 25% | 3rd 25% | 4th 25% |
| | 1. LANGUAGE ARTS | | | | | | |
| 8 | A. Vocabulary | 1. ______ | | | | | |
| 9 | | 2. ______ | | 15 | 10 | 5 | 0 |
| 10 | | 3. Teacher Estimate | | | | | |
| 11 | B. Reading | 1. ______ | | | | | |
| 12 | Comprehension | 2. ______ | | 15 | 10 | 5 | 0 |
| 13 | | 3. Teacher Estimate | | | | | |
| 14 | C. General Reading/ | 1. ______ | | | | | |
| 15 | Language Items | 2. ______ | | 15 | 10 | 5 | 0 |
| 16 | | 3. Teacher Estimate | | | | | |
| 17 | D. Language | 1. ______ | | | | | |
| 18 | Structure | 2. ______ | | 15 | 10 | 5 | 0 |
| 19 | | 3. Teacher Estimate | | | | | |
| 20 | E. Spelling | 1. ______ | | | | | |
| 21 | | 2. ______ | | 15 | 10 | 5 | 0 |
| 22 | | 3. Teacher Estimate | | | | | |
| 23 | | LANGUAGE ARTS SUBTOTAL | | | | | (to line 1) |
| | 2. COMMUNICATION | | | | | | |
| 24 | A. Speech | 1. ______ | | | | | |
| 25 | Intelligibility | 2. ______ | | 10 | 7 | 3 | 0 |
| 26 | | 3. Teacher Estimate | | | | | |
| 27 | B. Speechreading | 1. ______ | | | | | |
| 28 | | 2. ______ | | 10 | 7 | 3 | 0 |
| 29 | | 3. Teacher Estimate | | | | | |
| 30 | C. Speech Reception | 1. ______ | | | | | |
| 31 | | 2. ______ | | 10 | 7 | 3 | 0 |
| 32 | | 3. Teacher Estimate | | | | | |
| 33 | D. Attentiveness | 1. ______ | | | | | |
| 34 | | 2. ______ | | 10 | 7 | 3 | 0 |
| 35 | | 3. Teacher Estimate | | | | | |
| 36 | | COMMUNICATION SUBTOTAL | | | | | (to line 2) |

| Line | RATING AREA | RATING SOURCE | Grade/Score | Top 25% | 2nd 25% | 3rd 25% | 4th 25% |
|---|---|---|---|---|---|---|---|
| | 3. SUBJECT ACHIEVEMENT | | | | | | |
| 37 | A. Mathematical | 1. | | | | | |
| 38 | Computation | 2. | | 6 | 4 | 2 | 0 |
| 39 | | 3. Teacher Estimate | | | | | |
| 40 | B. Mathematical | 1. | | | | | |
| 41 | Concepts | 2. | | 6 | 4 | 2 | 0 |
| 42 | | 3. Teacher Estimate | | | | | |
| 43 | C. Mathematical | 1. | | | | | |
| 44 | Applications | 2. | | 6 | 4 | 2 | 0 |
| 45 | | 3. Teacher Estimate | | | | | |
| 46 | D. Science | 1. | | | | | |
| 47 | | 2. | | 6 | 4 | 2 | 0 |
| 48 | | 3. Teacher Estimate | | | | | |
| 49 | E. Social Science | 1. | | | | | |
| 50 | | 2. | | 6 | 4 | 2 | 0 |
| 51 | | 3. Teacher Estimate | | | | | |
| 52 | | SUBJECT ACHIEVEMENT SUBTOTAL | | | | (to line 3) | |
| | 4. INTELLECTUAL POTENTIAL | | | | | | |
| 53 | A. Verbal | 1. | | | | | |
| 54 | Intelligence | 2. | | 10 | 7 | 3 | 0 |
| 55 | | 3. Teacher Estimate | | | | | |
| 56 | B. Performance | 1. | | | | | |
| 57 | Intelligence | 2. | | 10 | 7 | 3 | 0 |
| 58 | | 3. Teacher Estimate | | | | | |
| 59 | | INTELLECTUAL POTENTIAL SUBTOTAL | | | | (to line 4) | |
| 60 | 5. SOCIALIZATION | 1. | | | | | |
| 61 | | 2. | | 25 | 18 | 8 | 0 |
| 62 | | 3. Teacher Estimate | | | | (to line 5) | |
| 63 | 6. PARENTAL | 1. | | | | | |
| 64 | SUPPORT | 2. | | 25 | 18 | 8 | 0 |
| 65 | | 3. Teacher Estimate | | | | (to line 6) | |

| Line | SOCIALIZATION RATING GUIDE | | | | |
|---|---|---|---|---|---|
| | CHARACTERISTICS | RATING POINTS | | | |
| | | Top 25% | 2nd 25% | 3rd 25% | 4th 25% |
| 66 | 1. Strong self concept. | 4 | 3 | 2 | 1 |
| 67 | 2. Able to accept criticism. | 4 | 3 | 2 | 1 |
| 68 | 3. Independent in actions. | 4 | 3 | 2 | 1 |
| 69 | 4. Makes appropriate decisions. | 4 | 3 | 2 | 1 |
| 70 | 5. Has own ideas. | 4 | 3 | 2 | 1 |
| 71 | 6. Encouraged by success. | 4 | 3 | 2 | 1 |
| 72 | 7. Pays close attention. | 4 | 3 | 2 | 1 |
| 73 | 8. On time with assignments. | 4 | 3 | 2 | 1 |
| 74 | 9. Careful with details. | 4 | 3 | 2 | 1 |
| 75 | 10. Work is organized. | 4 | 3 | 2 | 1 |
| 76 | 11. Able to draw conclusions. | 4 | 3 | 2 | 1 |
| 77 | 12. Able to generalize. | 4 | 3 | 2 | 1 |
| 78 | 13. Personable. | 4 | 3 | 2 | 1 |
| 79 | 14. Active participator. | 4 | 3 | 2 | 1 |
| 80 | 15. Thoughtful of others. | | | | |
| 81 | SOCIALIZATION SUBTOTAL | | ☐ | (to line 60) | |
| | Point distribution: 49 to 50 = 25 38 to 48 = 18 27 to 37 = 8 15 to 26 = 0 | | | | |

| Line | PARENTAL SUPPORT GUIDE | | | | |
|---|---|---|---|---|---|
| | CHARACTERISTICS | RATING POINTS | | | |
| | | Always | Mostly | Generally | Rarely |
| 82 | 1. Home language is English | 4 | 3 | 2 | 1 |
| 83 | 2. Ensure that homework is done. | 4 | 3 | 2 | 1 |
| 84 | 3. Assist with homework. | 4 | 3 | 2 | 1 |
| 85 | 4. Stimulate conversation. | 4 | 3 | 2 | 1 |
| 86 | 5. Expand vocabulary. | 4 | 3 | 2 | 1 |
| 87 | 6. Encourage community activity. | 4 | 3 | 2 | 1 |
| 88 | 7. Consult with teachers. | 4 | 3 | 2 | 1 |
| 89 | 8. Maintain hearing aids. | 4 | 3 | 2 | 1 |
| 90 | 9. Encourage reading. | 4 | 3 | 2 | 1 |
| 91 | 10. Maintain a positive view. | | | | |
| 92 | PARENTAL SUPPORT SUBTOTAL | | ☐ | (to line 63) | |
| | Point distribution: 32 to 40 = 25 23 to 33 = 18 15 to 22 = 8 10 to 14 = 0 | | | | |

# CHAPTER 10

# *Multihandicapped Hearing-impaired Students and Their Curriculum*

The multihandicapped hearing-impaired (MHHI) child presents an educational challenge of staggering proportions to those involved with this group and with hearing-impaired children in general. Previous chapters have outlined the difficulties inherent in working on reading, writing, mathematics, communication, and other areas with students who are denied the benefits of unimpaired hearing. No doubt exists that planning for the needs of this population taxes the resources of curriculum developers more than for most learners. When we add to this enervating disability the various learning problems associated with mental deficiency—learning disability, visual impairment, physical disability, or emotional disturbance—the size and complexity of the challenge increases dramatically. Experience has shown that this increase is not a simple doubling. The joining of these two results in interactions that give birth to unique educational needs not found in either handicap alone. The problem is so complex that, to date, those charged with developing appropriate programs for the MHHI child in general, or in any subgroup of this population, have met with markedly limited success.

This situation exists despite considerable effort, especially since the 1950s, to design and implement programs. Any survey of the literature on the MHHI population reveals at least three facts: (1) a variety of attempts have been made to design curricula and to implement programs to meet the educational needs of this group; (2) these attempts, while informative and partially successful, have not obtained generalizable success; and (3) the problem is growing in size rather than diminishing, as schools and programs accept more and more MHHI students. The mild successes achieved have documented the fact that the MHHI child can benefit from instruction. This fact alone will serve as sufficient reason for continued effort in this area. When contemporary legislative practice in the form of PL 94-142 in the United States or Bill 82 in Ontario, Canada, and the weight of relevant judicial judgments are added, it is assured that efforts will continue and increase in this area.

Educational attempts have yielded one major benefit. Research gathered from their successes and failures display a number of central questions that have emerged for consideration. It is necessary for those concerned with the MHHI, the group that Bryant (1983) has termed "a special population within a special population," to obtain a clear understanding of these issues before engaging in curricular design. Without such an understanding, any effort will be less successful than necessary.

Each of these issues will be addressed in some detail in the following pages. While it is presently unlikely that any new curricular attempt or reworking of an old approach will miraculously result in a generalizably successful program, it is likely that such efforts will reap richer harvests in educational terms. The questions to be addressed are:

1. What is meant by the term multihandicapped hearing impaired?
2. What are appropriate objectives to guide curriculum design?
3. What effect will level of severity have on curriculum design?
4. What role can curricula for other disabilities play in planning for the MHHI?
5. What changes in teacher preparation are required to deal with the MHHI population?
6. Are there any curricular models that appear more promising than others?

These six central questions will be discussed against the backdrop of program models discussed in the following section.

## PROGRAM MODELS

Alhough almost every school for the hearing impaired has attempted to program for the educational needs of the multihandicapped hearing impaired, few extensive program descriptions are available in the literature. Those available may be divided into three categories:

1. Omnibus programs that attempt to deal with all multihandicapping conditions.
2. Programs designed specifically for mentally retarded hearing-impaired individuals (MRHI).
3. Programs designed specifically for emotionaly disturbed hearing-impaired individuals (EDHI).

A fourth category is that of programs for deaf-blind individuals. Program models for this highly specialized population are not discussed in this chapter. Information on such programs may be found in McInnes and Treffry (1982), Orlansky (1982), Baud and Tweedie (1982), and Descarage (1982).

### An Omnibus Program Model

Bunch (1971) described a combined educational-vocational program for hearing-impaired students with additional handicaps. These handicaps included mental retardation, emotional disturbance, cerebral palsy, and physical disability. Most candidates for the program were selected from among students 12 years to 15 years of age experiencing significant difficulty with the regular program in a residential school for the hearing impaired. A number of candidates were selected from mental hospitals and programs for the retarded in which emotional problems and mental retardation originally had been considered their primary handicaps. The program emphasized appropriate levels of academic work, basic vocational activities, and socialization experiences. Program objectives were simply to work toward improvement in academic skills, vocational abilities, and behavior. No levels of improvement were projected.

Four principles guided design of the program. These were:

1. A low student-teacher ratio. No more than five students were assigned to a classroom to allow for development and implementation of individualized instructional plans.
2. A close association of academic areas and vocational areas. Larger-than-normal classroom areas (See Fig. 10-1) were selected to allow for a variety of work centers. A basic instructional method was to plan a vocational project in the academic areas, begin it in the vocational area, and then move back and forth from vocational area to academic area as necessary to explain and implement learning tasks as they arose. Relationships between reading, writing, computation, measurement, scientific principles, and the practical application of these skills were to be constantly and immediately emphasized within an individualized program format.
3. Realistic application of academic and vocational skills. A part of each student's day was spent in on-the-job training activities. Students were assigned to staff in various school departments as assistants. Work habits and the relationship of classroom activities and workplace requirements were stressed.

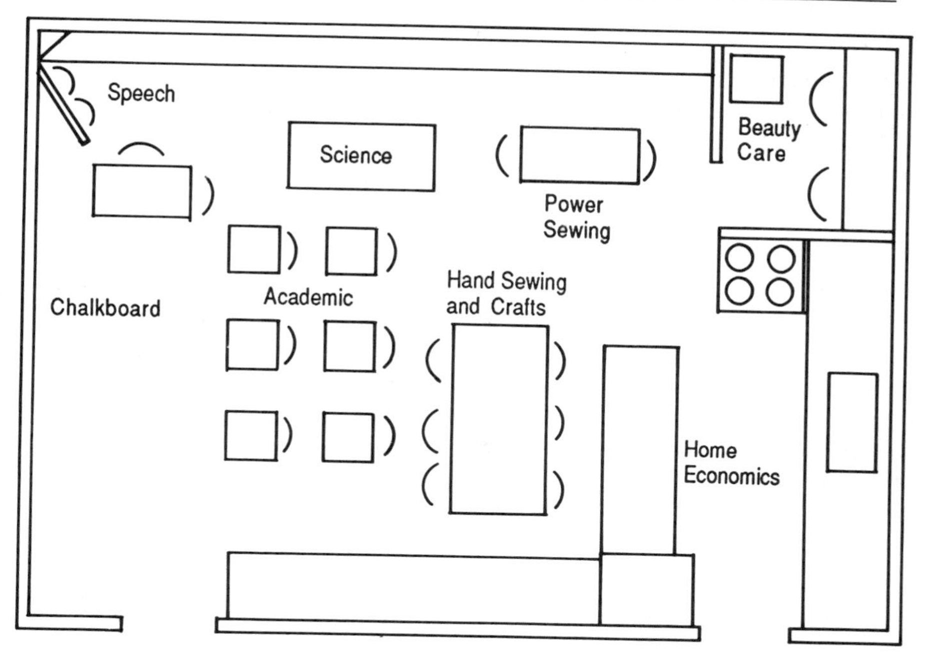


**Figure 10-1.** An omnibus model classroom incorporating academic and vocational areas.

4. Integration with other hearing-impaired students. Wherever and whenever possible students were placed in regular classrooms within the school. A specific focus on acceptable social behavior was built into the curriculum.

Bunch (1971) reported that considerable effort and care was expended in the selection and support of staff. Teachers working within the program were chosen on a volunteer basis. Two supervisory level staff were assigned the responsibility of working with the teaching staff in designing curricula, arranging timetables, implementing instructional methods, and generally supporting the teachers with all aspects of the program. Financial assistance was provided for teachers who wished to study areas of exceptionality in addition to hearing impairment. Teachers were not required to remain with the program more than 1 year if they desired a change. This staff support system was implemented with the rationale that those directly teaching multihandicapped hearing-impaired students were the most important people in the program, and the task for which they had volunteered was an exacting one. They must be supported directly and extensively for the program to succeed.

Program results were discussed in general terms. General progress in academic, vocational, and behavioral areas was claimed on the basis of teacher observation. No standardized test results were reported. A limited study of change in level of tested intelligence over a 2-year period in the program was noted. For 19 children assessed on the Wechsler Intelligence Scale for Children (WISC), initially, and then either on the WISC again or on the Wechsler Adult Intelligence Scale (WAIS), an average rise in tested level of intelligence from 70.00 points to 80.79 points was found. The increased ability to display intellectual potential is credited to program effect.

## A Program Model for MRHI Students

Naiman (1979, 1982) presented descriptions of a demonstration program for severely mentally retarded hearing-impaired adolescents. Candidates for the program were chosen among those living at home, those in custodial institutions, and those in school programs for the hearing impaired. Naiman noted that the demonstration project was designed for use in a range of settings, with a range of individuals, and across a number of degrees of retardation. The essential elements described by Naiman were:

**"NO ONE SETTING AND NO ONE CURRICULA COULD POSSIBLY MEET ALL NEEDS" OF THE CANDIDATES.** A variety of educational placements are necessary and movement from one setting to another be possible. Students should progress, if at all possible, toward the least restrictive and most normal environment within the full range of program offerings for hearing-impaired students. Out-of-school time should be spent in a family situation with parental support provided as necessary.

**A LOW STUDENT–TEACHER RATIO.** Each of five teachers were assigned six students. A graduate student assisted each teacher and a second adult drawn from among available teacher aides, parents, and volunteers worked in the classroom. Other support personnel including a curriculum specialist, an educational psychologist, and a parent counsellor were available within the school, while a physical therapist, speech therapist, medical coordinator, and peer tutors were available on a part-time basis.

**AN EDUCATIONAL MODEL OF ASSESSMENT—PRESCRIPTION–REASSESSMENT.** Assessment identified students' functional levels and an individual curriculum was designed on the basis of assessment information. Daily assessment was implemented in addition to initial and follow-up assessments focussed on general curricular objectives. The daily assessment instrument laid-out sequential steps leading to a curricular goal. This permitted easy and accurate determination of progress through tasks and effectiveness of learning.

**A CURRICULUM FOCUSSED ON MAXIMIZING SOCIAL COMPETENCE.** The primary thrust of the project was to promote independent living and social interaction skills. A curriculum must focus on these objectives and be sufficiently broad to allow for students at a basic self-care level as well as at higher levels. A social curriculum developed for mentally retarded individuals was adapted to meet the needs of the project population. This curriculum was comprised of three elements: perceptual-motor, concept formation, and social learning. It was based on a general task analytic model. This model was extended to a prevocational workshop that emphasized social skills and the world of work. Supporting the task analytic model was a token economy system reinforcing appropriate behavior.

**A VARIETY OF EXPERIENCES.** The handicap of impaired hearing isolates individuals from society and many experiences of society. Mental retardation has a similar effect. When these handicaps occur together, the social isolating and deprivation effect is heightened to a debilitating degree. To combat this effect, normal life experiences must become an integral and featured part of the educational program. Participants must learn to socialize with various groups, to function appropriately at home, school, and in public places, and to function appropriately in an individual situation.

Naiman emphasized that the above essentials are necessary in any project with MRHI students. In addition it is necessary to develop a vocational component and to develop communication skills through context and interpersonal communication. To promote appropriate use of the methodologies outlined in the instructional curriculum, specific attention must be paid to in-service training of all staff. Such training should orient on ways to develop communication, application of behavior modification principles, instructional strategies, materials development, interdisciplinary teamwork, assessment, and vocational needs and methods.

Naiman stated that clear evidence of progress was apparent in a "gradual, cumulative building of skills." (Naiman, 1982). This progress was sufficient in a number of instances for students to move from restricted learning environments to relatively less restricted environments.

## A Program Model for EDHI Students

Lennan (1973) described a comprehensive program for emotionally disturbed hearing-impaired children that has served as a model for other programs (Magill, 1973). A special unit of the Riverside School for the Deaf in California was set aside "to provide a basic educational program for severely multihandicapped educable deaf children between the ages of $5\frac{1}{2}$ and 18." Candidates were chosen from among students deemed inadmissable to regular classes in a school for the hearing impaired and students referred due to some type of severe learning, emotional, or behavioral problem. The goal for students with emotional or behavioral problems and average or better intellectual potential was "the level of adaptive behavior and academic achievement necessary for admission" to regular programs for the hearing impaired. The principles guiding development of this program were:

1. Concentration on communication skills (vocabulary, language, reading, manual communication) and mathematics. These areas were considered essential for admission to a regular class for hearing-impaired children.
2. A curriculum organized in performance objectives format with major categories of study (e.g., numbers and numerals) divided into subcategories (e.g., identifying numerals 0–9) with major objectives and subobjectives. Long range performance objectives for an eight week period guided development of biweekly lesson plans that also were couched in performance objective format.
3. A student staff ratio of approximately 4:1 with several teachers assigned to team-teaching in one classroom. A team-teaching model was chosen as it allowed newer teachers to work closely with more experienced staff, was considered to facilitate individualized instruction, provided for cooperative planning, professional growth, and leadership opportunities, and encouraged collegial reinforcement.
4. An engineered classroom design. Provision of teaching stations focussed on specific types of learning activities facilitated individual and small group instruction and fostered independent learning on follow-up tasks. The routine schedule of movement from teaching station-to-teaching station, with time and space provided for free play characteristic of an engineered classroom model was considered to provide security for the students and also to support behavior modification methodology.
5. A classroom management system based on behavior modification. Teachers were considered "behavioral engineers" with the basic task of shaping behaviors to facilitate learning. Student maladaptive behavior was defined in measurable terms on the basis of observation. Performance objectives were set and a token economy system established to reinforce appropriate behavior and task completion.

Lennan also discussed the experimental use of contingency contracting, reinforcement hierarchy, parent involvement, in-service training of staff, and extension of the behavior modification program to the dormitory. Program results were considered satisfactory with a number of students "graduating" to regular classes and a positive change in the behavior and learning of the majority of students observed (Lennan, 1967, 1968, 1970).

## Summary on Models

The three models discussed are typical of curricular attempts for the MHHI population. Even a cursory examination reveals that more similarities than differences exist. The following points are found in at least two of the models.

**A LOW STUDENT-TEACHER RATIO.** The task of teaching MHHI students is a task requiring individualized instruction and constant observation. No more than five students to one teacher was recommended. Where possible teacher aides or team teaching were advised to individualize instruction to the maximum degree.

**CLOSE ASSOCIATION OF ACADEMIC SKILLS, APPROPRIATE SOCIAL BEHAVIOR, AND APPROPRIATE WORK HABITS.** Many MHHI students are viewed as capable of securing employment in a sheltered situation or in regular employment. Active intervention is required to maximize the possibility of future employment.

**MHHI STUDENTS ARE TO BE INTEGRATED WHENEVER POSSIBLE.** Whereas it is considered necessary to segregate low-functioning students for specialized education at times, an objective of all programs was placement with less handicapped peers.

**AN ENGINEERED CLASSROOM DESIGN.** MHHI students learn best when specific areas are designated for specific types of learning tasks. This design promotes focussed learning and independence.

**A MAJOR CURRICULUM FOCUS ON APPROPRIATE SOCIAL BEHAVIOR.** One of the outstanding characteristics of the MHHI population is behavior that sets them apart from their peers. Teachers must plan for changes in social behavior at least as much as in academic behavior and possibly even more.

**A BEHAVIOR MODIFICATION AND PERFORMANCE-OBJECTIVE-BASED CURRICULUM.** MHHI students require reinforcement of appropriate behavior. While nontangible reinforcement systems are desirable, token economy systems are advisable for many. Since learning for MHHI students is especially difficult, curriculum planning must be unusually specific. A task analytic or performance objective approach best meets the needs for precision in planning.

Conversely, whereas certain common points, such as those above, emerge from an examination of model programs, other points emerge as well. These other points underline the fact that questions such as those posed earlier in this chapter remain unanswered. Should all MHHI students be grouped together for instruction? This is a question of definition of MHHI and severity of handicap. What are the purposes of MHHI programs? This is a question of curricular objectives. Is a particular service delivery model preferable to other models? This is a question of instructional design taking into consideration the unique relationships of hearing impairment and other disabilities. Finally there is the major question of teacher ability to deal with MHHI students. Are there teacher training needs yet unmet? These questions are addressed in the following pages.

## THE MEANING OF MHHI

An acceptable definition of the multihandicapped hearing-impaired student is difficult to establish. Yet without a workable definition it is impossible to prepare an appropriate curriculum. One of the first requirements in curriculum writing is to know the population of concern and its characteristics. In the case of MHHI students, determining this basic information is confounded by four factors:

1. The definition required is not the definition of a single handicap but the conjoining of at least two, and often more, handicaps. The existing definition for whatever handicaps are involved, plus their individual and shared characteristics, and the unique characteristics created by their conjoining must all be considered in any definition. Any definition of two handicaps (e.g., hearing impairment and mental retardation) is only a limited definition in that all other handicaps are ignored though any program will include students with more than two handicaps.
2. Severity of handicap must be considered. All handicaps run from mild to profound. In the case of the MHHI population, it is assumed that hearing impairment is the primary handicap. If the second handicap is primary, then the individual should be in a program focussed on that handicap. While this is simple to state, it is often difficult to determine primary handicap. Often even relatively minimal hearing loss is considered more educationally significant than a more significant other handicap.
3. Conflicting educational and medical models. In some sense all handicaps possess educational and medical significance. Hearing impairment is one that has been determined to hold greater educational than medical significance at all levels of severity. Such is not true of all other handicaps. The need to "care" in a custodial sense for individuals afflicted with mental retardation, emotional disturbance, and physical problems, for instance, at times overrides educational needs. Resolution of this point will determine the site of program delivery and the dominance of the educational or the medical model. However, it will not mean that medical or educational services should not be delivered in any situation, but, simply, which model leads and which follows.
4. Presence of an additional handicap which is occasioned by lack of appropriate education or educational opportunity. Improper educational placement or lack of any educationally relevant placement at all due to misdiagnosis, lack of facilities, or other causes is not uncommon. Indeed, some authorities condemn almost the entire educational system for the deaf as being inappropriate for many and for causing additional handicaps (Bond, 1979; Moores, 1982).

Various authorities have attempted to meet the need for a definition in various ways. One of these has been to deal with only one handicap in addition to hearing impairment. Thus, Stewart (1979) provided a definition for the developmentally delayed hearing impaired (DDHI), Lennan (1973) for the emotionally disturbed hearing impaired, and Naiman (1979, 1982) for the mentally retarded hearing impaired. To some degree this approach compensates for factor one, but hedges on factor two and ignores factors three and four. This approach allows the professional to isolate one additional handicap, group students for instruction, focus on personnel training in one new area, draw on teaching methods and materials from a relatively well-defined pool of resources, and get down to work in curriculum development. However, it does little to address the needs of those with other handicaps. It may be the approach of choice when a sufficient population of EDHI, DDHI, or MRHI exists within a school or program. Even then the degree of hearing impairment and degree of other handicap (e.g., mental retardation) when combined produce a number of possible combinations (See Fig. 10-2).

It is obvious that a mild hearing loss combined with a mild intellectual deficiency is far different than a profound hearing loss plus mild intellectual deficiency, or a mild hearing loss plus profound mental deficiency, and so on. The difference is one of primary handicap, educational placement, specialization of teachers and other staff, educational objectives, need for institutional care, and appropriate communication systems. There may well be additional differences. All must be considered in designing a curricula.

This simple two-handicap approach, however, does little for the most common situation, that of the school or program with a markedly heterogenous but small population of MHHI students; too small and too heterogenous to establish a series of programs for each combination of handicaps. Jones (1982, 1984) suggested that a preferred general method of attack for the multihandicapped hearing-impaired population would be to determine the educational significance of individual combinations of handicapping conditions and plan individualized programs on the basis of that determination. The concept of a noncategorical, individualized approach allowing grouping of students by educational need rather than handicap has considerable merit. In terms of the factors enumerated previously, factor one loses importance in a noncategorical system, factor two is considered directly, factor three is answered with an open preference for an educational model, and factor four is also directly addressed. In essence, the meaning of multiple handicaps is what effect they have on the learning of any individual. To the extent it is possible to assess learning needs and learning styles, it should be possible to design individual curricula taking them into consideration. A particular benefit of this approach is that it is adaptable to a broad range of handicaps and any size of population.

This method of dealing with the meaning of multihandicapping conditions has all the beauty and all the frustrations of apparent simplicity. Naturally, there are dynamics in educating MHHI students left unresolved by advancing the position that every MHHI student is an individual, and that associated educational problems can best be met by an individualized assessment programming approach. The major dynamics will be addressed in responses to the remaining central problems posed earlier. It cannot be denied, however, that such a model has many more plusses than minuses.

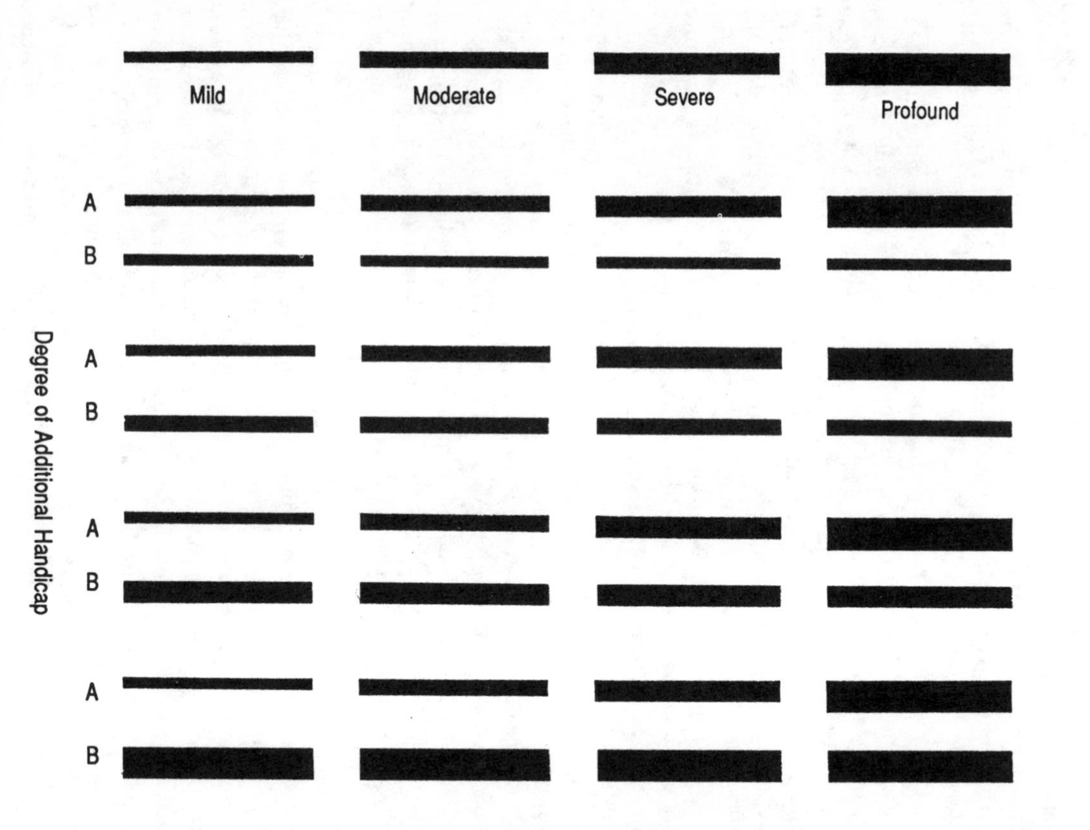


**Figure 10-2.** Relationship of degree of hearing impairment and degree of additional handicap with increasing severity.

## Curricular Objectives

The curricular objectives accompanying the models proposed by Bunch (1971), Lennan (1973), and Naiman (1979, 1982) have been reviewed briefly. Though each of these authors dwelt more on the general objectives for their programs than on the specific, it was noted that each followed an individualized program format, with Lennan and Naiman working from a base of task analytic or behavioral objective principles. It is the author's experience that many programs for MHHI students do not do much more than state general objectives and then leave it up to individual teachers to develop their own more specific objectives following a system of their choice. This approach has been defended on the grounds of teacher independence, program flexibility, and immediate response to needs. In talented hands this practice can be effective. In less talented hands it is educational anarchy.

Acceptable educational practice mandates the statement of long-range general curricular objectives reinforced by short-term objectives stated in a systematic fashion by teachers trained in a particular method. The need for careful delineation of curricular objectives in programs for MHHI students was underlined by Arkell (1979) when she stated, "The myriad of educational problems typically seen in deaf students with multiple involvements necessitates a systematic structuring of the educational programming process, if instructional intervention with these students is to be successful." The need for systematic structuring is even more pronounced when the population of learners in question are unusually difficult to teach and plan for, and for whom progress is painstakingly won.

In some sense, it is not any one specific long-range or short-term objective being pursued that is important, as much as it is the relationship of such an objective to the determined educational needs of an individual student, and to other objectives designed to meet similar needs. The MHHI student's needs are different only in extent from those of other learners. Objectives are similar to those for less handicapped students but, typically, require longer periods of time to reach, begin at a more fundamental level, and require division into a greater number of intermediate objectives. To many, these requirements mean writing objectives according to a behavioral objective format. This position has considerable merit but also a major possible pitfall. Some of those who practice behaviorally based educational methods appear to value the objective more than the learner. Education at the expense of the humanness of the learner is never acceptable.

As noted earlier it is necessary that teachers be trained to design programs for the multihandicapped students they teach. Such a statement may appear too obvious to even bother making. Unfortunately, available research suggests that many teachers of MHHI children are neither trained for the job nor are they working with such students by choice. Moores (1982), in reviewing a study of qualifications of teachers of MRHI students stated, "In sum, a majority of teachers of deaf retarded students in residential schools for the deaf are not trained to teach mentally retarded deaf children, did not choose to teach such children, and would prefer not to teach such children." It is difficult to see how such teachers would exert the cognitive energy required to produce appropriate curricular objectives. That many do so is a tribute to their professionalism, which is, nonetheless, not a sufficient substitute for training. Programs will be effective only to the degree that appropriate individualized long-range and short-range objectives are determined and pursued by well-trained staff.

## Level of Severity

As is evident from previous discussion level of severity differs significantly from student to student (see Fig. 10-2). Mild and even moderate degrees of additional handicap pose no insuperable obstacles in most programs for hearing-impaired students and for most teachers, no matter what the degree of hearing loss. Basic methods found appropriate for hearing-impaired children are sufficiently flexible and effective for those with additional handicaps of relatively minor degree. Conjoining of handicapping conditions such as those illustrated below may be dealt with through the regular curriculum within a normal classroom situation.

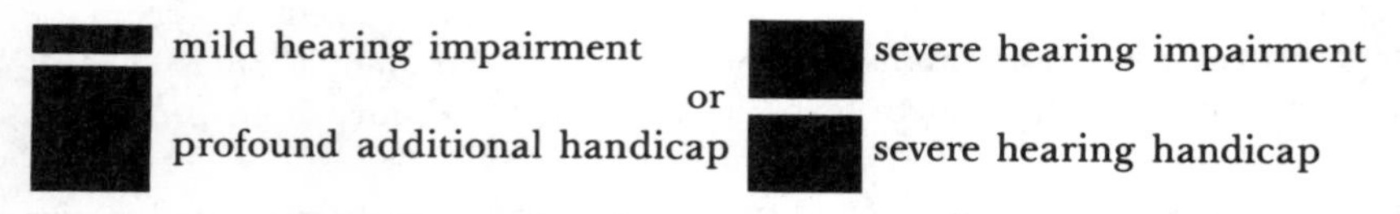


It is only when degree of additional handicap becomes severe and profound that level of severity becomes of substantial importance.

At this level alternative curricula become necessary and grouping of MHHI students of like educational needs becomes appropriate. These two points are the major effects of increased levels of severity in additional handicapping conditions. Severe and profound mental retardation, emotional disturbance, or visual impairment demand attention to their particular disabling characteristics. This attention must be translated in curricular terms, appropriate environments, and teachers and other staff trained in both hearing impairment and other handicapping conditions of concern.

## Curricula and Other Disabilities

Few programs in hearing impairment make use of curricula developed for other disabilities. The routine approach is to adapt curricula developed for hearing impairment or to engage in an exercise of developing specially designed curricula in-house. As Stewart (1979) noted such adaptations or new curricula focus on hearing impairment and its characteristics. "Schools for deaf children have traditionally organized their program of services around the educational and communication needs generated by moderate to profound deafness. Little attention has been given by these schools to the special needs of deaf persons who are also emotionally disturbed, developmentally disabled, or otherwise multiply disabled." Notwithstanding the example of those who have reached beyond hearing impairment for materials and techniques (Hicks, 1983; Lennan, 1973; Naiman, 1979, 1982), and the logic of reaching beyond hearing impairment for curricular materials and methods aimed at additional handicaps, most educators appear to believe, as Vockell, Vockell, and Mattick (1973) commented in their study on Project LIFE materials, that "teaching methods used with deaf children should be considered as the primary teaching procedures. These should be adapted to meet the specific needs precipitated by the learning disability or the degree of retardation."

This approach suffers from the limitations of being excessively categorical, ignoring the fact that the additional handicap may hold more educational significance than does hearing impairment for the individual, and the fact that a blending of curricular materials and methods from a number of handicapping areas may be more powerful in educational terms than stolid reliance on any one single approach. The favored approach should be to assess the educational needs and strengths of the individual, group those individuals with similar needs and strengths, delineate appropriate educational objectives for this group of individuals, and then to select materials and techniques to pursue these objectives from among the array of resources available in hearing impairment and additional handicapping conditions. The six phases for program development suggested by Arkell (1979) are helpful in this regard.

1. Begin with child observation and assessment period
2. Pinpoint target behaviors
3. Develop instructional objectives
4. Perform task analysis
5. Determine appropriate instructional program
6. Determine appropriate evaluative system

This child-centered approach utilizing techniques such as behavioral objective writing, task analysis, and programming components from a variety of handicapping areas appears most promising.

### Teacher Preparation

The approach suggesting incorporation of curricula from other areas of handicap also suggests that teachers become familiar with these disciplines. Without such familiarity little progress toward a non-categorical approach based on the actual educational needs and strengths of the MHHI population can be expected.

Existing teacher education programs in hearing impairment do not deal extensively with other exceptionalities and vice versa. Though the need for opportunities to study other areas has been recognized among teachers of the hearing impaired, few programs doing so exist (Moores, 1982; Jones & Holzhauer, 1983; Bunch, in press). Curtis and Tweedie (1985) discussed the limitations of teacher training with specific reference to curricula in their general overview of curricular planning for the MHHI student. They identified lack of training in a sufficient number of areas, the doctrinaire approach of many programs, differences in communication philosophy in the oral versus manual sense, conflicts between individual teacher and educational program orientations, and individual differences in educational orientation as salient difficulties in curricular planning in this area.

Jones and Holzhauer (1983) reported on additional handicaps of relatively lesser or greater training concern for teachers in MHHI programs and those preparing for such programs. The areas considered in most need of intense teacher preparation were:

1. Severe cerebral palsy
2. Visual impairment, mental retardation, and cerebral palsy
3. Severe emotional or behavioral impairment
4. Severe mental retardation
5. Profound mental retardation
6. Blindness
7. Visual motor learning disabilities
8. Mental retardation and cerebral palsy

Need for training was noted in the mild and moderate ranges of these disabilities as well, but to lesser degrees.

Studies such as that by Jones and Holzhauer (1983) have provided basic structural parameters for teacher preparation in the MHHI area. To date, few programs have developed extensive training. Concerned and active teachers have studied other exceptionalities on their own initiative and in isolation from hearing impairment. Such a stop-gap approach is insufficient to meet needs already apparent and likely to increase. Fortunately, a limited number of programs offering integrated training in education of MHHI students, notably that at Gallaudet College in the United States, have been established. Until such programs are generally available and knowledge of MHHI needs and strategies more commonplace, teacher education in hearing impairment will continue to suffer from a serious deficiency in this important area.

## A SUGGESTED CURRICULAR MODEL

Two choices for a program model are apparent. The first is a specialized model focussed on one handicap in addition to hearing impairment. The second is an omnibus model designed to service a variety of handicapping conditions in addition to hearing impairment. This latter model would be of the greatest general benefit. The majority of programs for hearing-impaired students do not have sufficiently large populations to set-up all of the specialized programs necessary to handle all combinations of hearing impairment and one other handicap. Thus, the following are guidelines for a suggested omnibus curricular model.

**THE CURRICULUM MUST BE SUFFICIENTLY FLEXIBLE TO ACCOMMODATE THE NEEDS OF A VARIETY OF HANDICAPPING CONDITIONS.** A program with students exhibiting a variety of handicaps cannot, almost by definition, afford a categorical or subject bias. Such a program must address itself to common educational needs. A student centered curricular approach designed to assess individual needs and to group students for instruction on the basis of those needs is desirable.

**THE CURRICULUM MUST PERMIT THE DEVELOPMENT OF PROGRAMS FOCUSSED ON INDIVIDUAL NEEDS.** Any individualized program should have as a central feature a sophisticated student assessment system. It is necessary to develop detailed knowledge of the strengths and weaknesses of each student to design appropriate programs. Without such an on-going evaluative system, it is unlikely that meaningful and successful programs can be designed.

**THE CURRICULUM MUST INCLUDE A PROCESS FOR CONTINUOUS EVALUATION.** Curricular objectives either of long-term or short-term nature are derived from the on-going assessment process. Delineation of these goals for MHHI students must be more precise than for many other students due to their need for step-by-step instruction and difficulty following holistic types of instructional strategies.

**OBJECTIVE SETTING MUST BE PRECISE (A BEHAVIORAL OBJECTIVE OR TASK ANALYTIC MODEL IS SUGGESTED).** Objectives will reflect learning needs arising from various handicapping conditions. To a considerable degree these needs have been considered in the development of methods and materials for children with mental retardation, emotional disturbance, among others, as single handicaps. Teachers in programs for MHHI students should be prepared to use such methods and materials.

**CURRICULA SHOULD INCORPORATE METHODS AND MATERIALS DESIGNED FOR HANDICAPPING CONDITIONS OTHER THAN HEARING IMPAIRMENT.** One of the most significant needs of MHHI students is preparation for future employment. At present many such students encounter greater than necessary difficulty obtaining employment. They have not received the benefits of a long-term program focussed on prevocational preparation and on-the-job training. To be successful, any program for the MHHI population must work toward preparing students for the workplace but not at the expense of academic preparation.

**CURRICULA MUST INCLUDE SPECIFIED PREPARATION OF A PREVOCATIONAL AND VOCATIONAL NATURE CLOSELY ALLIED WITH ACADEMIC PREPARATION.** To function successfully in the world of work and in society in general the MHHI student must have the opportunity to meet and to share experiences with less handicapped and nonhandicapped peers. Curricula must be devised so that opportunities for mainstreaming are available and so that individual students may receive the benefits of educational and social placement in increasingly less-restricted environments.

**CURRICULA MUST BE SUFFICIENTLY FLEXIBLE TO PERMIT ANY STUDENT'S PLACEMENT TO BE ALTERED IN THE PURSUIT OF INCREASINGLY NORMAL EXPERIENCES IN A SERIES OF LESS RESTRICTIVE ENVIRONMENTS.** Any curriculum for MHHI students should reflect these basic principles. Individual programs will vary but the philosophical and functional bases underlying programs in general should be consistent. Actual areas of emphasis within a program will be defined by the nature of the students involved in a program and by what competent professionals see as their needs. Guidelines for program development and curricular suggestions are plentiful, if not collected in one place. Among those who have written in this area are Appell (1982), Arkell (1979, 1982), Brill (1974), Bryant (1983), Colasuonno (1982), Curtis and Tweedie (1985), Downey (1983), Gates (1982), Hicks (1983), Hyde and Engle (1977), Hundert and Buller (1978), Mavilya (1982), Powers and Harris (1982), Proctor (1984), Restaino (1982), and Stewart (1979). The information contained in these books and articles will serve to assist in the development of programs emphasizing a number of possible topics.

The essential ingredient lacking in many programs is a decision to plan and implement with a well-defined and well-supported curriculum for MHHI students. Once this decision is made and resources allocated, significant benefit for MHHI students can be realized. The problems noted and suggestions made throughout this chapter will serve as useful points for consideration in any endeavor in this area.

## REFERENCES

Appell, M.W. (1982). Early education for the severely handicapped/hearing-impaired child. In R. Campbell and V. Baldwin (Eds.), *Severely handicapped/hearing-impaired students.* Baltimore, MD: Brookes, pp. 98-114.

Arkell, C. (1979). Educational programming for multiply involved deaf students. *Volta Review, 81,* 25-34.

Arkell, C. (1982). Functional curriculum development for multiply involved hearing-impaired students. *Volta Review, 84,* 198-208.

Baud, H., & Tweedie, D. (1982). Future trends in deaf-blind education—Revisited. *Directions, 3*(2), 35-37.

Bond, D.E. (1979). Aspects of psycho-educational assessment of hearing-impaired children with additional handicaps. *Journal of the British Association of Teachers of the Deaf, 3*, 76-79.

Brill, R. (1974). *Education of the deaf: Administrative and professional developments* (2nd ed.). Washington, DC: Gallaudet College Press.

Bryant, P.A. (1983). Curriculum for the multihandicapped prevocational student. In F. Solano, J. Egelston-Dodd, & E. Costello (Eds.), *Focus on infusion* (pp. 161-166). Silver Spring, MD: Convention of American Instructors of the Deaf.

Bunch, G.0. (1971). An academic-vocational program for multiply handicapped deaf students. *Volta Review, 73*, 417-425.

Bunch, G.0. (in press). Teacher preparation in hearing impairment: A proposed model. *Canadian Journal of Education*.

Colasuonno, T. (1982). The special education unit model at the Lexington School for the Deaf. *Directions, 3*(2), 26-28.

Curtis, W.S., & Tweedie, D. (1985). Content and process in curriculum planning. In E. Cherow (Ed.), *Hearing-impaired children and youth with developmental disabilities*. Washington, DC: Gallaudet College Press, pp. 246-269.

Descarage, S.M. (1982). Training for life: A living and work program for deaf-blind youth. *Directions, 3*(2), 53-59.

Downey, N. (1983). Career development: Prevocational training for multiply handicapped hearing-impaired adolescents. In F. Solano, J. Egelston-Dodd, & E. Costello (Eds.), *Focus on Infusion* (Vol. II). Silver Spring, MD: Convention of American Instructors of the Deaf.

Gates, C.F. (1982). Early intervention with multihandicapped children. In D. Tweedie & E.M. Shroyer (Eds.), *The multihandicapped hearing impaired: Identification and instruction*. Washington, DC: Gallaudet College Press, pp. 95-102.

Hicks, W. (1983). Educational disorders: An approach to programming for student needs. *Directions, 3*(4), 36-39.

Hundert, J., & Buller, G.I. (1978). The special individualized program: A unit for the integration of students with severe emotional problems. *ACEHI Journal, 5*, 11-17.

Hyde, S., & Engle, D. (1977). The Potomac program: A curriculum for the severely *handicapped deaf — hearing impaired — non-verbal*. Beaverton, OR: Dormac.

Jones, T.W. (1982). Multihandicapped hearing-impaired students: Problems in identification and definition. *Directions, 3*(2), 6-11.

Jones, T.W. (1984). A framework of identification, classification, and placement of multihandicapped hearing-impaired students. *Volta Review, 86*, 142-151.

Jones, T.W., & Holzhauer, E. (1983). Preparing teachers of multihandicapped hearing-impaired students. *Directions, 3*(3), 52-57.

Lennan, R.K. (1967). Report of a pilot project in the education of emotionally disturbed deaf boys. *Report of the Proceedings of the 43rd Meeting of the American Instructors of the Deaf, 43*, 280-291.

Lennan, R.K. (1968). A pilot project for emotionally disturbed deaf boys. *Volta Review, 70*, 513-516.

Lennan, R.K. (1970). Report on a program for emotionally disturbed deaf boys. *American Annals of the Deaf, 115*, 469-480.

Lennan, R.K. (1973). The deaf multihandicapped unit at the California School for the Deaf, Riverside. *American Annals of the Deaf, 118*, 439-445.

Magill, C. (1973). A programme for multiply handicapped deaf children: Our attempt. In G. Bunch (Ed.), *Proceedings: First National Conference of Canadian Teachers of the Deaf.* Belleville, Ont.: Association of Canadian Educators of the Hearing Impaired, pp. 66-73.

Mavilya, M. (1982). Assessment, curriculum, and intervention strategies for hearing-impaired mentally retarded children. In D. Tweedie & E.H. Schroyer (Eds.), *The Multihandicapped hearing impaired*. Washington, DC: Gallaudet College Press, pp. 113-123.

McInnes, J.M., & Treffry, J.A. (1982). *Deaf-blind infants and children: A developmental guide.* Toronto, Ont.: University of Toronto Press.

Moores, D.F. (1982). *Educating the deaf: Psychology, principles, and practices* (2nd ed.). Boston: Houghton Mifflin.

Naiman, D. (1979). Educating severely handicapped deaf children. *American Annals of the Deaf, 124*, 381-396.

Naiman, D. (1982). Educational programming for hearing impaired mentally retarded adolescents. In D. Tweedie & E.H. Schroyer (Eds.), *The multihandicapped hearing impaired*. Washington, DC: Gallaudet College Press, pp. 148-161.

Orlansky, M.D. (1982). The education and placement of deaf-blind students: Current issues and recommendations. *Directions, 3*(2), 29-34.

Powers, A.R., & Harris, A.R. (1982). Strategies for teaching language and/or learning disabled hearing impaired children. In D. Tweedie & E.H. Schroyer (Eds.), *The multihandicapped hearing impaired*. Washington, DC: Gallaudet College Press, pp. 249-263.

Proctor, L.A. (1984) *Multihandicapped deaf adults: A manual for instruction of independent living skills.* Washington, DC: Gallaudet College Press.

Restaino, L.C.R. (1982). A curriculum development project for the multihandicapped hearing impaired child ten years later. In D. Tweedie & E.H. Schroyer (Eds.), *The multihandicapped hearing impaired*. Washington, DC: Gallaudet College Press, pp. 162-182.

Stewart, L.G. (1979). *Hearing impaired developmentally disabled persons* (Final Report). Tucson, AZ: University of Arizona, Rehabilitation Center, College of Education.

Vockell, K., Vockell, E.L., & Mattick, P. (1973). Language for mentally retarded deaf children: Project LIFE. *Volta Review, 75*, 431-439.

# INDEX